# SECONDARY HYPERTENSION

# CLINICAL HYPERTENSION AND VASCULAR DISEASES

WILLIAM B. WHITE, MD

*SERIES EDITOR*

***Secondary Hypertension:*** *Clinical Presentation, Diagnosis, and Treatment, edited by George A. Mansoor, MD, 2004*

***Pediatric Hypertension,*** *edited by Ronald J. Portman, MD, Jonathan M. Sorof, MD, and Julie R. Ingelfinger, MD, 2004*

# SECONDARY HYPERTENSION

## *Clinical Presentation, Diagnosis, and Treatment*

*Edited by*

GEORGE A. MANSOOR, MD, FRCP (EDIN)

*Section of Hypertension and Clinical Pharmacology, University of Connecticut School of Medicine, Farmington, CT*

HUMANA PRESS
TOTOWA, NEW JERSEY

999 Riverview Drive, Suite 208
Totowa, New Jersey 07512

**humanapress.com**

For additional copies, pricing for bulk purchases, and/or information about other Humana titles, contact Humana at the above address or at any of the following numbers: Tel.: 973-256-1699; Fax: 973-256-8341, E-mail: humana@humanapr.com; or visit our Website: www.humanapress.com



All articles, comments, opinions, conclusions, or recommendations are those of the author(s), and do not necessarily reflect the views of the publisher.

Due diligence has been taken by the publishers, editors, and authors of this book to assure the accuracy of the information published and to describe generally accepted practices. The contributors herein have carefully checked to ensure that the drug selections and dosages set forth in this text are accurate and in accord with the standards accepted at the time of publication. Notwithstanding, as new research, changes in government regulations, and knowledge from clinical experience relating to drug therapy and drug reactions constantly occurs, the reader is advised to check the product information provided by the manufacturer of each drug for any change in dosages or for additional warnings and contraindications. This is of utmost importance when the recommended drug herein is a new or infrequently used drug. It is the responsibility of the treating physician to determine dosages and treatment strategies for individual patients. Further it is the responsibility of the health care provider to ascertain the Food and Drug Administration status of each drug or device used in their clinical practice. The publisher, editors, and authors are not responsible for errors or omissions or for any consequences from the application of the information presented in this book and make no warranty, express or implied, with respect to the contents in this publication.

Production Editor: Robin B. Weisberg.
Cover Illustration: (Foreground) From Chapter 13, "Biochemical Diagnosis and Localization of Pheochromocytoma," by Emmanuel L. Bravo. (Background) From Chapter 4, "Diagnostic Evaluation for Patients With Renovascular Hypertension," by Sumeska Thavarajah and William B. White.
Cover design by Patricia F. Cleary.

This publication is printed on acid-free paper. ∞
ANSI Z39.48-1984 (American National Standards Institute) Permanence of Paper for Printed Library Materials.



Printed in the United States of America. 10 9 8 7 6 5 4 3 2 1
1-59259-757-2 (e-ISBN)

Library of Congress Cataloging-in-Publication Data

Secondary hypertension : clinical presentation, diagnosis, and treatment / edited by George A. Mansoor.
p. ; cm. -- (Clinical hypertension and vascular diseases)
Includes bibliographical references and index.
ISBN 1-58829-141-3 (alk. paper)
1. Hypertension.
[DNLM: 1. Hypertension--etiology. 2. Hypertension--diagnosis. 3. Hypertension--therapy. WG 340 S445 2004] I. Mansoor, George A. II. Series.
RC685.H8S43 2004
616.1'32--dc22 2003022071

# Series Editor's Introduction

Secondary forms of hypertension are not uncommon in clinical practice, but they are often overlooked or forgotten by clinicians in many fields of medicine. Dr. George Mansoor's volume on *Secondary Hypertension* is an important contribution to the field of clinical hypertension and vascular diseases, since it brings up to date the numerous diagnostic and therapeutic advances in the evaluation for secondary types of hypertension. In the past, textbooks usually stated that an etiology could be determined in less than 5% of patients presenting with newly diagnosed hypertension. We now know this is far too low a proportion (e.g., primary hyperaldosteronism alone may account for hypertension in 5% of patients presenting with chronic elevations in blood pressure).

*Secondary Hypertension* has been thoughtfully organized into chapters evaluating screening and diagnosis, as well as medical and/or surgical intervention of the well-known etiologies of secondary hypertension in adults and children. Additional coverage is given to such exogenous or lesser appreciated causes of secondary hypertension as obstructive sleep apnea and drugs. These sections make this book novel because in the past little attention has been paid to the effects of noncardiac drugs that interfere with antihypertensive therapy or to exogenous substances that might induce refractory hypertension.

As series editor of *Clinical Hypertension and Vascular Diseases,* I was delighted to learn of the superb authors recruited by Dr. Mansoor during the development of this volume. Each chapter has been written by an authority in his or her field. *Secondary Hypertension* will be of great value to all students and physicians interested in hypertension research, education, and practice for the years to come.

**William B. White,** MD
*Professor of Medicine*
*University of Connecticut School of Medicine,*
*Farmington, CT*

# Preface

*Secondary Hypertension: Clinical Presentation, Diagnosis, and Treatment* reviews the essential clinical, diagnostic, and treatment aspects of secondary hypertension. The need for such a book is great as knowledge in this field has progressed rapidly and new and unique forms of secondary hypertension are being described on a regular basis. However, such traditional disorders as renal artery stenosis, aldosteronism, and pheochromocytoma have remained major considerations when secondary hypertension is suspected and still occupy a significant part of our time as specialists in hypertension. The discovery of secondary hypertension is important; it provides a potential cure for the patient, but at other times provides physiological information on which the clinician can base drug therapy. This book, therefore, covers in detail the forms of secondary hypertension likely to be considered in persons with suggestive clinical features or resistant hypertension.

Our knowledge regarding most forms of secondary hypertension has grown significantly and our conventional impressions of some of these have certainly changed. The availability of magnetic resonance imaging has helped us in the evaluation of coarctation of the aorta and renal artery stenosis. Reliable biochemical tests allow us to screen relatively easily for a variety of endocrine causes of hypertension. In terms of treatment, we have a vast array of drugs available to treat hypertension, but also interventional therapy directed at the form of secondary hypertension, e.g., surgery or anti-aldosterone drugs. Finally, it is becoming clear that some disorders contribute more often to hypertension than previously believed; this is the case with obstructive sleep apnea and possibly primary aldosteronism. There is a need for a book collating and updating knowledge in this area; the causes and management of secondary hypertension span several traditional disciplines, including internal medicine, nephrology, cardiovascular medicine, endocrinology, and pulmonology. Each chapter gives a concise approach to its topic and therefore can be read on its own.

Chapter 1 discusses the most common reason that an evaluation for secondary hypertension is performed: refractory hypertension. With today's lower goals for blood pressure, we may need to re-examine how we define refractory hypertension. In Chapter 2, Dr. Ehud Grossman and Dr. Franz Messerli consider the exogenous causes of hypertension. They review old and new culprit substances that raise blood pressure and discuss possible mechanisms for their undesirable actions.

Part II reviews renal disease and secondary hypertension. In Chapter 3, Dr. Robert Toto tackles the area of renal disease and hypertension. Hypertension is almost universally found in the presence of renal disease and may have a role in the progression of intrinsic renal disorders. Dr. Toto reviews current approaches to evaluating and managing hypertension in this setting. Dr. Sumeska Thavarajah and Dr. William White (Chapter 4) provide a comprehensive account of diagnostic strategies for renovascular hypertension and renal artery stenosis. Chapter 5 is devoted to the role of interventional therapies such as balloon angioplasty and stenting in the management of renovascular hypertension. In Chapter 6, Dr. Vincent Canzanello reviews important information regarding the medical treatment of renovascular hypertension and emphasizes that the majority of patients can be controlled medically. A debate continues in the literature about the relative merits of medical vs interventional treatments for renovascular hypertension. Finally, secondary hypertension caused by excessive renin production, as in renin-producing tumors, is reviewed by Dr. Timothy Reudelhuber in Chapter 7.

Part III covers adrenal medullary and cortical causes of secondary hypertension. Dr. William Young (Chapter 8) reviews expertly the diagnostic strategy for primary aldosteronism, and Dr. Emmanuel Bravo (Chapter 9) reviews the treatment aspects of primary aldosteronism. They emphasize the advantages of ambulatory screening of hypertensive patients without hypokalemia as well as the fact that most patients with bilateral adrenal hyperplasia can enjoy excellent blood pressure control with medical treatment. The laparoscopic surgical removal of aldosteronomas is detailed by Dr. Mihir Desai and Dr. Inderbir Gill (Chapter 10) so as to make it understandable to both physicians and surgeons. In Chapter 11, Dr. William Kendrick, Dr. Jean-Michel Achard, and Dr. David Warnock then review the other forms of low-renin hypertension, including monogenic forms. They emphasize the fact that all these disorders cause hypertension through sodium retention. The last chapter in this section, by Dr. Judith Whitworth, Dr. George Mangos, and Dr. John Kelly (Chapter 12), reviews the mechanisms, clinical evaluation, and treatment of hypertension from Cushing's syndrome, resulting from a variety of pathological entities.

Part IV on adrenal medulla and hypertension is given detailed consideration because pheochromocytoma can be a malignant condition. This section not only considers pheochromocytoma, but other disorders mimicking it. In Chapter 13, Dr. Emmanuel Bravo leads the reader through a superlative account of when to suspect and how to screen for pheochromocytoma. Dr. Carl Malchoff, Dr. Dougald MacGillivray, and Dr. Steven Shichman (Chapter 14) review the current management of pheochromocytoma, including preoperative management and care of advanced cases. In Chapter 15, Dr. Otto Kuchel reviews a number of conditions that may mimic pheochromocytoma, so-called pseudo-pheochromocytoma, and also reviews the differentiating features of these disorders.

In their chapter, Dr. Empar Lurbe and Dr. Joseph Redon (Chapter 16) provide an excellent review of secondary hypertension in children and adolescents. Obviously, the younger a child with hypertension is, the more likely that a secondary form of hypertension will be discovered. Finally, Chapter 17 by Dr. Thomas Pickering and Dr. Mona Yacoub reviews the normal hemodynamic and other changes during sleep, considers the relationship of sleep apnea to hypertension and its complications, and brings us up to date on its clinical features, diagnosis, and treatment.

We have invited contributors who are easily recognizable as leaders in the field of hypertension. They have worked hard to expertly and concisely review traditional and established causes of secondary hypertension as well as new and less well known ones. Each chapter merits multiple reads and can act as a starting point for anyone seeking an up-to-date, scientifically accurate review of a particular area in secondary hypertension. Of course, we are grateful to the authors who have worked hard on this book and provided us with excellent work. Special thanks to Diane Webster from the editorial office of Blood Pressure Monitoring at the University of Connecticut Health Center for helping with chapter preparation.

We also thank Paul Dolgert at Humana Press for recognizing the importance of this book and the need for it. We hope you find *Secondary Hypertension: Clinical Presentation, Diagnosis, and Treatment* enjoyable and scientifically current.

**George A. Mansoor,** *MD, FRCP (EDIN)*

# Contents

# Contributors

Jean-Michel Achard, MD, PhD • *Department of Physiology, University Hospital, Limoges, France*

Emmanuel L. Bravo, MD • *Department of Nephrology and Hypertension, The Cleveland Clinic Foundation, Cleveland, OH*

Vincent J. Canzanello, MD • *Division of Hypertension and Internal Medicine and Division of Nephrology and Internal Medicine, Mayo Clinic and Mayo Medical School, Rochester, MN*

Mihir M. Desai, MD • *Section of Laparoscopic and Minimally Invasive Surgery, Urological Institute, Cleveland Clinic Foundation, Cleveland, OH*

Inderbir S. Gill, MD • *Section of Laparoscopic and Minimally Invasive Surgery, Urological Institute, Cleveland Clinic Foundation, Cleveland, OH*

Ehud Grossman, MD • *Department of Internal Medicine, The Chaim Sheba Medical Center, Tel-Hashomer, Israel*

William T. Kendrick, MD • *Departments of Medicine and Physiology & Biophysics, and Nephrology Research and Training Center, University of Alabama at Birmingham, Birmingham, AL*

John J. Kelly, MD • *Departments of Medicine and Renal Medicine, St. George Hospital, The University of New South Wales, Kogarah, Australia*

Otto Kuchel, MD, DSc • *University of Montreal and Clinical Research Institute of Montreal, Montréal, Québec, Canada*

Empar Lurbe, MD • *Pediatric Nephrology Unit, Hospital General, University of Valencia, Valencia, Spain*

Carl D. Malchoff, MD, PhD • *Department of Medicine, University of Connecticut Health Center, Farmington, CT*

Dougald MacGillivray, MD • *University of Vermont Department of Surgery at Maine Medical Center, Portland, ME*

George J. Mangos, MD • *Departments of Medicine and Renal Medicine, St. George Hospital, The University of New South Wales, Kogarah, Australia*

George A. Mansoor, MD, FRCP (EDIN) • *Section of Hypertension and Clinical Pharmacology, University of Connecticut School of Medicine, Farmington, CT*

Franz H. Messerli, MD • *Ochsner Clinic Foundation, New Orleans, LA*

THOMAS G. PICKERING, MD, DPHIL • *Behavioral Cardiovascular Health and Hypertension Program, Columbia Presbyterian Hospital, New York, NY*

JOSEP REDON, MD • *Hypertension Clinic, Internal Medicine, Hospital Clinic, University of Valencia, Valencia, Spain*

TIMOTHY L. REUDELHUBER, PhD • *Laboratory of Molecular Biochemistry of Hypertension, Clinical Research Institute of Montreal, Montréal, Québec, Canada*

STEVEN SHICHMAN, MD • *Department of Urology, Hartford Hospital, Hartford, CT and Department of Urology, University of Connecticut Health Center, Farmington, CT*

SUMESKA THAVARAJAH, MD • *Section of Hypertension and Clinical Pharmacology, University of Connecticut Health Center, Farmington, CT*

ROBERT D. TOTO, MD • *Division of Nephrology, University of Texas Southwestern Medical Center, Dallas, TX*

DAVID G. WARNOCK, MD • *Division of Nephrology, University of Alabama at Birmingham, Birmingham, AL*

WILLIAM B. WHITE, MD • *Section of Hypertension and Clinical Pharmacology, University of Connecticut School of Medicine, Farmington, CT*

JUDITH A. WHITWORTH, MD, PhD • *John Curtin School of Medical Research, The Australian National University, Canberra, Australia*

MONA YACOUB, MD • *Division of General Medicine, Columbia Presbyterian Hospital, New York, NY*

WILLIAM F. YOUNG, JR., MD • *Division of Endocrinology and Metabolism, Mayo Clinic and Medical School, Rochester, MN*

# I

# Introduction

# 1 Refractory Hypertension

*George A. Mansoor,* MD, FRCP (EDIN)

*Contents*



## INTRODUCTION

The terms *refractory hypertension or drug-resistant hypertension* have become entrenched in clinical medicine and are used interchangeably in this chapter. The traditional definition of refractory hypertension specifies that treatment of the patient with two or more antihypertensive agents at moderate or high doses is necessary and that goal blood pressure (BP) is not achieved *(1–6)*. However, some authors use the term refractory or resistant hypertension when a diuretic has been incorporated into the treatment regimen that includes two or more antihypertensive

From: *Secondary Hypertension: Clinical Presentation, Diagnosis, and Treatment*
Edited by: G. A. Mansoor © Humana Press Inc., Totowa, NJ

drugs at moderate to high doses. Hence, the definition of refractory hypertension used in the literature has varied in the number and types of antihypertensive drugs and levels of BP.

Today, our definition must be appropriately modified as new and diverse pharmacological agents for hypertension treatment have become available and as our methods for evaluating patients with hypertension have been refined. Certainly, the treating clinician has a vast and expanding armamentarium of drug therapy targeting various body systems that initiate or maintain hypertension in patients. All prior definitions have relied on office BP measurements without reference to home or ambulatory BP readings. These additional methods of measuring and monitoring BP may be useful in our management of patients with refractory hypertension.

A definition of refractory hypertension must also be tempered by the progressive lowering since the 1990s of goal BP, which has the potential to increase the number of "uncontrolled" hypertensive patients. To illustrate these lower BP goals, the Sixth Joint National Committee on the Prevention, Detection, Evaluation and Treatment of High Blood Pressure recommended a target office BP of less than 140 mmHg for systolic and less than 90 mmHg for diastolic readings *(7)* for the hypertensive person without comorbidity. However, in persons with diabetes mellitus or other vascular diseases, the committee recommended a target office BP less than 130 mmHg systolic and less than 85 mmHg for diastolic BP. For patients with renal disease and proteinuria in excess of 1 g, a goal BP of less than 125 mmHg systolic and less than 75 mmHg for diastolic BP was set. Such ambitious goals for BP control place more patients in the refractory hypertension category if achievement of BP goals is part of the definition.

These practical issues in deciding which patients should be labeled as having refractory hypertension are important for several reasons. First, patients with refractory hypertension are usually targeted for further evaluation including identifying possible underlying secondary causes of hypertension. Second, refractory hypertension that is uncorrected confers added risk to that patient, and aggressive control of concomitant cardiovascular risk factors is mandatory. Third, many patients with persistent refractory hypertension will be referred to a hypertension specialist for evaluation and treatment *(8)*. All these factors, therefore, not only place the patient with refractory hypertension in a high-risk category but also target the patient for costly and potentially invasive evaluation. Therefore, it is important that the working definition of refractory hypertension be widely agreed on. An acceptable and pragmatic working

Table 1
Criteria for Refractory Hypertension

| |
|---|
| * Treatment with at least two drugs in moderate to high doses |
| * Treatment with a diuretic type appropriate to the level of renal function |
| * Office BP significantly above goal |
| * Follow-up of at least 3 to 6 months |

definition includes treatment with at least two drugs in moderate to high doses in combination with a diuretic and BP remaining significantly above goal as measured by office methods over a 2- to 3-month period (Table 1).

Despite the availability of newer antihypertensive drugs, the number of patients with resistant hypertension is probably higher than in the 1990s because of the tighter goals of BP. In hypertension clinics, as many as 20–40% of patients are referred because of refractory or resistant hypertension *(1–2)*. The rate of refractory hypertension is probably lower in general medical clinics and the general population and is estimated at 5 to 10% of the hypertensive population.

## BLOOD PRESSURE ELEVATION NOT REFLECTIVE OF PERSISTENT HYPERTENSION

### *Errors and Misleading BP Measurements*

Many factors affect the measurement of office BP, making elevated readings possible when 24-hour BP is normal. Because there is no absolute diagnostic test for hypertension, the actual BP measurement is the key diagnostic step. Unfortunately, this measurement is frequently done in an unstandardized way and with minimal regard for proper methodology. Measuring BP according to standard guidelines *(9)* would go a long way to correcting poor techniques by health care providers. Equipment for measuring BP should be maintained in working order and clinicians should be trained and retrained at regular intervals in measuring BP. Such maintenance applies to mercury, aneroid, and oscillometric devices. Widespread agitation to reduce mercury in medical institutions may lead to a variety of devices being introduced for BP measurement that are likely to be inferior to the conventional mercury manometer. In one institution where all mercury manometers were replaced by aneroid devices *(10)*, having a routine maintenance protocol was shown to be better than not having routine maintenance. Making sure that the observer's hearing is normal may help to ensure accurate readings. Talking by either the physician or nurse taking the BP or the patient or both parties can raise BP significantly in hypertensive and normotensive subjects and should be avoided. Use of a small cuff relative to arm circumference may also artifactually raise BP.

When the measurement of BP is performed correctly, erroneously high readings may still be seen. Some patients exhibit persistently high BP readings without commensurate organ damage and on intra-arterial measurement have normal BP *(11)*. That is, the intra-arterial BP is normal, although simultaneous clinical auscultation indicates severely elevated BP. This situation has been termed *pseudohypertension*. Patients with pseudohypertension commonly have calcified blood vessels and the high BP reading is presumably an artifact of the difficulty in compressing the calcified artery with a cuff. Pseudohypertension has been described in patients with chronic renal failure *(12)*, scleroderma *(13)*, and Williams' syndrome *(14)*, and in the elderly *(15)*. Treatment in these patients is difficult and may precipitate hypotension unless the normalcy of intra-arterial pressure is recognized. The use of Osler's maneuver to predict the presence of pseudohypertension has limited utility and intra-arterial readings are essential to document the disorder *(16)*. Pseudohypertension should be suspected in patients with chronic renal failure or medical states predisposing to arterial calcification and extremely high BP with little clinical damage evident. The differences between clinical and intra-arterial readings can be dramatic and often higher than 100 mmHg *(17)*. An added clinical problem is the patient who has pseudohypertension but is also hypertensive on intra-arterial measurements but at a much lower level than indicated by auscultation. Such patients should be treated, but monitoring their treatment is problematic because of the unreliability of mercury measurements. Oscillometric devices may perform better in these patients with pseudohypertension and are an option for following BP over time.

### *Elevated Office BP Is Not Reflective of Persistent Hypertension*

An important question is whether patients who are suspected of a pressor effect as a cause of refractory BP elevation should undergo ambulatory BP monitoring. Several consensus documents recommend ambulatory BP monitoring in patients with refractory hypertension *(18)*, but this can be logistically difficult to accomplish. The high readings (at times close to 180–200 mmHg), especially in patients with persistent hypertension on ambulatory monitoring, make the procedure uncomfortable because of the need for repeated high inflation pressures. Although demographic factors identifying such patients lack sensitivity and specificity, it would be prudent to consider ambulatory monitoring for patients with labile BP who report much lower home BP readings. Ambulatory monitoring does provide additional risk stratification for patients with refractory hypertension *(19)*.

Redon *(19)* and colleagues recruited 86 clinical outpatients who had a clinic diastolic BP over 100 mmHg on three clinical visits and who were receiving three or more drugs for hypertension, with at least one being a diuretic. This group of patients had an average office BP of 170–180/105–110 mmHg and had creatinine clearances over 60 mL/min/1.73m$^2$. Patients with diabetes mellitus or with known secondary hypertension were excluded. The group was studied with ambulatory BP monitoring and then followed for 48 months to document cardiovascular complications. The patients' hypertension was treated and BP lowered during the observation period according to routine clinical practice. The authors divided patients into tertiles of initial daytime BP for analysis (daytime diastolic <88 mmHg, daytime diastolic 88–97 mmHg, and daytime diastolic >97 mmHg) and compared event-free survival curves in the three groups. The extent of office BP reduction over the follow-up period was similar in the three groups. There were 21 new events during the follow-up period (11 patients with coronary events, 5 patients with cerebral events, 4 patients with congestive heart failure, and 1 patient with a hypertensive emergency). The subjects in the lowest tertile had a significantly lower event rate than the subjects in either the middle or upper tertile. The middle and upper tertile groups were not statistically different. The results were similar when subjects with no prior cardiovascular complications were analyzed separately. Therefore, in patients with defined refractory hypertension, ambulatory BP was an independent marker for new events above and beyond office readings. Not all patients with refractory hypertension are therefore at equal risk. Indeed, in one study of patients referred for ambulatory BP monitoring *(20)*, 28% of patients with resistant hypertension (three or more drugs for hypertension) were found to have a daytime BP less than 135/85 mmHg, indicating that their hypertension was not really "resistant" and was an artifact of the office setting. The authors suggested that 24-hour BP monitoring be the next logical step in evaluating persons with apparent drug-resistant hypertension.

## CAUSES OF REFRACTORY HYPERTENSION

Once the issues raised here regarding BP measurement itself are considered, it is necessary to examine the underlying causes of refractory hypertension. The main categories to be considered include nonadherence to the prescribed treatment regimen, a suboptimal drug combination, exogenous ingestions increasing BP, demographic or biological factors promoting hypertension, and remediable or secondary causes of hypertension. Often, multiple causes are present in the same patient (e.g., an obese patient who is taking low doses of antihypertensive drugs and who is also ingesting a high sodium diet and taking nonsteroidal anti-inflammatory drugs). In one study of refractory hypertension from a referral center *(3)*, it was reported that suboptimal treatment was the cause in 40%, nonadherence to treatment in 10–50%, white coat hypertension in 4%, and secondary causes in 10%.

## NONADHERENCE TO LIFESTYLE MODIFICATIONS AND DRUG THERAPY

Nonadherence is an issue affecting the treatment of all chronic diseases such as hypertension and diabetes mellitus. It represents a failure of the physician–patient relationship and can lead to unwanted consequences for the patient. Physician, medical process, and patient factors such as cost and motivation may play crucial roles in adherence *(21)*. One way to improve adherence in hypertensive patients is to empower them with BP goals, self-monitoring, and their own ability to influence their disease as well as involvement of other health care team members *(22,23)*. It is not possible to predict, based on demographic factors, which patients are following the prescribed regimen. Patients who fail to keep appointments, or do not refill their medications on time, or have unhealthy lifestyles are more likely not to follow a prescribed regimen. Strategic reminder systems using pill boxes, magnets, computer logs, or automatic electronic calendar scheduling may improve adherence when it is hindered by memory deficits *(24)*. Above all, a systematic time of taking prescribed drugs is important for consistent drug intake.

Unfortunately, too many patients with refractory hypertension do not follow even moderate sodium restriction, partially mitigating the effects of drug therapy. However, few, if any, patients with hypertension are ever appropriately educated regarding sources of sodium and ways to lower sodium intake. The "I don't add salt" mantra seems to absolve patients of excessive sodium intake, whereas salt content of food is hardly ever discussed. Furthermore, the general debate about salt and BP in the public media has indicated to patients that the evidence for sodium worsening hypertension is weak. Several antihypertensives show synergistic effects on reducing BP when used together with sodium reduction.

A powerful tool is measurement of 24-hour urinary sodium as an indicator of sodium intake in patients with refractory hypertension.

Clinicians must accept some responsibility for the issue of nonadherence to drugs. Drug-dosing frequency, cost of drugs, side effects, and other issues important to patients must be discussed and minimized to prevent nonadherence. Frequently, sexual dysfunction in a young male with hypertension leads to discontinuation of medications. A carefully measured empathic approach by the physician can reveal such problems and can lead to their prompt resolution.

Although widely believed to be a major factor in patients with resistant hypertension, nonadherence has not been well studied. Two recent studies have provided contradictory evidence on whether compliance is a major cause in resistant hypertension. In a recent study from Switzerland *(25)*, electronic medical event monitoring systems were used to study 110 patients with treatment-responsive hypertension and another group with treatment-resistant hypertension. All patients were studied using ambulatory BP monitoring, and medication compliance was monitored over a 4-week period. Patients with 80% or greater doses removed from medication bottles were considered adherent to prescribed therapy. The study group averaged 64 years of age and 10% were current smokers. Based on the electronic pill counts, 86 patients were considered adherent. These two groups were well matched for demographic factors and hypertension history. When the hypertension responsiveness was based on ambulatory daytime BP less than 135/85 mmHg, no differences were seen in mean or median doses of pills taken. Patients who were prescribed twice daily dosing had a lower compliance than those prescribed once daily dosing. The actual monitoring itself did not influence compliance as judged by ambulatory BP averages that were unchanged after the study. In this somewhat selected population, noncompliance with treatment was not more common among patients with resistant hypertension. This study has several shortcomings including the short duration and lack of an active intervention. In contrast to these findings, a prospective study of 41 patients with resistant hypertension was performed to assess compliance (*26*). Patients were told their medication intake would be assessed using an electronic monitor. Without changing drug treatment, this step alone reduced BP and normalized in one-third of subjects. The authors suggested that objective monitoring of compliance may be a useful step in refractory hypertension. Undoubtedly, issues of adherence need to be considered in patients with refractory hypertension.

Table 2
Substances That Can Increase BP or Antagonize Drug Therapy

* Nonselective nonsteroidal anti-inflammatory drugs
* Selective nonsteroidal anti-inflammatory drugs (cyclooxygenase 2 inhibitors)
* Ethanol
* Cocaine and other amphetamine-like drugs
* Oral contraceptive pill
* Over-the-counter nasal decongestants with sympathomimetic agents
* Licorice
* Cyclosporine and tacrolimus
* Corticosteroids and anabolic steroids
* Excessive ingestion of caffeine
* Erythropoietin
* Mono-oxidase inhibitors when mixed with foods containing tyramine
* Supplements containing ephedrine
* Appetite suppressants
* Newer antidepressants

## SUBSTANCES MITIGATING THE RESPONSE TO THE DRUG REGIMEN

A multitude of supplements, herbal substances, illicit substances, and prescription drugs can interfere with the action of antihypertensive drugs (Table 2). The most prevalent of these substances seen in clinical practice are nonsteroidal anti-inflammatory drugs (NSAIDs), alcohol, and cocaine. Newer cyclooxygenase selective inhibitors (COX-2 inhibitors) also raise BP in predisposed individuals.

### *NSAIDs*

The widespread access to and use of NSAIDs in society make it likely that many hypertensive patients are ingesting these drugs on a regular basis. NSAIDs raise BP by causing sodium and water retention, by increasing intravascular volume, and by also directly inhibiting renal-dilating prostaglandins. Even if NSAIDs raised BP minimally in individual patients, they could have a large impact on the population's BP; the attributable effect would be large. The BP-raising effect of such therapy has been reported as being anywhere from 3.3 to 5 mmHg in hypertensive patients with some drugs (e.g., indomethacin causing more of an effect while aspirin and sulindac appear to have a smaller effect

*[27]*). One meta-analysis suggested that patients taking β-adrenoceptor blockers and angiotensin-converting enzyme inhibitors were more likely to have interference in BP control *(27)*.

The newer selective COX-2 inhibitors appear to cause fewer gastric side effects than traditional nonselective drugs. The effects on BP are not well studied but it does appear that these new drugs can increase BP in patients taking antihypertensives *(28)*. Logically, they may be postulated to interfere mostly with the classes of drugs that work to lower BP via vasodilating prostaglandins.

## *Alcohol and Hypertension*

Ethanol is widely ingested throughout the world and increased consumption has been firmly linked to increased levels of BP in multiple epidemiological studies *(29)*. Ethanol appears to have an effect on BP within a few hours of ingestion and a dose-response effect has been observed on BP. Removal of ethanol generally leads to lower BP levels, which implicates it with little doubt as a pressor agent when ingested in moderate amounts. However, clinical trial data regarding the effects on BP have been obtained largely in small trials in which reduction of alcohol intake resulted in lower BP. Every patient with refractory hypertension must be questioned about alcohol intake and the effects of excess alcohol on BP must be explained.

The Prevention and Treatment of Hypertension Study (PATHS) was the largest randomized trial *(30)* to examine the effects of alcohol reduction on BP. PATHS enrolled 641 moderate to heavy drinkers with diastolic BP of 80–99 mmHg. Randomization was to a sustained reduction in alcohol intake or no intervention. The study was designed to approximate a difference between the two groups of at least two drinks. A difference of only 1.3 drinks per day was observed between the two groups up until 24 months of follow-up because a larger than expected reduction in alcohol use was seen in the control group. A nonsignificant reduction in BP of 0.9/0.6 mmHg was therefore observed. Other randomized studies with a larger reduction in alcohol intake showed larger BP declines in although they generally had fewer participants.

## *Cocaine and Hypertension*

The use of cocaine is associated more with episodic increases in BP with hypertensive emergencies, myocardial infarction, seizures, cardiac arrhythmias, and stroke. It is unclear whether chronic sustained hypertension may be associated with cocaine use *(31)*. However, in many clinical scenarios where hypertension is resistant or labile, cocaine use must be considered as a contributing factor.

### *Cyclosporine, Tacrolimus, and Hypertension*

Cyclosporine and tacrolimus, both calcineurin inhibitors, are increasingly used to treat various immunological and dermatological diseases in addition to their use in renal diseases and clinical transplantation. Their administration is associated with either rapid onset of hypertension or gradual increases over several weeks to months *(32)*. There remains considerable discussion about the mechanism of hypertension in persons receiving cyclosporine. In brief, renal, neural, and vascular effects have been proposed to explain the increases in BP seen in patients on calcineurin inhibitors. Early studies showed that cyclosporine hypertension was particularly salt sensitive. Other studies have suggested vascular constriction as a factor in the development of hypertension. Finally, activation of the central and renal sympathetic nervous systems probably plays a role as well. Tacrolimus appears to produce less vasoconstriction than cyclosporine and probably causes smaller increases in BP. Consideration should be given to dose reduction of these agents if the clinical situation allows in a patient with refractory hypertension. Dihydropyridine calcium channel blockers have been touted as important drugs to use in this setting.

## OPTIMAL DRUG REGIMEN AND RESISTANT HYPERTENSION

Perhaps the largest contribution of a hypertension specialist is the ability to optimize drug therapy in patients receiving multiple agents. In one series where a cause of resistant hypertension was attributed *(2)*, suboptimal therapy was the cause in 43% of patients. In the majority of these patients, BP lowering was observed with alterations in therapeutic regimens. The changes made included adding a diuretic, increasing drug doses or drug-dosing frequency, or selecting a suitable drug combination with a synergistic effect on lowering BP. The appropriate diuretic should be chosen for the level of renal function, with loop diuretics being preferred in patients with impaired renal function. It has been suggested *(33)* that a rational method to treat hypertension and achieve control is to evaluate each person's renin system, stratify them according to whether they are low or high renin, and then treat accordingly (diuretics for patients with low renin, and antirenin and anti-angiotensin therapies for those with high renin). Of course, the extremes of renin also provide a clue to some forms of secondary hypertension. In 73 patients with hypertension resistant to one or more agents subjected to this analysis and subsequent treatment, BP was lowered by 23/11 mmHg and patients were taking fewer medications *(33)*.

## SECONDARY HYPERTENSION

Inevitably, if BP remains above goal, consideration is given to the possibility that the patient has secondary hypertension. Certainly, any hypertensive patient whose clinical history examination or laboratory data suggest a secondary cause should be thoroughly evaluated (Tables 3 and 4). Otherwise, there is much variability in the evaluation for secondary hypertension in patients with refractory hypertension. Some practitioners perform a minimal evaluation including screening for renal parenchymal disease, thyroid disease, primary hyperaldosteronism, and renal artery stenosis in truly resistant patients. The cost effectiveness of this approach has not been studied.

### *Primary Aldosteronism As a Cause of Refractory Hypertension*

There has been a marked increase in the frequency of diagnosis of primary aldosteronism and a realization that many patients do not have hypokalemia *(34–36)*. Various reports now estimate that 2–10% of patients with resistant hypertension may have primary aldosteronism *(36)*. Although this is likely an overestimate because of excessive reliance on the aldosterone-to-renin ratio as a diagnostic tool, there is little debate that aldosteronism is considered routinely in patients with resistant hypertension. The pathophysiology of the disorder is usually either an adenoma or bilateral adrenal hyperplasia causing inappropriately high and nonsuppressible aldosterone levels. This anomaly leads to sodium and water retention and hypertension with suppressed plasma renin activity. This avid return of sodium in the distal convoluted tubules leads to excessive potassium loss that can be detected in the urine. However, it appears that the disorder spans a spectrum and it may be difficult to distinguish low-renin hypertension from aldosteronism *(37)*. It is easy to see why the prescribed antihypertensive drugs or dietary sodium intake may mask hypokalemia.

Although there is continuing debate about the optimal diagnostic approach to aldosteronism, clinicians typically proceed sequentially through screening, confirmation, subtype determination, and then treat-

Table 3
Clinical Clues to Secondary Hypertension

| |
|---|
| *Historical factors pointing to secondary hypertension* |
| Early or late onset of hypertension |
| Sudden increase in BP |
| Hypertension associated with complications |
| Refractory hypertension |
| Excessive BP lowering with certain antihypertensive drugs |

Table 4
Typical Symptoms and Signs of Certain Forms of Secondary Hypertension

| *Symptoms and signs* | *Type of secondary hypertension suggested* |
|---|---|
| Multiple vascular risk factors, abdominal bruit, unexplained renal insufficiency, resistant hypertension | Renal artery stenosis |
| Proteinuria, renal dysfunction, nocturia, peripheral edema | Renal parenchymal disease |
| Hypokalemia, nocturia, cramps, family history | Primary aldosteronism |
| Hematuria, large flank masses, family history of renal disease | Autosomal dominant polycystic kidney disease |
| Daytime fatigue, sleepiness, snoring, large neck size, apnea | Sleep apnea |
| Proximal weakness, diabetes, truncal obesity, striae, hypokalemia | Cushing's disease |
| Early onset hypertension, reduced or delayed pulses in the legs, disparity in arm BP | Aortic coarctation |
| Headache, palpitations, sweating, pallor, tachycardia | Pheochromocytoma |

ment. Screening involves the measurement of a simultaneous serum aldosterone level and a plasma renin activity in an ambulatory patient. If this ratio is significantly elevated (>30) and the serum aldosterone is 15 ng/dL or greater, then formal salt suppression testing is performed, if it is clinically safe to do so. Salt suppression protocols have generally been developed in patients not receiving antihypertensive therapy but today these tests are done while patients ingest antihypertensive drugs. The short intravenous 4-hour suppression protocol or an outpatient oral salt-loading protocol can be used. At times, the results of these two tests disagree, making it problematic for the clinician. Lack of suppression of aldosterone to normal levels on either test confirms inappropriate autonomous aldosterone secretion, the hallmark of aldosteronism. There is a need for agreement on the appropriate thresholds for the diagnosis when using the different salt suppression protocols.

An important, although relatively rare, subtype *(38)* is glucocorticoid remediable hyperaldosteronism, which is associated with resistant hypertension at a young age *(39)*. In this variant of aldosteronism, a chimeric gene causes the synthesis of aldosterone to be under the control of the glucocorticoid arm of the pituitary–adrenal axis. There is usually a history of early onset moderate to severe hypertension, with family members also developing hypertension at an early age. One unfortunate complication that may be elicited in the history is cerebral hemorrhage, which occurs at a mean age of 32 years. The cause of this complication appears to be the presence of intracranial aneurysms. Hence, screening for cerebral aneurysms every 5 years is recommended for patients with this disorder after they achieve puberty. Serum potassium levels are in the normal range in systematically studied patients with this disorder *(39)*.

There is little doubt that primary aldosteronism can cause refractory hypertension *(40)* and even malignant hypertension *(41,42)*. A review of several recent case series of patients with primary aldosteronism *(43–45)* reveals that in general prior to diagnosis and appropriate treatment, patients have BP readings over 160–170 mmHg for systolic and over 100 mmHg for diastolic BP. Clinical practice also indicates that refractory hypertension is indeed a common clue to the presence of primary aldosteronism.

### *Pheochromocytoma and Refractory Hypertension*

Excessive circulating catecholamines, the hallmark of symptomatic pheochromocytoma, cause not only paroxysmal and often impressive symptoms but also chronic hypertension with periodic worsening. These paroxysms may be provoked by changes in posture, exercise, or medications. Frequently, attacks are sudden in onset and slowly dissipate. These circulating catecholamines are effective promoters of cardiovascular complications and are typically secreted by an intra-abdominal tumor (98%) with the possibility of malignancy. Therefore, although a rare cause of secondary hypertension, pheochromocytoma deserves attention as a diagnosis not to be missed. Most tumors secrete a preponderance of norepinephrine and, less so, epinephrine, but either catecholamine alone or dopamine only secretion has been reported. Over half the patients have sustained hypertension that fluctuates *(46)*. It is not clear whether all patients with resistant hypertension should be screened for pheochromocytoma. Patients with any suggestive symptoms or signs or associated genetic diseases (e.g., von Hippel-Lindau or multiple endocrine neoplasia), however, should be screened *(47)*.

### *Renal Artery Stenosis and Refractory Hypertension*

In the paper by Setaro et al. on resistant hypertension in a tertiary care clinic *(1)*, 4% of patients had renal artery stenosis. Indeed, the disorder is usually screened for when hypertension is resistant, or renal function deteriorates, or recurrent bouts of flash pulmonary edema are seen. In the large Dutch renal artery stenosis trial *(48)*, resistance to two drugs was considered a criterion for angiography. Among 41% of patients receiving either enalapril or amlodipine along with a diuretic and whose diastolic BP remained over 95 mmHg, 20% were found to have renal artery stenosis on angiography. Consideration should be given to atherosclerotic renal artery stenosis in older patients with vascular risk factors and to the fibromuscular dysplastic variant in younger persons with hypertension. The latter is significantly benefited in terms of BP cure from revascularization, whereas in the former some improvement is seen although cure is rare.

### *Sleep Apnea and Resistant Hypertension*

It is generally accepted that a relationship exists between obstructive sleep apnea (OSA) and hypertension but cause and effect is still debated *(49)*. The two disorders, however, share a number of other demographic parameters that may explain their relationship. Significant OSA clearly raises BP during sleep but the effects on BP throughout the rest of the day are unknown. Furthermore, it is unclear if OSA can cause daytime hypertension to be resistant and unresponsive to treatment.

In one study of patients referred to a sleep laboratory *(50)*, an attempt was made to examine whether OSA contributes to resistant hypertension. A total of 1485 patients were diagnosed with OSA during a 10-year period and were not being treated with positive nasal pressure. The effectiveness of antihypertensive drug therapy and the presence of OSA was examined by analyzing only treated hypertensive patients ($N = 393$). The group was further divided into effectively treated ($n = 183$, BP <140/90 mmHg) and ineffectively treated ($n = 74$, BP 140/90 mmHg). BP was measured three times each in the morning and evening on the night of polysomnographic study. The apnea–hypopnea index was higher in the ineffective group after adjusting for gender, age, and neck circumference. This was confirmed in a logistic regression analysis using predictor variables of age, body mass index, gender, pack-years of smoking, and apnea–hypopnea index. Logan added some data on this issue *(51)* by performing polysomnographic studies on 41 subjects with uncontrolled hypertension despite a three or more drug regimen at maximal doses and preferably including a diuretic. The patients were drawn from a specialty hypertension clinic and underwent ambulatory BP monitoring and polysomnography. OSA was defined as 10 or more obstructive apneas and hypopneas per hour of sleep. Overall, 83% of these selected patients had OSA, with 96% in males and 65% in females. Similarly, Kraiczi et al. *(52)* compared BP and cardiac structure in 81 patients with varying severities of sleep apnea. They found that the apnea–hypopnea index was predictive of office daytime and nighttime diastolic BP and office systolic and nighttime systolic BP.

An intriguing question is whether certain drugs are more effective in patients with both OSA and hypertension *(53)*. Forty patients with OSA and hypertension were treated in sequence with two of five antihypertensive agents (atenolol, amlodipine, enalapril, hydrochlorothiazide, Losartan) for 6 weeks with 3 weeks of washout. Office diastolic BP was most effectively lowered by atenolol with no differences in reductions of systolic BP. Additionally, atenolol and hydrochlorothiazide both lowered nocturnal systolic and diastolic BP more than the other agents.

## SUMMARY

The numbers of patients not achieving goal BP despite treatment with two or more drugs challenge every clinician. However, a methodological approach is necessary to avoid repeated changes in therapy with no improvement in BP. Serious consideration should be given early to the possibility that office BP may not reflect average BP, and home or ambulatory readings should be considered. Patient adherence needs to be reinforced and any barriers to this exposed and remedied. Ingestions of other substances that may directly or indirectly keep BP levels elevated must be consciously inquired about and removed if possible. An optimal regimen including the use of diuretics and also consideration given to secondary causes of hypertension may be better directed by a hypertension specialist. Discovery of certain forms of secondary hypertension can lead to specific disease-targeted intervention or drug selection. Refractory hypertension will nevertheless continue to be a challenge to physicians.

## REFERENCES


1. Setaro JF, Black HR. Refractory hypertension. N Engl J Med 1992;20;327: 543–547.
2. Alderman MH, Budner N, Cohen H, Lamport B, Ooi WL. Prevalence of drug resistant hypertension. Hypertension 1988;11:II71–75.
3. Yakovlevitch M, Black HR. Resistant hypertension in a tertiary care clinic. Arch Intern Med 1991;151:1786–1792.
4. Oparil S, Calhoun DA. Managing the patient with hard-to-control hypertension. Am Fam Physician 1998;57:1007–1014.
5. Vidt DG. Contributing factors in resistant hypertension: truly refractory disease is rarely found in a properly conducted workup. Postgrad Med 2000;107:57–70.
6. Alper AB Jr, Calhoun DA. Contemporary management of refractory hypertension. Curr Hypertens Rep 1999;5:402–407.
7. Joint National Committee on Prevention, Detection, Evaluation and Treatment of High Blood Pressure. The sixth report of the Joint National Committee on Prevention, Detection, Evaluation and Treatment of High Blood Pressure. Arch Intern Med 1997;157:2413–2446.
8. Krakoff LR. Hypertension specialists: ready or not, here we come. Am J Hypertens 1999;12:242–243.
9. American Society of Hypertension. Recommendations for routine blood pressure measurement by indirect cuff sphygmomanometry. Am J Hypertens 1992;5: 207–209.
10. Canzanello VJ, Jensen PL, Schwartz GL. Are aneroid sphygmomanometers accurate in hospital and clinic settings? Arch Intern Med 2001;161:729–731.
11. Messerli FH, Ventura HO, Amodeo C. Osler's maneuver and pseudohypertension. N Engl J Med 1985;312:1548–1551.
12. Kuriyama S, Tomonari H, Utsunomiya Y, Kinoshita N, Matsumoto H. Pseudohypertension in hemodialyzed arteriosclerotic patients. Nephron 1994;66:479–480.
13. Rosner MH, Okusa MD. Pseudohypertension in a patient with diffuse scleroderma. Am J Kidney Dis 2001;37:E32.
14. Bastianon V. Pseudohypertension and Williams syndrome. Pediatr Cardiol 1996;17:132.
15. Anzal M, Palmer AJ, Starr J, Bulpitt CJ. The prevalence of pseudohypertension in the elderly. J Hum Hypertens 1996;10:409–411.
16. Belmin J, Visintin JM, Salvatore R, Sebban C, Moulias R. Osler's maneuver: absence of usefulness for the detection of pseudohypertension in an elderly population. Am J Med 1995;98:42–49.
17. Massay RJ, Mansoor GA. A case of pseudohypertension. West Indian Med J 1990;39:114–117.
18. Pickering TG. A review of national guidelines on the clinical use of ambulatory blood pressure monitoring. Blood Press Monit 1996;1:151–156.
19. Redon J, Campos C, Narciso ML, Rodicio JL, Pascual JM, Ruilope LM. Prognostic value of ambulatory blood pressure monitoring in refractory hypertension: a prospective study. Hypertension 1998;31:712–718.
20. Brown MA, Megan LM, Martin A. Is resistant hypertension really resistant? Am J Hypertens 2001;14:1263–1269.
21. Hill MN. Comprehensive hypertension care in young urban black men: an example of a program of nursing research that integrates genetic science, clinical interventions, and patient outcomes. Nurs Clin North Am 2000;35:773–793.

22. Rogers MA, Small D, Buchan DA, et al.Home monitoring service improves mean arterial pressure in patients with essential hypertension: a randomized, controlled trial. Ann Intern Med 2001;5;134:1024–1032.
23. Mehos BM, Saseen JJ, MacLaughlin EJ. Effect of pharmacist intervention and initiation of home blood pressure monitoring in patients with uncontrolled hypertension. Pharmacotherapy 2000;20:1384–1389.
24. Bertholet N, Favrat B, Fallab-Stubi CL, Brunner HR, Burnier M. Why objective monitoring of compliance is important in the management of hypertension. J Clin Hypertens (Greenwich) 2000;2:258–262.
25. Nuesch R, Schroeder K, Dieterle T, Martina B, Battegay E. Relation between insufficient response to antihypertensive treatment and poor compliance with treatment: a prospective case-control study. BMJ 2001;323:142–146.
26. Burnier M, Schneider MP, Chiolero A, Stubi CL, Brunner HR. Electronic compliance monitoring in resistant hypertension: the basis for rational therapeutic decisions. J Hypertens 2001;19:335–341.
27. Johnson AG, Nguyen TV, Day RO. Do nonsteroidal anti-inflammatory drugs affect blood pressure? a meta-analysis. Ann Intern Med 1994;15;121:289–300.
28. Whelton A, Fort JG, Puma JA, Normandin D, Bello AE, Verburg KM; SUCCESS VI Study Group. Cyclooxygenase-2–specific inhibitors and cardiorenal function: a randomized, controlled trial of celecoxib and rofecoxib in older hypertensive osteoarthritis patients. Am J Ther 2001;8:85–95.
29. Beilin LJ. Alcohol and hypertension. Clin Exp Pharmacol Physiol 1995;22:185–188.
30. Cushman WC, Cutler JA, Hanna E, et al. Prevention and treatment of hypertension study (PATHS): effects of an alcohol treatment program on blood pressure. Arch Intern Med 1998;158:1197–1207.
31. Brecklin CS, Gopaniuk-Folga A, Kravetz T, et al. Prevalence of hypertension in chronic cocaine users. Am J Hypertens 1998;11:1279–1283.
32. Taler SJ, Textor SC, Canzanello VJ, Schwartz L. Cyclosporin-induced hypertension: incidence, pathogenesis and management. Drug Saf 1999;20:437–449.
33. Blumenfeld JD, Laragh JH. Renin system analysis: a rational method for the diagnosis and treatment of the individual patient with hypertension. Am J Hypertens 1998;11:894–896.
34. Stowasser M. Primary aldosteronism: rare bird or common cause of secondary hypertension? Curr Hypertens Rep 2001;3:230–239.
35. Young WF Jr. Primary aldosteronism: a common and curable form of hypertension. Cardiol Rev 1999;7:207–214.
36. Fardella CE, Mosso L, Gomez-Sanchez C, et al. Primary hyperaldosteronism in essential hypertensives: prevalence, biochemical profile, and molecular biology. J Clin Endocrinol Metab 2000;85:1863–1867.
37. Ganguly A. Prevalence of primary aldosteronism in unselected hypertensive populations: screening and definitive diagnosis. J Clin Endocrinol Metab 2001; 86:4002–4004.
38. Gates LJ, Benjamin N, Haites NE, MacConnachie AA, McLay JS. Is random screening of value in detecting glucocorticoid-remediable aldosteronism within a hypertensive population? J Hum Hypertens 2001;15:173–176.
39. Dluhy RG, Anderson B, Harlin B, Ingelfinger J, Lifton R. Glucocorticoid-remediable aldosteronism is associated with severe hypertension in early childhood. J Pediatr 2001;138:715–720.
40. Schamess A, Bernik T, Tenner S. Refractory hypertension due to Conn's syndrome. Postgrad Med 1994;95:199–206.

41. Murphy BF, Whitworth JA, Kincaid-Smith P. Malignant hypertension due to an aldosterone producing adrenal adenoma. Clin Exp Hypertens A 1985;7:939–950.
42. Zarifis J, Lip GY, Leatherdale B, Beevers G. Malignant hypertension in association with primary aldosteronism. Blood Press 1996;5:250–254.
43. Magill SB, Raff H, Shaker JL, Brickner RC, Knechtges TE, Kehoe ME, Findling JW. Comparison of adrenal vein sampling and computed tomography in the differentiation of primary aldosteronism. J Clin Endocrinol Metab 2001;86:1066–1071.
44. Rossi GP, Sacchetto A, Chiesura-Corona M, et al. Identification of the etiology of primary aldosteronism with adrenal vein sampling in patients with equivocal computed tomography and magnetic resonance findings: results in 104 consecutive cases. J Clin Endocrinol Metab 2001;86:1083–1090.
45. Blumenfeld JD, Sealey JE, Schlussel Y, et al. Diagnosis and treatment of primary hyperaldosteronism. Ann Intern Med 1994;121:877–885.
46. Bravo EL. Evolving concepts in the pathophysiology, diagnosis, and treatment of pheochromocytoma. Endocr Rev 1994;15:356–368.
47. Pacak K, Linehan WM, Eisenhofer G, Walther MM, Goldstein DS. Recent advances in genetics, diagnosis, localization, and treatment of pheochromocytoma. Ann Intern Med 2001;134:315–329.
48. van Jaarsveld BC, Krijnen P, Derkx FH, et al. Resistance to antihypertensive medication as predictor of renal artery stenosis: comparison of two drug regimens. J Hum Hypertens 2001;15:669–676
49. Leung RS, Bradley TD. Sleep apnea and cardiovascular disease. Am J Respir Crit Care Med 2001;164:2147–2165.
50. Lavie P, Hoffstein V. Sleep apnea syndrome: a possible contributing factor to resistant hypertension. Sleep 2001;24:721–725.
51. Logan AG, Perlikowski SM, Mente A, et al. High prevalence of unrecognized sleep apnoea in drug-resistant hypertension. J Hypertens 2001;19:2271–2277.
52. Kraiczi H, Peker Y, Caidahl K, Samuelsson A, Hedner J. Blood pressure, cardiac structure and severity of obstructive sleep apnea in a sleep clinic population. J Hypertens 2001;19:2071–2078.
53. Kraiczi H, Hedner J, Peker Y, Grote L. Comparison of atenolol, amlodipine, enalapril, hydrochlorothiazide, and losartan for antihypertensive treatment in patients with obstructive sleep apnea. Am J Respir Crit Care Med 2000;161: 1423–1428.

# 2 Iatrogenic and Drug-Induced Hypertension

*Ehud Grossman, MD*
*and Franz H. Messerli, MD*

*CONTENTS*



From: *Secondary Hypertension: Clinical Presentation, Diagnosis, and Treatment*
Edited by: G. A. Mansoor © Humana Press Inc., Totowa, NJ

## INTRODUCTION

A variety of drugs and chemical substances have been shown to elevate blood pressure (BP). Most often, the increase in BP is transient and of questionable clinical significance. However, more sustained hypertension and even accelerated hypertensive cardiovascular disease have occasionally been documented to occur after exposure to certain chemical substances. Of note, a variety of drugs also make "essential" hypertension more resistant to antihypertensive therapy. An accurate and detailed medical history should, therefore, include specific inquiries concerning foods, poisons, and medications. This is particularly important with regard to such things as over-the-counter drugs, nutritional supplements, diets, and health foods, which are often not considered to be drugs and, therefore, are frequently omitted from the history.

Identification of such substances is important because their elimination can obviate the need for unnecessary, costly, and potentially dangerous evaluations and/or treatments. When drug- or chemical-induced hypertension is identified, discontinuation of the causative agent should be recommended. When it is not possible to discontinue agents that cause hypertension, institution of appropriate antihypertensive treatment is indicated. In the absence of specific treatment guidelines for drug-induced hypertension, the recommended initial antihypertensive therapy should be directed to neutralize the specific mechanism causing hypertension (Table 1).

## STEROIDS

### *Corticosteroids*

Hypertension occurs in about 20% of patients treated with high doses of synthetic corticosteroids. Oral cortisol increases BP in a dose-dependent fashion. At a dose of 80–200 mg/day, the peak increases in systolic pressure are of the order of 15 mmHg. This increase in BP is apparent within 24 hours. The mechanism of glucocorticoid (GC)-induced hypertension remains uncertain and it seems to be multifactorial. GC-induced hypertension occurs often in elderly patients and is more common in patients with positive family history of essential hypertension. Hemodynamically, corticosteroids increase BP through increasing circulatory volume, cardiac output, and peripheral resistance. Certain exogenous compounds such as liquorice, phenylbutazone, carbenoxolone, 9-α fluoroprednisolone, and 9-α fluorocortisol have mineralocorticoid activity and, when ingested in excessive quantities, may produce arterial hypertension characterized by the clinical picture of "pseudohyperaldosteronism" with increased exchangeable sodium and blood volume, hypokalemia with metabolic alkalosis, and suppressed plasma renin and aldosterone levels. Prolonged use of high-dose ketoconazole may alter enzymatic degradation of steroids, leading to mineralocorticoid-related hypertension. Skin ointments, antihemorrhoidal preparations, ophthalmic drops, and nasal sprays may contain substances with mineralocorticoid activity (9-$\alpha$ fluoroprednisolone) and sympathetic amines. Their excessive use may even cause severe arterial hypertension. Discontinuation of these substances is recommended to lower BP. However, when steroid treatment is mandatory, a diuretic is the drug of choice, because volume overload is the main mechanism by which steroids raise BP; careful monitoring of potassium is necessary.

### *Sex Hormones*

Oral contraceptives (OCs) induce hypertension in approximately 5% of users of high-dose compounds that contain at least 50 mg estrogen and 1 to 4 mg progestin, and small increases in BP have been reported even among users of modern low-dose formulations. Women with a history of high BP during pregnancy; those with a family history of hypertension; cigarette smokers; those who are obese, black, or diabetic; and those with renal diseases may respond with a greater increase in BP. Compared with women who had never used OCs, users of OCs have an increased risk of developing hypertension (risk ratio = 1.8; 95% CI = 1.5–2.3). However, only in a small percentage could hypertension be attributed to OC use. Risk of hypertension decreased quickly with cessation of OCs, and past users appeared to have only a slightly increased risk. The increase in BP is usually minimal; however, severe hypertensive episodes, including malignant hypertension, have been reported. Postmenopausal estrogen replacement therapy (ERT) decreases BP slightly, and rare cases of estrogen-induced hypertension represent an idiosyncratic reaction to ERT. Cessation of ERT is recommended when hypertension develops. However, if ERT should be continued, a diuretic is the most appropriate treatment because the contraceptives estrogen and androgen increase BP via fluid retention.

Men receiving estrogen to treat prostatic cancer may also exhibit an increase in BP.

Danazol, a semisynthetic androgen that is used to treat endometriosis and hereditary angioedema, was reported to induce hypertension through fluid retention.

Table 1
Management of Drug-Induced Hypertension

| *Ingredient* | *Management* | *Notes* |
|---|---|---|
| **Steroids** | | |
| Glucocorticoids | Discontinue. If not possible start diuretics | Monitor potassium |
| Mineralocorticoids | Discontinue. If not possible start diuretics | Monitor potassium |
| Sex Hormones | | |
| **Anesthetics and narcotics** | | |
| Ketamine hydrochloride | Initial therapy: clonidine, α-blockers | |
| Desflurane | Initial therapy : α-blockers, α+β-blockers | |
| Naloxone | Initial therapy : α-blockers | |
| Sevoflurane | Clonidine, or combination of diltiazem and nicardipine | |
| **Drugs affecting the sympathetic nervous system** | | |
| Ophthalmic solutions | Initial therapy : α-blockers, α+β-blockers | Avoid β-blockers |
| Antiemetic agents | | Transient increase in BP |
| Yohimbine hydrochloride | Discontinue | Avoid in hypertensive patients and in those treated with tricyclic antidepressants |
| Glucagon (only in patients with pheochromocytoma) | Initial therapy : Intravenous phentholamin, oral phenoxybenzamine, or α1-blockers | |
| Cocaine | Initial therapy : α-blockers, nitroglycerin and verapamil | Most patients do not require treatment |

| | | |
|---|---|---|
| Anorexics | Discontinue treatment | |
| Nasal decongestant | Initial therapy : α+β-blockers | |
| Cough medications | Discontinue treatment | |
| Sibutramine | Discontinue sibutramine or modify antihypertensive therapy | In obese hypertensive patients, the BP reduction achieved by weight loss negates the potential increase related to the drug |
| Clozapine | Discontinue. If not possible, start α-blockers or nifedipine | |
| **Antidepressant agents** | | |
| MAOIs | Initial therapy : α-blockers | |
| Tricyclic antidepressants | Initial therapy : α-blockers | |
| Serotonin agonist | Initial therapy : α-blockers | |
| **Miscellaneous** | | |
| Cyclosporine | Discontinue, or switch to tacrolimus, if not possible start calcium antagonists. Other drugs are also effective. | Calcium antagonists may increase cyclosporine blood levels. Multidrug therapy may be necessary |
| Tacrolimus | Discontinue, if not possible start calcium antagonists. Other drugs are also effective. | |
| r-HuEPO | Lower the dose, if unsuccessful start calcium antagonists or α-blockers. Diuretics and ACE inhibitors may be less effective. | Dialysis with conventional antihypertensive treatment may be effective. Phlebotomy may rapidly lower BP |
| Bromocriptine disulfiram | | Avoid use for suppression of lactation |
| Alcohol | Moderate alcohol intake | |
| NSAID | Calcium antagonists | Assess the risk of an increase in BP against the expected benefit. Among COX-2 inhibitors, celecoxib affects BP less than rofecoxib |

## ANESTHETICS AND NARCOTICS

Ketamine hydrochloride has been reported to severely increase BP. In one study, clonidine that suppresses sympathetic activity was effective in reducing the hypertensive response to ketamine.

Desflurane may induce hypertension via stimulation of the sympathetic nervous system. Sympatholytic agents such as α-blockers and α+β blockers may lower BP.

Sevoflurane may increase BP during anesthesia. Treatment with clonidine or a combination of diltiazem and nicardipine may blunt the BP increase.

The simultaneous use of vasoconstrictors (felypressin) with topical cocaine can result in severe hypertension. At least one case was treated successfully with labetalol.

Hypertensive responses to naloxone (opiate antagonist), especially during attempted reversal of narcotic-induced anesthesia in hypertensive patients, have also been reported. Naloxone seems to acutely reverse the antihypertensive effects of clonidine and can thereby cause an acute hypertensive emergency.

## DRUGS AFFECTING THE SYMPATHETIC NERVOUS SYSTEM

Phenylephrine, a sympathomimetic agent with a potent vasoconstrictor activity, has been reported to severely increase BP following its administration in an ophthalmic solution. Dipivalyl adrenaline, an adrenaline prodrug used topically in the management of chronic simple glaucoma, can also increase BP in treated hypertensive patients.

The concomitant use of sympathomimetic agents and β-blockers can severely increase BP because of unopposed α-adrenergic vasoconstriction. The substitution of α-blockers or agents such as labetalol or carvedilol, which block both α- and β-adrenergic receptors, should prevent this detrimental reaction.

Antiemetic agents such as metoclopramide, alizapride and prochlorperazine have been reported to increase BP transiently in patients treated with cisplatin.

Yohimbine hydrochloride—an $\alpha_2$-adrenoceptor antagonist that is approved (but of questionable efficacy) for treatment of impotence—may significantly increase BP in hypertensive patients. Yohimbine should be avoided or used intermittently only in hypertensive patients and in those undergoing concurrent treatment with tricyclic antidepressants.

Glucagon may induce severe hypertension in patients with pheochromocytoma. Blocking the α-adrenoceptors by either intravenous phentolamine or oral agents such as phenoxybenzamine or doxazosin may prevent catastrophic cardiovascular events.

Cocaine intoxication is characterized by α-adrenergic overactivity often associated with increased BP. Cocaine use is associated with acute but not chronic hypertension. Severe hypertension has been reported to occur in subjects treated with propranolol. Most patients with cocaine-related hypertension do not require pharmacological therapy, but if treatment is necessary, α-adrenergic receptor antagonists would seem a logical choice for initial treatment. β-Blockers can be useful in the management of cardiac dysrhythmias, but they should be used with caution because of the possibility of exacerbating hypertension resulting from unopposed α-receptor activity. Nitroglycerin and verapamil reverse cocaine-induced hypertension and coronary arterial vasoconstriction and therefore are the agents of choice in treating patients with cocaine-associated chest pain. One case of hypertensive encephalopathy secondary to cocaine abuse was treated successfully with nitroprusside and captopril.

### *Sibutramine*

Sibutramine is a novel serotonin and noradrenaline reuptake inhibitor anti-obesity drug. Sibutramine reduces food intake by enhancing the physiological response of post-ingestive satiety and increases energy expenditure. By activating the sympathetic nervous system, the drug increases heart rate and BP in obese normotensive subjects. In obese patients whose hypertension is well controlled with a β-blocker or angiotensin-converting enzyme (ACE) inhibitor, sibutramine achieves weight loss without compromising good BP control. It seems that in obese hypertensive patients the BP reduction achieved by weight loss negates the potential BP increase related to the drug. Nevertheless, obese patients being treated with sibutramine should be monitored periodically for changes in BP. If BP becomes elevated, sibutramine should be withdrawn.

### *Clozapine*

Clozapine is an antipsychotic agent that is used for schizophrenic symptoms in patients refractory to classical antipsychotics. This drug may raise BP by sympathetic activation. Several case reports of pseudopheochromocytoma syndrome associated with clozapine have been described. BP and sympathetic overactivity were normalized upon treatment discontinuation. In one case, nifedipine controlled clozapine-induced hypertension. However, α-adrenergic receptor antagonists would seem a more appropriate choice for initial treatment.

## IMMUNOSUPPRESSIVE AGENTS

Cyclosporin A—a potent, orally active immunosuppressive drug—may induce arterial hypertension. The incidence of cyclosporin-associated hypertension (CAH) varies with the patient population under evaluation. The greatest experience to date has been with patients undergoing organ transplantation, with kidney recipients representing the largest single group.

However, CAH is also common in patients with autoimmune disease and dermatologic disorders. The risk of CAH is unrelated to sex or race, but it is dose-related and it increases with age of the patient and with preexisting hypertension or high serum creatinine levels. Although most patients present with mild to moderate asymptomatic BP elevation, others may rapidly develop severe hypertension and encephalopathy. BP usually falls after the withdrawal or substitution of cyclosporine immunosuppression but may not remit completely. Unfortunately, it is often not possible to discontinue therapy. Calcium antagonists have been used successfully but they can increase cyclosporin blood levels. ACE inhibitors, labetalol, β-blockers, clonidine, and diuretics are also effective in some patients. Diuretic therapy should be used with caution because of the risk of prerenal azotemia and electrolyte abnormalities. Usually, multidrug therapy is necessary to control CAH.

Tacrolimus, another immunosuppressive agent that inhibits calcineurin, may also induce hypertension. However, it produces less hypertension than cyclosporin A, and therefore switching to tacrolimus may be considered in patients with CAH.

Rapamycin, a novel immunosuppressive agent that does not inhibit calcineurin, has not been reported to produce nephrotoxicity and/or hypertension.

## OVER-THE-COUNTER DRUGS

Most nonprescription anorexics contain combinations of an antihistamine and an adrenergic agonist (usually phenylpropanolamine [PPA], ephedrine, pseudoephedrine, or caffeine). All act by potentiating presynaptic norepinephrine release and by directly activating adrenergic receptors. α-Adrenergic intoxication induced by nasal decongestant and cough medications containing massive doses of oxymetazoline hydrochloride, phenylephrine hydrochloride, and ephedrine hydrochloride has been reported to result in severe hypertension. Labetalol may be an effective treatment in these cases.

Until recently, PPA was the active ingredient in most diet aids and many decongestant agents and was also used as a substitute for amphetamine. Use of excessive doses may result in severe hypertension.

Caffeine can acutely and transiently increase BP by increasing peripheral resistance. The reaction to caffeine is more pronounced in males than females, and in those with a positive family history of hypertension than in those with a negative family history. Concomitant medications, such as monoamine oxidase inhibitors (MAOIs), antihypertensive drugs, OCs, and nonsteroidal anti-inflammatory drugs (NSAIDs) seem to increase the risk of hypertension.

## ANTIDEPRESSANT AGENTS

MAOIs can induce severe hypertension when patients consume foods containing tyramine. However, there are some reports of MAOIs causing severe hypertensive reaction even without use of concomitant medications. Among the various MAOIs, tranylcypromine is the most hazardous, whereas moclobemide and brofaromine seem to be the least likely to induce hypertensive reaction. These drugs exert their effects by delaying the metabolism of sympathomimetic amines and 5-hydroxytryptophan, and by increasing the store of norepinephrine in postganglionic sympathetic neurons. $\alpha$-Adrenergic receptor antagonists would seem an appropriate choice for initial treatment.

Tricyclic antidepressants block the reuptake of the neurotransmitters in the synapse in the central nervous system. There are some reports that these agents increase BP, mainly in patients with panic disorders.

Buspirone, a serotonin receptor type 1$\alpha$ agonist, has also been reported to increase BP. It is speculated that buspirone increases BP by its metabolite 1-2 pyrimidinyl piperazine which is an $\alpha_2$-adrenoceptor antagonist and therefore should not be used concomitantly with an MAOI. A small but sustained and dose-dependent increase in arterial pressure seems to occur with other serotonin agonists as well. Venlafaxine has a dose-dependent effect on BP that is clinically significant at high doses. Episodes of severe hypertension were described in patients treated with other antidepressant agents such as fluoxetine, fluoxetine plus selegiline, and thioridazine.

## ANTINEOPLASTIC AGENTS

Several alkylating agents can increase BP. In one series, 15 of 18 patients treated with multiple alkylating agents following autologous bone marrow transplantation developed hypertension. Hypertensive reactions associated with paclitaxel treatment has been reported.

## RECOMBINANT HUMAN ERYTHROPOIETIN

Recombinant human erythropoietin (r-HuEPO) has revolutionized the treatment of anemia in renal failure patients, both in the pre- and postdialysis phase. Not only does the treatment improve well-being, but it also positively influences cardiac function and permits cardiac hypertrophy to regress. However, r-HuEPO therapy can lead to an increase in BP. The increase in BP associated with r-HuEPO therapy appears to be dose-related. Systemic hypertension has been reported to develop, or to worsen, in 20–30% of patients treated with r-HuEPO worldwide. In hemodialysis patients with systemic hypotension, r-HuEPO usually induces a 10% increase in BP, with no significant change in the frequency of hypotensive episodes. Hypertension may develop in some patients as early as 2 weeks and in others as late as 4 months after the start of r-HuEPO treatment.

In general, hypertension has not proved to be a serious general problem in the r-HuEPO-treated patient; however, few cases of hypertensive crisis with encephalopathy have been reported.

Several risk factors for the development, or worsening, of hypertension after r-HuEPO therapy have been identified. They include the presence of pre-existing hypertension, rapid increase in hematocrit, a low baseline hematocrit before r-HuEPO administration, high doses and intravenous route of administration, and the presence of native kidneys. There are several potential mechanisms by which r-HuEPO therapy may increase BP in hemodialysis patients. They include increased blood viscosity; the loss of hypoxic vasodilation; the activation of neurohumoral systems (catecholamines, the renin-angiotensin system); and especially a direct vascular effect. This last mechanism is supported by several studies, and many factors may be involved in its pathogenesis (an increased cell calcium uptake; an imbalance in local vasoactive agents, with increased synthesis of ET-1; a mitogenic effect; and a platelet-dependent mechanism). By optimizing dialysis treatment, paying close attention to volume regulation, giving r-HuEPO subcutaneously and in a fashion to increase hematocrit gradually, the occurrence of BP increases can be minimized.

Hemodynamically, r-HuEPO increases BP by a marked increase in peripheral resistance associated with only a mild decrease in cardiac output. Vasodilators such as calcium antagonists, and α-adrenergic receptor antagonists should therefore be effective in lowering BP. Diuretics, ACE inhibitors, and angiotensin type 1 receptor antagonists may be less effective because blood volume has been shown to be unchanged, and both plasma renin activity and angiotensin II are suppressed in r-HuEPO-treated patients. The hypertension associated with r-HuEPO has not generally been too difficult to control. In one study, 42% of the patients with r-HuEPO-induced hypertension had their BP controlled with a single agent. BP can usually be managed with a combination of fluid removal with dialysis and conventional antihypertensive therapy. If these measures are unsuccessful, the dose of r-HuEPO should be lowered or therapy should be held for several weeks. Phlebotomy of 500 mL of blood may rapidly lower BP in refractory patients.

## BROMOCRIPTINE

Bromocriptine mesylate is commonly used for prolactin inhibition and suppression of puerperal lactation. Although bromocriptine often has a hypotensive effect, severe hypertension with subsequent stroke has been reported in the postpartum period. Patients with pregnancy-induced hypertension are at increased risk to develop hypertension. The suppression of lactation is no longer a Food and Drug Administration-approved use for bromocriptine.

## DISULFIRAM

Disulfiram is commonly used as a pharmacologic adjunct in the treatment of alcoholism. Administration of 500 mg/day of disulfiram for 2 to 3 weeks has been reported to increase BP slightly. A low dose of 125 mg per day of this agent may also increase BP. It seems that changes in peripheral or central noradrenergic activity are responsible for the increase in arterial pressure.

## ALCOHOL

Excessive chronic alcohol use has clearly been shown to raise BP and can also increase resistance to antihypertensive therapy. Pathogenesis of alcohol-related hypertension seems to be multifactorial and related to direct vasculotoxicity, symphathetic activity, salt water logging, and activation of the renin angiotensin system.

Thc BP effects of alcohol are independent from obesity, salt intake, cigarette smoking, and potassium intake. There is a dose–response relationship for the hypertensive effects of alcohol. Abstinence or at least moderation of alcohol intake is recommended as an initial therapy for mild hypertension. A reasonable approach is to limit daily alcohol consumption to no more than approximately 1–2 ounces of alcohol.

## NONSTEROIDAL ANTI-INFLAMMATORY DRUGS

NSAIDs can induce an increase in BP and interfere with antihypertensive treatment, nullifying its effect. Two meta-analyses have demonstrated that, after pooling data drawn from published reports of randomized trials of younger adults, NSAID use produces a clinically significant increment in mean BP of 5 mmHg. Recent NSAID users had a 1.7-fold higher risk of requiring the initiation of antihypertensive therapy compared with nonusers; NSAID users also had a 40% increased risk of receiving a diagnosis of hypertension compared with nonusers. Elderly patients, those with pre-existing hypertension, salt-sensitive patients, patients with renal failure and patients with renovascular hypertension are at a higher risk to develop severe hypertension when treated with NSAIDs. The mechanisms whereby NSAIDs raise BP are not fully understood. Inhibiting the synthesis of prostaglandins from arachidonic acid via cyclooxygenase (COX)-1 and COX-2, the 2 isoforms of COX, is probably the main mechanism of action. Interference with both the control of vascular resistance and the regulation of extracellular volume homeostasis has been incriminated, but several other putative mechanisms such as moderation of adrenergic activity or resetting of the baroreceptor response may also be involved. NSAIDs may interact with some antihypertensive agents such as diuretics, beta-blockers and ACE inhibitors but do not interact with calcium antagonists and central acting drugs, the antihypertensive efficacy of which is apparently unrelated with production of PGs. NSAIDs vary considerably in their effect on BP. Stratification by NSAID type revealed that indomethacin, piroxicam and naproxen were associated with the largest increases in BP, whereas sulindac and aspirin have little effect on BP. Low dose aspirin has no effect on BP control in hypertensive patients. The new orally-effective specific COX-2 inhibitors, rofecoxib and celecoxib, increase BP in a dose-dependent manner as the traditional NSAIDs. However, there is evidence that patients receiving celecoxib experience less destabilization of BP compared with those receiving rofecoxib. Because COX-2 inhibitors are usually given for a prolonged period of time, the risk of an increase in BP must be assessed against the expected benefit of treatment. In patients who take NSAIDs, calcium antagonists would appear to be a preferred choice to other antihypertensive agents.

## HEAVY METALS

Several studies show that cumulative exposure to lead, even at low levels sustained by the general population, may increase the risk of hypertension. Some reports suggest that arsenic or cadmium exposure also may induce hypertension in humans. However, in a recent study, environmental exposure to cadmium was not associated with higher conventional BP or 24-hour ambulatory BP measurements.

## SCORPIONS AND BLACK WIDOWS

Venoms of scorpions (especially the South American species) and black widows commonly produce a clinical picture of profuse perspiration, lacrimation, vomiting, convulsion, and cardiovascular collapse. However, occasionally hypertension and bradycardia occur. Hypertension is mediated by a massive discharge of catecholamines into the circulation produced by the venom, and therefore β- or α-blockade is effective in this condition.

## AMPHOTERICIN B

Amphotericin B (AmB) is the mainstay of therapy for serious fungal infections. A few cases of severe hypertension associated with the use of AmB deoxycholate have been reported in the literature, and recently one case report of hypertension associated with a lipid-containing preparation of the medication has been described.

## ANTI-HIV TREATMENT

One case report of severe hypertension and renal atrophy associated with the protease inhibitor indinavir has been described. Hypertensive crisis secondary to phenylpropanolamine interacting with triple-drug therapy for HIV prophylaxis has also been reported. Additionally, potential drug interactions exist between antiretroviral medications, particularly the protease inhibitors and antihypertensive medications.

## CONCLUSIONS

A myriad of therapeutic agents or chemical substances can induce either transient or sustained hypertension, exacerbate well-controlled hypertension, or antagonize the effects of antihypertensive therapy. Careful evaluation of a patient's drug regimen may identify so-called chemically induced hypertension and prevent or minimize the need for lifelong antihypertensive therapy. Whenever chemically induced hypertension has been identified, the causative agent should be discontinued. However, when discontinuation is not possible, institution of appropriate and targeted antihypertensive therapy is indicated. In the absence of specific treatment guidelines for drug-induced hypertension, the recommended initial antihypertensive therapy should be directed toward neutralizing the specific mechanism by which the chemical agent causes hypertension.

## SUGGESTED READINGS


1. Grossman E, Messerli FH. High Blood Pressure. A side effect of drugs, poisons, and food. Arch Intern Med 1995;155:450–460.
2. Clyburn EB, DiPette DJ. Hypertension induced by drugs and other substances. Semin Nephrol 1995;15:72–86.
3. De Leeuw PW. Nonsteroidal anti-inflammatory drugs and hypertension: the risks in perspective. Drugs 1996;51:179–187.
4. Bursztyn M, Zelig O, Or R, Nagler A. Isradipine for the prevention of cyclosporine-induced hpertension in allogeneic bone marrow transplant recipients: a randomized, double-blind study. Transplantation. 1997;63:1034–1036.
5. Chasan-Taber L, Willett WC, Manson JE, et al. Prospective study of oral contraceptives and hypertension among women in the United States. Circulation 1996;94: 483–489.
6. Bennet WM, Porter GA. Cyclosporine-associated hypertension. Am J Med 1988;85:131–133.
7. Levin N. Management of BP changes during recombinant human erythropoietin therapy. Semin Nephrol 1989;9(1 Suppl 2):16–20.
8. MacMahon S. Alcohol consumption and hypertension. Hypertension 1987;9: 111–121.
9. Pope JE, Anderson JJ, Felson DT. A meta-analysis of the effects of nonsteroidal anti-inflammatory drugs on blood pressure. Arch Intern Med 1993;153: 477–484.
10. Frishman WH. Effects of nonsteroidal anti-inflammatory drug therapy on blood pressure and peripheral edema. Am J Cardiol 2002;89(6A):18D–25D.
11. Whelton A, Fort JG, Puma JA, Normandin D, Bello AE, Verburg KM. Cyclooxygenase-2—specific inhibitors and cardiorenal function: a randomized, controlled trial of celecoxib and rofecoxib in older hypertensive osteoarthritis patients. Am J Ther 2001;8:85–95.
12. White WB, Faich G, Whelton A, et al. Comparison of thromboembolic events in patients treated with celecoxib, a cyclooxygenase-2 specific inhibitor, versus ibuprofen or diclofenac. Am J Cardiol 2002;89:425–430.
13. Brem AS. Insights into glucocorticoid-associated hypertension. Am J Kidney Dis 2001;37:1–10.
14. Cheng Y, Schwartz J, Sparrow D, Aro A, Weiss ST, Hu H. Bone lead and blood lead levels in relation to baseline blood pressure and the prospective development of hypertension: the Normative Aging Study. Am J Epidemiol 2001;153:164–171.
15. Sibutramine: new preparation. Slight weight loss; but also a slight rise in blood pressure... Prescrire Int 2001;10:140–145.
16. McMahon FG, Weinstein SP, Rowe E, et al. Sibutramine is safe and effective for weight loss in obese patients whose hypertension is well controlled with angiotensin-converting enzyme inhibitors. J Hum Hypertens 2002;16:5–11.

17. Sramek JJ, Leibowitz MT, Weinstein SP et al. Efficacy and safety of sibutramine for weight loss in obese patients with hypertension well controlled by beta-adrenergic blocking agents: a placebo-controlled, double-blind, randomised trial. J Hum Hypertens 2002;16:13–19.

# II
# Renal Disease and Secondary Hypertension

# 3 Hypertension in Chronic Kidney Disease

*Robert D. Toto,* MD

CONTENTS



## INTRODUCTION

Hypertension occurs in more than 90% of patients with chronic kidney disease (CKD) during the course of their disease. Hypertension can directly injure the kidney and it is a recognized risk factor for development of end-stage renal disease (ESRD) and accounts for nearly 30% of new cases of ESRD in the United States. Moreover, ESRD attributed to hypertensive nephrosclerosis has been increasing annually about 8% per year, despite reductions in death caused by stroke and myocardial infarction during the same time period. Diabetes and hypertension account for nearly three-fourths of the nearly 400,000 persons currently under treatment for ESRD by dialysis or kidney transplant. It is now recognized that of the factors contributing to hypertensive renal injury, the renin-angio-

From: *Secondary Hypertension: Clinical Presentation, Diagnosis, and Treatment*
Edited by: G. A. Mansoor © Humana Press Inc., Totowa, NJ

tensin-aldosterone system (RAAS) plays a key role in the development and progression of CKD caused by hypertension, diabetes, and glomerulonephritis. Recent advances in the pathogenesis and treatment of hypertension in CKD are the subject of this chapter.

## CHRONIC KIDNEY DISEASE AND END-STAGE RENAL DISEASE

CKD is defined as a chronic impairment in kidney function and/or structural damage in association with increased risk for progression to ESRD. ESRD is a catastrophic illness characterized by life-threatening cardiovascular morbidity and multiorgan system dysfunction. The life span of an average patient with ESRD treated by dialysis is approximately seven years and the annual mortality rate of the U.S. hemodialysis population is about 20% per year *(1)*. Quality of life on dialysis is poor, characterized by high morbidity and hospitalization rates. Moreover, 60% of deaths in the hemodialysis population are attributed to cardiovascular causes. Non-renal cardiovascular diseases such as congestive heart failure, myocardial infarction, sudden death, and stroke are important comorbidities in the ESRD population. Type II diabetes mellitus is now the most common cause of ESRD and the vast majority of these patients are hypertensive *(1)*. Furthermore, African-Americans and Mexican-Americans have a threefold higher incidence of ESRD attributed to type II diabetes as compared to non-Hispanic whites. African-Americans also experience a fivefold higher incidence of hypertensive nephrosclerosis compared to non-Hispanic whites and Mexican-Americans *(2–5)*. Therefore, finding ways to prevent or stall the onset of ESRD is a high priority.

However, ESRD represents the tip of the iceberg of CKD. It is estimated that more than 7 million Americans have or are at risk for CKD, and most of them are hypertensive *(2)*. These individuals are widely distributed among the population and, if they are receiving care are managed by primary care physicians. Early identification and treatment of hypertension in CKD by primary care providers is becoming an increasingly important component of medical practice. Therefore, practitioners need to understand the progressive nature of renal disease and how to manage hypertension in CKD.

## HYPERTENSION AND CHRONIC KIDNEY DISEASE

### *Hypertension As an Important Risk Factor for ESRD*

Approximately 90% of patients who progress to ESRD are hypertensive during the course of renal disease *(6)*. Moreover, uncontrolled hypertension accelerates the rate of progression in these individuals regardless of the cause of CKD. Data from large clinical trials and epidemiological studies indicate that hypertension is an important risk factor for progressive kidney disease *(7–10)*. Among screenees of the Multiple Risk Factor Intervention Trial (MRFIT) the relative risk for ESRD increases with increasing systolic BP (SBP) independent of diastolic BP (DBP) (Fig. 1). Over a 16-year period, 847 of the 361,000 male screenees either died of or were treated for ESRD. Elevated SBP was a strong and independent risk factor for the development of ESRD, with a graded relationship between risk and SBP. In fact, a relatively small increase in SBP doubled the risk of ESRD. Furthermore, mild to moderate elevations of SBP correlated with kidney disease. A similar relationship between elevated SBP and risk for progression of diabetic nephropathy has been demonstrated *(11)*.

## *Hypertension Control Is Suboptimal in Patients With CKD*

Blood pressure control among hypertensives (SBP ≥ 140 mmHg or DBP ≥ 90 mmHg) in general and among CKD patients in particular is suboptimal *(12,13)*. Thus, most individuals with hypertension are either unaware of their hypertension or have inadequate treatment to control their BP. In older individuals systolic hypertension is the most prominent finding in BP measurement. This is important because the median age of patients developing ESRD in the United States is 64, and systolic hypertension is an independent predictor of developing ESRD. Among hypertensives with CKD or at risk for CKD (serum creatinine ≥ 1.5 mg/dL), only 11% surveyed in the National Health and Nutrition Examination Survey III had BP controlled to the level recommended by the sixth report of the Joint National committee on Prevention Detection, Evaluation and Treatment of High Blood Pressure (JNC VI) (Fig. 2). This finding represents an important challenge to the medical community, especially to the primary care provider.

## *Pathophysiology*

### General Mechanisms

Two major factors contribute to elevated BP in patients with most forms of CKD peripheral vasoconstriction and volume expansion (Fig. 3). Treatment of hypertension in CKD is based on these two major pathophysiological mechanisms. Drugs that inhibit the RAAS and block sympathetic nerve traffic are very effective in lowering BP, as are vasodilators and diuretics. Angiotensin II (AngII), hypertension, and proteinuria are linked in patients with CKD and represent major modifiable risk factors. The following section focuses on the role of these three factors in CKD.

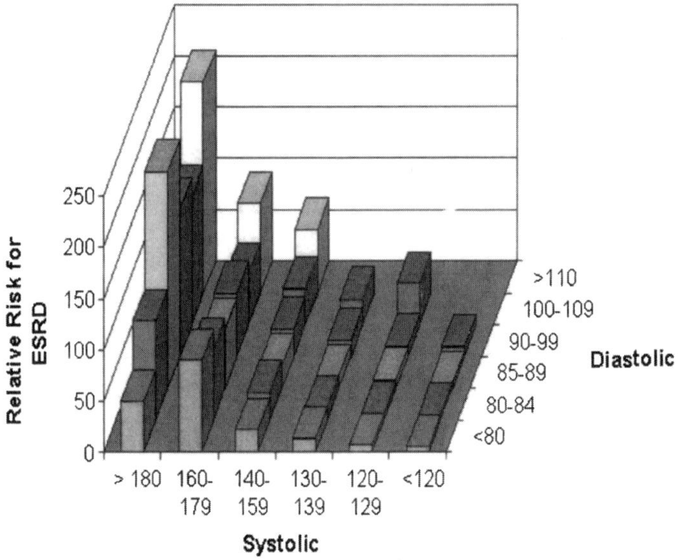


**Fig. 1.** Hypertension and end-stage renal disease (ESRD): MRFIT screenees ($N$ = 361,000) (from ref. *8*).

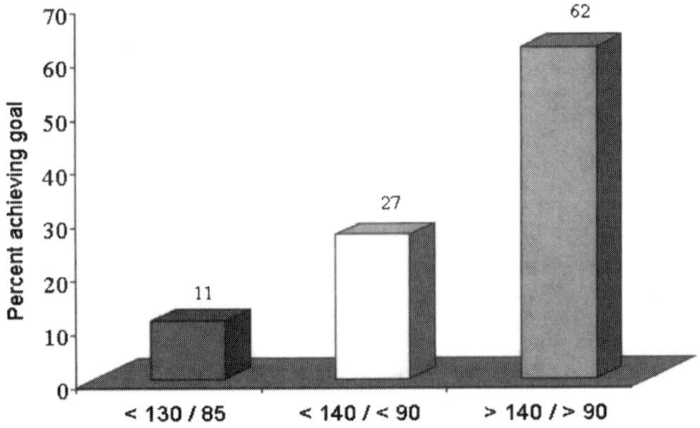


**Fig. 2.** Blood pressure control among hypertensive individuals with renal disease (Scr ≥ 1.5 mg/dL): NHANES III ($N$ = 16,589) (from ref. *13*).

## Role of Ang II

Ang II can be produced by angiotensin-converting enzyme (ACE) and non-ACE pathways in many tissues as well as in the circulation.

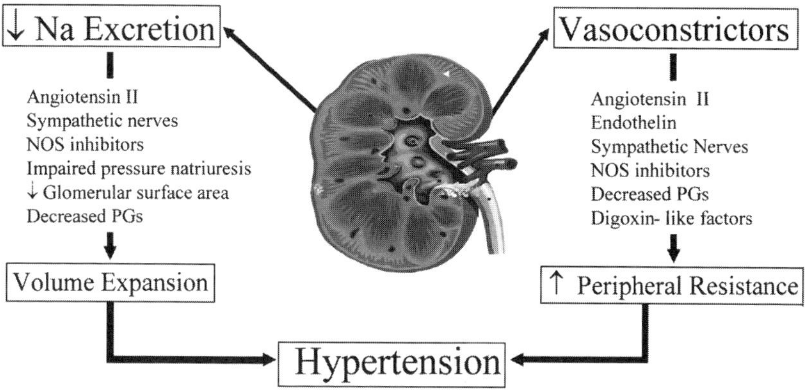


**Fig. 3.** Basic mechanisms by which the kidney can cause hypertension.

Physiological effects of Ang II in humans are conferred by its binding to the Ang II subtype 1 ($AT_1$) receptor present in kidney, heart, brain, systemic vasculature, adrenal gland, liver and other tissues. Ang II binds to the angiotensin subtype 1 receptor on the cell surface resulting in sodium reabsorption and vasoconstriction of the efferent arteriole in the kidney, aldosterone release from the adrenal gland, increased inotropy and chronotropy in the heart, and proliferative, hypertrophic, and proinflammatory effects (increased tissue and plasma plasminogen activator inhibitor type [PAI]-1 and transforming growth factor [TGF]-β levels) in many tissues. The importance of Ang II binding to the angiotensin subtype 2 receptor in humans is unknown. However, in some animal models, Ang II binding to subtype 2 receptors causes vasodilation and natriuresis, effects opposite of those observed with subtype 1 receptor activation *(15)*.

In animal models of human disease, Ang II causes glomerular capillary hypertension caused by relative vasoconstriction of the efferent arteriole *(14,15)*. Ang II also has nonhemodynamic effects in the kidney including activation of nicotinamide adenine dinucleotide phosphate(NADPH) oxidase (increases free radicals), inhibition of nitric oxide, and increased production of sclerosis-producing factors TGF-β and PAI-1 (Fig. 4). These effects conspire to produce sclerosis, fibrosis, and chronic irreversible kidney damage.

Ang II plays a prominent role in the development and progression of common hypertensive kidney diseases including diabetes, hypertensive nephrosclerosis, glomerulonephritis and polycystic kidney disease

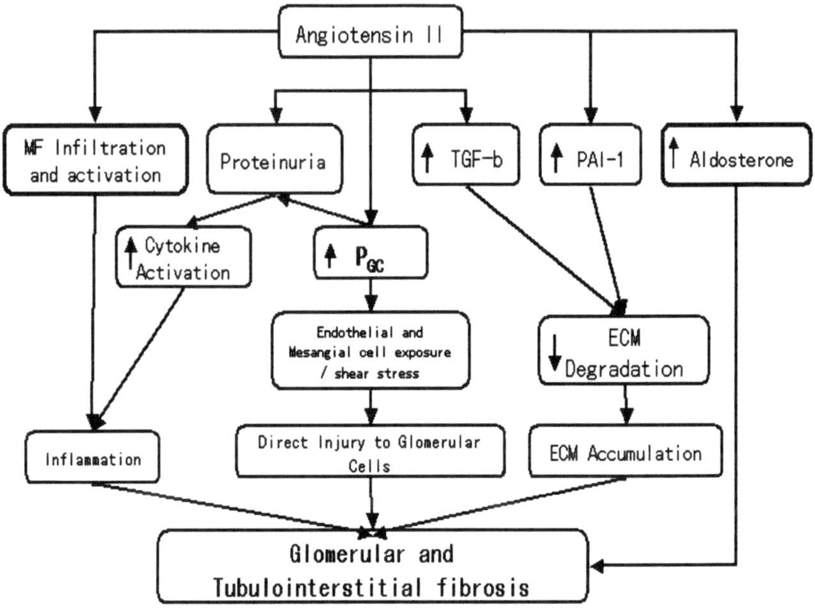


**Fig. 4.** Central role of angiotensin II in chronic renal failure (from ref. *15*).

*(14,15)*. Thus, ACE inhibitors (ACEIs) and Ang II type I receptor blockers (ARBs) slow renal disease progression and improve outcomes in patients with CKD *(15)*. Intrarenal Ang II production is important in humans with kidney disease. Moreover, dissociation between plasma Ang II concentration (which returns to pre-ACE therapy level) and kidney and cardiovascular outcomes during chronic administration of ACE inhibitors suggest that tissue Ang II concentration/action predominates *(16)*.

## Effects of ACEIs and ARBs in Experimental Renal Disease

Figure 5 illustrates the typical hemodynamic picture observed during micropuncture studies of rats with kidney failure caused by renal ablation, diabetes mellitus, glomerulonephritis *(17)*. As shown in the left panel, afferent arteriolar resistance is markedly reduced and efferent resistance is slightly reduced in part because of increased Ang II activity and/or action. Consequently, glomerular pressure ($P_{GC}$) is increased. In the presence of systemic hypertension, glomerular hypertension is aggravated and glomerular barrier function is impaired. The latter allows passage of protein from the capillary lumen into Bowman's space and subsequently into the urine. Treatment with an ACEI inhibitor or an ARB decreases efferent resistance, glomerular pressure, and proteinuria.

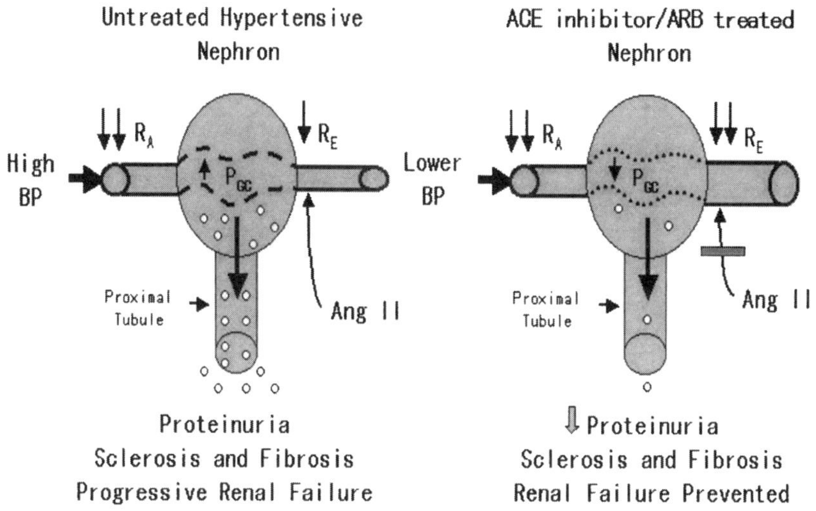


**Fig. 5.** In experimental animal models inhibition blockade of aII prevents or ameliorates hypertensive renal disease.

Additionally, glomerular structure and function are preserved and tubulointerstitial fibrosis is markedly attenuated *(9,16,17)*. If these agents are administered at the time of renal injury, these functional alterations and the structural injury can be completely prevented. Furthermore, when they are administered after the onset of renal injury, proteinuria is reduced and disease progression is slowed. However, it is important to note that lowering capillary pressure in animals or humans with renal disease may also lower glomerular filtration rate (GFR). Thus, it is quite common for clinicians to observe a small and persistent increase in serum creatinine concentration as a consequence of lowering ($P_{GC}$) and hence GFR after lowering BP with ACEIs or ARBs.

### Reducing Proteinuria

**Detecting Abnormal Albumin Excretion Rate.** Excessive excretion of albumin in the urine becomes apparent by reagent test strips when there is 300 mg/L or 300 mg albumin /g or more creatinine in the urine (Table 1). If the dipstick test is negative, albumin and creatinine in a random ("spot") urine sample should be sent to the lab *(18,19)*. The recommended method for quantifying albuminuria and longitudinal follow-up is the urinary albumin to creatinine ratio obtained from a random urine sample. A normal urine albumin excretion rate is less than 30 mg albumin/g creatinine. Microalbuminuria is defined as an albumin excretion in the range of more than 30 to less than 300 mg/g creatinine

Table 1
Definition and Clinical Implications of Albuminuria*

| | *Microalbuminuria* | *Macroalbuminuria (Overt Nephropathy)* |
|---|---|---|
| Routine dipstick | No | Yes |
| Urine albumin | 30–300 mg Alb/g Cr | ≥ 300 mg Alb/g Cr |
| Renal significance | Marker of incipient diabetic nephropathy | Marker of progressive renal disease |
| Increased CV risk | Yes | Yes |

*Random (spot) urine, preferably morning sample
*Random urine albumin creatinine ratio

and is not detected by the routine dipstick method (which detects albumin, not other proteins such as light chains). Macroalbuminuria is defined as an albumin excretion rate of 300 mg/g or more of creatinine. Albuminuria is a marker for both progression of nephropathy and cardiovascular death risk in patients with type I and type II diabetes *(20–26)*.

Proteinuria has been extensively studied as a marker for progression of kidney disease *(20,27–50)*. In clinical trials, patients with impaired kidney function and high-grade (>1 g/d) proteinuria progress at a faster rate than those with low-grade (<1 g/d) proteinuria *(51)*. For example, in both diabetic and nondiabetic patients with proteinuric kidney disease, acceleration of kidney disease progression correlates with the level of baseline proteinuria. Even in patients with controlled essential hypertension and no evidence of kidney disease, the onset of proteinuria may be a marker of future decline of kidney function *(21,22,24,52)*. The Modification of Diet in Renal Disease (MDRD) study of a lower protein diet and BP in CKD patients demonstrated that baseline proteinuria was an independent risk factor for kidney disease progression *(28–30)*. Meta-analysis of clinical trials in nondiabetic CKD suggests that higher grade proteinuria at baseline predicts greater benefit from ACEI inhibitor therapy *(51)*.

#### Hypertension

Most large clinical trials of antihypertensive therapy have focused on cardiac and cerebrovascular endpoints. Consequently, only a few clinical trials have examined the effect of BP lowering on the progression of kidney disease in both diabetic and nondiabetic patients. Early clinical trials in hypertensive patients with kidney insufficiency failed to show a significant benefit of BP lowering on decline in GFR *(52,53)*. However, the target level of BP control in these studies was relatively high by today's standard. In contrast, more recent clinical trials with lower target BP levels have demonstrated that lowering BP in hypertensive patients at risk for or with already established kidney disease preserves kidney function. For example, the MDRD study, which included 800 subjects with CKD of diffuse pathophysiological origin, demonstrated that subjects with higher grade proteinuria (i.e. ≥ 1.0 g/d) randomized to a lower BP goal of 125/75 mmHg had significantly slower rate of decline in GFR as compared to those randomized to a higher BP goal of about 139/89 mmHg *(54)*. Figure 6 illustrates the mean rate of decline in GFR plotted as a function of mean controlled systolic BP in nine clinical trials of both diabetic *(55–57)* and nondiabetics with CKD *(29,47,58–60)*. Lower SBP was associated with slower rate of decline in GFR *(61)*. For example, in a hypertensive patient with Type II diabetic nephropathy, with a creatinine of 2 mg/dL (GFR of about 50 mL/min), systolic BP of 150 mmHg is associated with a GFR decline at a rate of about 8 mL/min/year. At this rate the patient will be on dialysis (GFR of 10 mL/min) in 5 years (8 mL/min/year × 5 = 40). In contrast, if the SBP level is controlled in the range of 130–135 mmHg, GFR is predicted to decline at about –2 mL/min/yr. In this case, the patient would still reach ESRD in 20 years.

## THE IMPORTANCE OF LOWERING BLOOD PRESSURE AND PROTEINURIA WITH DRUGS THAT INHIBIT THE RENIN-ANGIOTENSIN SYSTEM

### *CKD Caused by Nondiabetic Renal Disease*

Several clinical trials have shown that ACEI-based regimens are superior to non-ACEI-based regimens in nondiabetic patients with hypertensive CKD *(51)*. In a meta-analysis of 11 controlled clinical trials including 1,860 patients, Jafar et al demonstrated that for any level of SBP the risk for developing ESRD was lower in those treated with ACEI as compared to the patients not treated with *(51)*. The degree of risk reduction for ESRD was linearly related to SBP within the range of 100–120 mmHg, consistent with the recommendation for achieving an SBP goal of 120–130 mmHg in CKD. Moreover, the beneficial effect of ACE inhibition to reduce the risk for ESRD was greatest in subjects who had the highest baseline proteinuria. However, for subjects with < 1.0 g/day or less of proteinuria in this analysis, superiority of ACEI therapy could not be demonstrated. After adjusting for baseline and followup proteinuria and SBP, the relative risk reduction for ESRD during ACEI therapy was 30% compared to non-ACEI therapy. That is, after control-

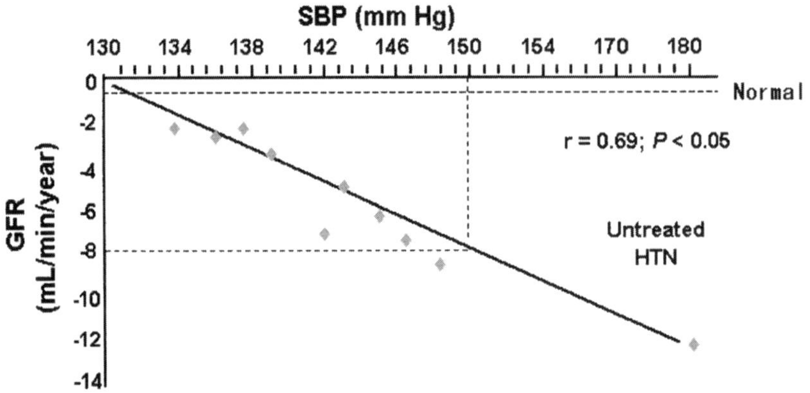


**Fig. 6.** The impact of blood pressure lowering on progression of renal disease (from ref. *11*).

ling for effects of lowering BP and proteinuria, the renoprotective effect of ACEI persisted. These data indicate that antihypertensive regimens including ACEI are more effective than regimens not including an ACE inhibitor; beneficial effects of ACEI go beyond lowering BP and proteinuria, and ACEI are indicated in the treatment of nondiabetic patients with CKD and proteinuria.

### *CKD Caused by Hypertensive Nephrosclerosis*

End-stage kidney disease attributed to hypertension occurs at rates fivefold higher in African-Americans compared to both non-Hispanic whites and Hispanics. Lowering BP in hypertensive nephrosclerosis is associated with a slow rate of decline in GFR in African-Americans *(61)*. The African-American Study of Hypertension and Kidney Disease (AASK Trial) demonstrated that lowering BP with ACE-based regimens is superior to non-ACE-based regimens for renoprotection in African-Americans with hypertensive nephrosclerosis. In the AASK Trial, 1094 hypertensive African-Americans with CKD (GFR 20–65 mL/min) caused by hypertensive nephrosclerosis were randomized to one of two different levels of BP control (1) mean arterial pressure (MAP) less than 92 mmHg or (2) MAP equal to 102–107 mmHg. In addition, participants were randomly assigned to one of three antihypertensive drug regimens consisting of an ACEI (ramipril), a dihydropyridine calcium channel blocker (DHP CCB) (amlodipine), or a β-blocker (Metoprolol XL). Diuretics, α-blockers, clonidine, and vasodilators were added to each drug group as needed to achieve and maintain BP control *(62)*.

In comparing BP control groups, there were no significant differences in overall rate of decline in GFR (primary outcome) or composite clinical outcome of rapid decline in GFR (50% decrease from baseline ESRD or death [secondary outcome]). However, in those with a baseline urine protein excretion rate of more than 300 mg/day, GFR decline was significantly slower in the ramipril group compared to the amlodipine group. Moreover, there was a 38% risk reduction for the ramipril versus amlodipine groups in the clinical composite outcome. Also, proteinuria increased by 60% in participants in the amlodipine group and declined by 20% in the ramipril group during the first 6 months of the study. This difference was significant and persisted throughout the followup period of 3 years. Most important, these differences were not explained by differences in BP control level. Three important conclusions emerged from this study: (a) BP control to currently recommended levels can be achieved in hypertensive African-Americans with CKD; (b) initial antihypertensive therapy with an ACEI offers greater benefit in slowing deterioration of kidney function than a DHP CCB in patients with CKD; and (c) ACEIs are renoprotective particularly in patients with a urine protein/creatinine ratio of more than 300 mg/g creatinine or a value of more than 0.22.

## *CKD Caused by Diabetic Nephropathy*

Diabetic nephropathy is the leading cause of ESRD and is driving the rising tide of ESRD. Approximately 30–40% of type I and type II diabetes patients develop progressive CKD leading to ESRD. Evidence from large-scale multicenter clinical trials indicate that ACEIs and ARBs are the preferred first-line therapy for diabetics with early and late nephropathy.

### Type I Diabetes

ACEIs are known to reduce the risk of onset of overt nephropathy in type I diabetics with microalbuminuria. Meta-analysis of more than 20 clinical trials confirm that type I diabetics with microalbuminuria should be treated with an ACEI to reduce the risk of progression of proteinuria to overt renal disease *(63)*. In addition, ACEIs have been shown to lower BP, preserve renal function, and reduce risk for developing ESRD in patients with type I diabetic nephropathy *(64)*. As shown in Fig. 7, the rate of doubling of serum creatinine was significantly reduced during treatment with captopril as compared to placebo-treated patients in a trial of 409 type I diabetics with nephropathy (>500 mg protein excretion per day). It is important to note that BP reduction was similar but reduc-

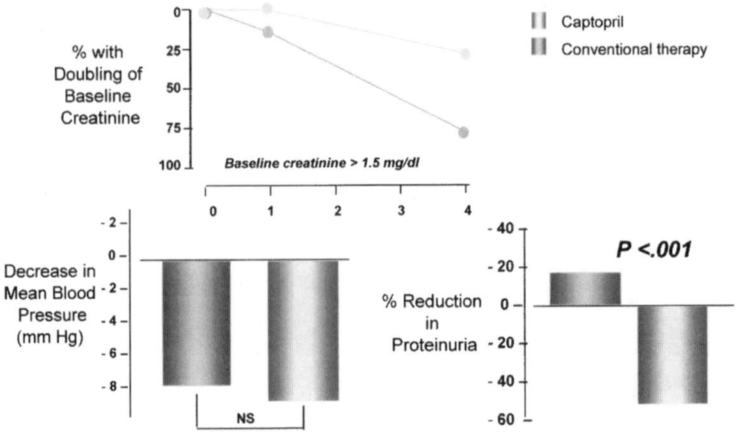


**Fig. 7.** Captopril treatment of type I diabetics with nephropathy.

tion in proteinuria was markedly different between the groups. Two important findings emerged from this study and deserve emphasis: (a) the benefit of captopril as compared to placebo control was observed only in patients with an elevated serum creatinine at baseline (> 1.5 mg/dL), and (b) captopril, but not the placebo, significantly lowered urine protein excretion despite the fact that mean reduction in BP was similar between treatment groups and did not explain the difference in outcome.

### Type II Diabetes

Type II diabetes accounts for the majority of cases of diabetic ESRD, and this trend is expected to increase in the future. However, in contrast to type I diabetes, there are no large-scale trials using ACEIs to prevent kidney failure. Several small clinical trials in patients with microalbuminuria and overt nephropathy in the setting of type II diabetes mellitus demonstrated reduction in proteinuria and/or slowing of GFR decline; however, until now there have been no randomized controlled trials examining outcomes such as doubling serum creatinine, ESRD, and death in type II diabetes *(11)*. However, ACEIs have been applied to the type II diabetes population with established or suspected diabetic nephropathy through extrapolation from studies performed in type I diabetics with nephropathy *(64)*.

**Early Nephropathy.** In a recently published trial, the ARB irbesartan, as compared to either amlodipine or conventional antihypertensive therapy, was demonstrated to reduce the risk of onset of overt nephropathy in hypertensive type II diabetics with microalbuminuria by 71% *(100)*. BP control was similar among the three treatment arms of this study and the risk reduction for irbesartan in a once-daily dose of 300 mg was 71% compared to conventional therapy *(65)*.

**Late Nephropathy.** Two large-scale multicenter clinical trials involving 3230 patients with type II diabetes and overt nephropathy have demonstrated that ARBs reduce proteinuria and reduce the risk of progression of renal disease as compared to non-ACE antihypertensive drug therapy *(65,66)*. The Reduction in Endpoints in Non-insulin Dependent Diabetes Mellitus with the Angiotensin II Antagonist Losartan (RENAAL) Trial was a multinational, double-blind, randomized placebo-controlled trial evaluating the kidney protective effects of losartan in 1513 patients with type II diabetes and nephropathy who were followed for an average of 3.4 years *(65)*. Participants were maintained on conventional therapy at baseline and then randomized to either placebo or losartan 50–100 mg administered once daily to achieve a target BP goal of less than 140/90 mmHg. The primary outcome was a composite of doubling serum creatinine, ESRD, or death. The results showed that losartan treatment reduced the risk of the primary composite outcome by 16%. Risk reductions were 25% for doubling serum creatinine, 28% for ESRD, and 20% for combined endpoint of ESRD or death. There was no significant difference in all-cause mortality in losartan-treated patients. Losartan-treated participants had a 32% risk reduction for first hospitalization for heart failure and a 35% reduction in proteinuria compared to the placebo-treated participants. Also, the rate of decline in estimated GFR was significantly slower during losartan treatment compared to placebo. Importantly, there was no significant difference in BP level between groups: 140/74 mmHg for losartan and 142/74 mmHg for placebo. There was also a 32% risk reduction in subsequent development of ESRD in those patients who had already reached a doubling of serum creatinine endpoint but continued on blinded study medication—further evidence of renoprotection with losartan. Clinical and laboratory adverse events were similar between the losartan and placebo groups. In this trial, 80% of participants in both groups were concomitantly treated with a CCB (80% DHP) in order to achieve BP control. The fact that losartan treatment remained superior to placebo suggests that this maneuver does not prevent the antiproteinuric and renoprotective effects of losartan.

In summary, the RENAAL trial demonstrated that treatment of type II diabetic nephropathy with losartan alone or in combination with conventional antihypertensive therapy reduces proteinuria, slows progression of kidney disease, and reduces the incidence of hospitalization for heart failure beyond BP lowering.

The Irbesartan in Diabetic Nephropathy Trial (IDNT) was performed contemporaneously with the RENAAL trial in a nearly identical patient population of 1715 Type 2 diabetics with hypertension and overt proteinuria *(66)*. The same primary composite endpoint as with RENAAL was used, and the study design and baseline patient characteristics were similar. However, the IDNT is unique in that it randomized participants in double-blind fashion to once-daily doses of irbesartan, or amlodipine, or conventional antihypertensive therapy excluding ACEIs, CCB and other ARBs. Conventional therapy was employed in the irbesartan and amlodipine groups to achieve a goal BP of less than systolic 135/less than diastolic 85 mmHg. The average followup was about 3 years. The results indicated that irbesartan compared to amlodipine and in conventional groups reduced the risk for the primary composite endpoint of doubling serum creatinine, ESRD, or death by 20%, and relative risk for doubling of serum creatinine was reduced by 39%. Proteinuria was significantly reduced by irbesartan as compared to placebo or amlodipine groups, and BP control was similar among the groups, indicating that the beneficial effects of irbesartan on kidney outcomes were independent of the BP lowering effects. In summary, the IDNT demonstrated that Irbesartan is renoprotective in hypertensive proteinuric type 2 diabetics beyond BP lowering compared to both amlodipine and placebo on the background of conventional therapy.

It is important to note the common themes found in recent clinical trials of both nondiabetic and diabetic patients with CKD. First, drugs that inhibit the renin-angiotensin system were found to be superior to those that do not. Second, multiple-drug therapy was required to reach the target BP goals in patients with kidney disease. Third, the most striking (kidney) benefits were observed in patients with abnormally elevated baseline serum creatinine and protein excretion rates. Moreover, these beneficial effects were accompanied not only by a reduction in BP but also by a reduction in proteinuria. This means that the elevated serum creatinine concentration per se is not a contraindication to the use of an ACEI or Ang II receptor antagonists, but quite the contrary. The weight of the evidence indicates that it is patients with elevated baseline serum creatinine who benefit most. Therefore, optimal care of the patient with progressive CKD caused by diabetic and nondiabetic nephropathies should include an ACEI or ARB.

Taken together, three large double-blind, placebo-controlled clinical trials involving 3361 type 2 diabetics with either early (microalbuminuric) or late (macroalbuminuric) nephropathy demonstrate that

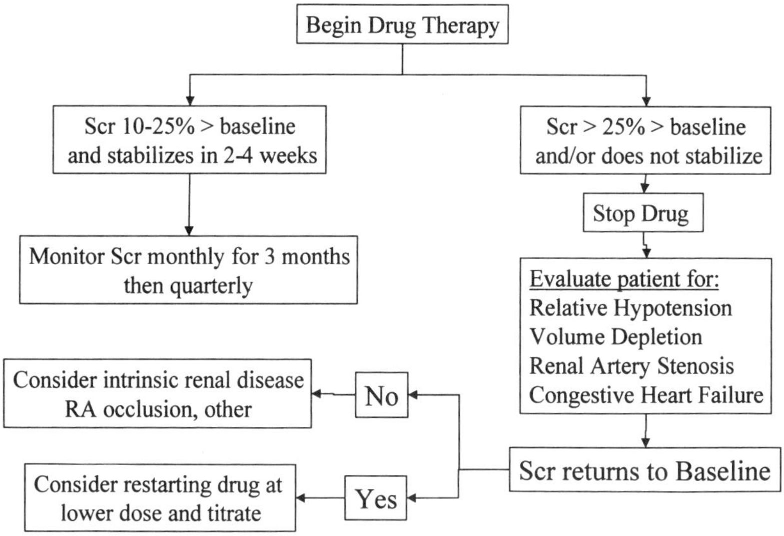


**Fig. 8.** Management of hypercreatininemia after initiation of ACEI, ARB, or other antihpertensive agent.

treatment with an ARB lowers BP, reduces proteinuria, and slows progression of renal disease.

### *Who Should Not Receive an ACEI or an ARB?*

Reasons to avoid initiation of therapy with either ACEIs or ARBs include (1) Hyperkalemia (potassium ≥ 5.3 mEq/L) (2) known allergy (e.g., rash, angioedema, cough, etc.); and (3) known or suspected critical bilateral renal artery stenosis. The observation that serum creatinine often increases after administration of an ACEI or Ang II receptor antagonist in patients with nephropathy is common and, as alluded to earlier, is expected on the basis of the known intrarenal hemodynamic effects of inhibition of AII production or action. Figure 8 illustrates an algorithm for managing elevation of serum creatinine after initiation of an ACEI or ARB in a patient with CKD.

## RECOMMENDATIONS FOR ACHIEVING AND MAINTAINING BP GOAL OF 120–130/70–80 MMHG IN HYPERTENSIVE CHRONIC KIDNEY DISEASES

### *General Approach*

The average number of medications required to achieve BP control in hypertension trials, including patients with and without kidney disease, ranges from two to five. Thus, when treating patients with hypertensive kidney diseases one must anticipate the need for multidrug therapy. An approach recommended by the National Kidney Foundation for hypertensive diabetics is illustrated in Fig. 9. The first step in this regimen is the use of an ACEI combined with a diuretic. Subsequent steps in the algorithm may be flexible in various patient groups. Maintaining the BP within the control range is possible for prolonged periods of time but requires frequent followup. Achieving these goals in diabetics and nondiabetics has not been shown to increase morbidity or mortality compared to higher BP control levels *(67,68)*. Home BP monitoring may facilitate management, and BP devices for home use are now relatively inexpensive. Furthermore, most patients can be taught how to use BP devices to their advantage in long-term treatment. Patients with CKD and hypertension should be encouraged to purchase a BP measuring device, record their BP daily and use these values as a guide to keep their pressure under control.

## *Antihypertensive Choices*

### ACEIs

ACEIs are recommended as first-line antihypertensive therapy for patients with CKD. These agents not only preserve kidney function but also have beneficial effects on the cardiovascular system overall. Once-daily ACEIs are preferred for compliance purposes, but the effect is a class effect and there is no evidence of superiority of one agent over another as far as kidney disease is concerned. The starting dose of the ACEI should depend on the BP and desired goal. For proteinuric patients the dose should generally be titrated to the maximal tolerable dose, whether or not additional antihypertensive therapy is needed. The maximal dose for an ACEI in CKD has not been established, and most studies have used moderate doses (e.g., type I diabetes trial used 75 mg/day of captopril). Therefore, additional dose-titration studies targeted at antiproteinuric and renoprotective effects are needed.

### ARBs

The role of ARBS in treatment of kidney disease patients has not been clearly defined. However, these agents have been shown to be equivalent to ACEIs for both BP and proteinuria reduction. To date, long-term outcome trials in nephropathy with these agents have not been published. Two large multicenter clinical trials in hypertensive diabetics with nephropathy are in the final phase at the time of this writing. However, the results are not yet known. As a group, the ARBs are generally better tolerated than ACEIs. Because of ARBs' known efficacy for BP

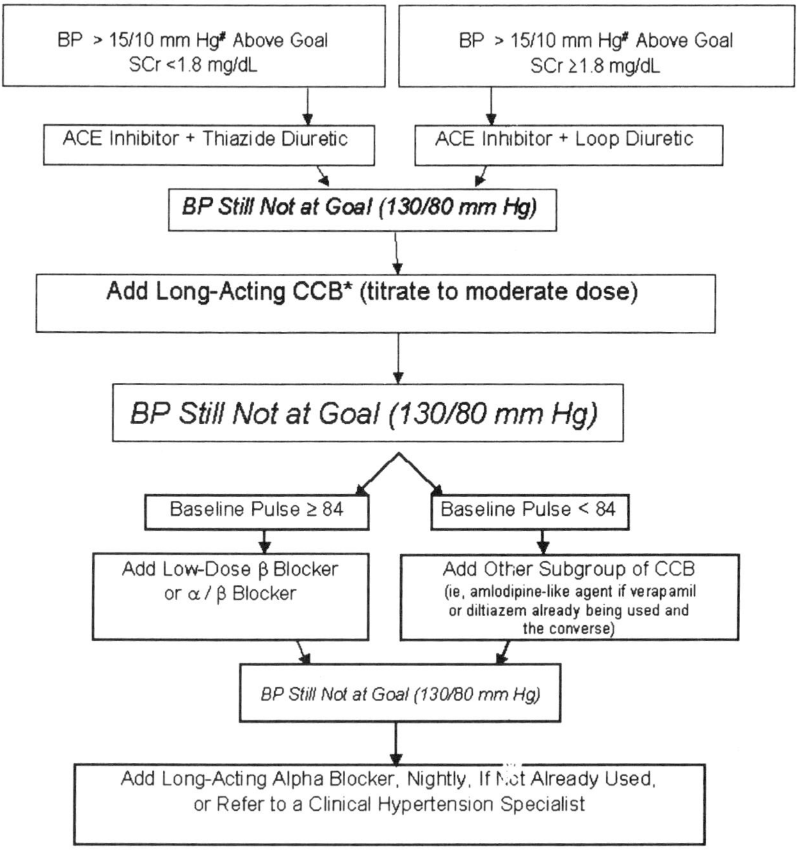


**Fig. 9.** Algorithm for blood pressure control in hypertensive renal diseases (from ref. *11*).

and proteinuria lowering and their effect of antagonizing Ang II, many practicing clinicians prescribe these agents for ACEI-intolerant patients. These agents are not recommended as first-line therapy at this time, primarily because of the lack of outcome studies. Many once-daily ARBs are available and starting doses should be tailored to individual BP and BP goal as noted for ACEIs. As described above for ACEIs the maximal dose for ARBs in CKD is not known and additional dose titration studies are needed to examine effects on proteinuria and renoprotection.

### Diuretics

A diuretic is recommended as the second agent because BP elevation in kidney failure is in part mediated by volume expansion even in the absence of overt edema. Diuretics are particularly important for patients with severe hypertension and kidney failure, especially those with edema. For patients with serum creatinine less than 1.8 mg/dL, thiazide diuretics may suffice. However, for more advanced kidney disease, loop diuretics should be used. Furosemide should be administered at least twice daily, whereas torsemide once daily may suffice.

### CCBs

Third line agents to achieve the goal include CCBs. An important question is whether to use a DHP versus non-DHP. Some small studies in diabetic kidney disease suggest that non-DHP CCBs are superior to DHP CCBs for reducing proteinuria *(69)*. In nondiabetics with proteinuric nephropathies, long-term treatment with DHP CCBs may increase proteinuria if BP goal is not achieved. In the AASK study, ACE inhibition as compared to DHP CCBs improved outcomes in patients with hypertensive nephrosclerosis and more than 300 mg/day of proteinuria. However, the agents were not combined *(70)*. In contrast, a CCB was administered to 80% of patients in RENAAL and did not offset the renoprotective effect of losartan. On the basis of current evidence in hypertensive proteinuric CKD patients, CCBs should be added to an ACEI- or ARB-based regimen if BP is not yet at goal.

### β-Blockers

β-Blockers are effective antihypertensives in patients with CKD. Moreover, because of the high incidence of cardiac disease in this patient population β-blockers are increasingly employed to manage hypertension in both diabetic and nondiabetic patients with CKD. Additionally, in the AASK trial the long-acting β-blocker metoprolol was associated with a significant 37% risk reduction for the secondary combined outcome of rapid decline in GFR or ESRD or death as compared to the DHP CCB (amlodipine) in patients with elevated baseline proteinuria (R. Toto, unpublished observation). Additionally, β-blockers may be used in conjunction with CCBs and ACEIs particularly in diabetic patients with kidney disease. However, adding β-blockers to ACEI and/or ARB therapy should prompt measurement of serum potassium because these agents added together could cause or worsen existing hyperkalemia.

### α-Blockers and Centrally Acting α-2 Antagonists

α-blockers and centrally acting α-2 antagonists have received little attention in the treatment of kidney disease but are not considered first- or second-line therapy. Most protocols, including the AASK study and the algorithm for treatmenting the hypertensive diabetic recommended by the National Kidney Foundation, suggest use of this class after ACEIs, diuretics, CCBs, and/or β-blockers have been added. These agents can be extremely effective adjunctive agents in patients with kidney disease.

### Vasodilators

Hydralazine and minoxidil are still useful agents for managing severe hypertension in kidney disease. These drugs are used in many clinical trials and in clinics for this purpose. They are generally considered last in line for administration to patients with kidney disease following titration of the above-noted drug classes.

### Mineralocorticoid Receptor Antagonists

Spironolactone 25 mg once daily can reduce BP and proteinuria in hypertensive patients with overt proteinuria when added to ACEI therapy *(71)*. Animal studies have demonstrated that a blockade of mineralocorticoid receptors may attenuate renal scarring independent of BP effects; however, there are no outcomes trials in CKD *(72)*. If mineralocorticoid antagonists are added to other antihypertensive agents in CKD patients, serum potassium must be monitored closely because the risk for hyperkalemia can be markedly increased at a dose of 25 mg once daily.

## SUMMARY

In summary, end-stage kidney disease incidence and prevalence are increasing and type II diabetes mellitus has emerged as the major cause of ESRD. Lowering BP preserves kidney function in patients with common hypertensive kidney diseases including hypertensive nephrosclerosis and diabetes. The clinician should focus on achieving a goal BP of 120–130 systolic and 70–80 diastolic with the emphasis on BP "goal" rather than "control." Optimal management of hypertension in this setting should include either an ACEI or Ang II receptor antagonist as part of the antihypertensive regimen.

## REFERENCES

1. NIH. U.S. Renal Data System, USRDS 2000 annual data report. 12th annual report. 6-10-0200. Bethesda, MD, National Institute of Diabetes and Digestive and Kidney Diseases.
2. Jones CA, McQuillan GM, Kusek JW, et al. Serum creatinine levels in the U.S. population: third National Health and Nutrition Examination Survey [published erratum appears in Am J Kidney Dis 2000 Jan;35(1):178]. Am J Kidney Dis 1998;32(6):992–999.
3. The fifth report of the Joint National Committee on Detection, Evaluation and Treatment of High Blood Pressure (JNC V). Arch Int Med 1993;153:154–183.

4. Wright, JT, Kusek, JW, Toto, RD, et al. Design and baseline characteristics of participants in the African American Study of Kidney Disease and Hypertension (AASK) Pilot Study. Control Clin. Trials 1996;17:3S–16S.
5. Joint National Committee on Prevention EaToH. The sixth report of the Joint National Committee on Prevention, Detection, Evaluation and Treatment of High Blood Pressure. Arch Int Med 1997;157:2413–2446.
6. Mailloux LU, Levey AS. Hypertension in patients with chronic renal disease. Am J Kidney Dis 1998;32(5 Suppl 3):S120–S141.
7. Shulman NB, Ford CE, Hall WD, et al. Prognostic value of serum creatinine and effect of treatment of hypertension on renal function: results from the Hypertension Detection and Follow-up study. Hypertension 1989;13(suppl I):I 80–I 93.
8. Klag MJ, Whelton PK, Randall BL, et al. Blood pressure and end-stage renal disease in men. N Engl J Med 1996;334(1):13–18.
9. Klag MJ, Whelton PK, Randall BL, et al. Blood pressure and end-stage renal disease in men. N Engl J Med 1996;334(1):13–18. Au Ref 9 duplicates ref 8. Delete ref 9 and renumber here and in text or provide new new ref.
10. Shulman NB. Epidemiology of hypertension in blacks. In: Hall WD, Saunders E, Shulman NB, ed. Hypertension in Blacks: Epidemiology, pathophysiology and treamtent. Chicago: New York Medical Publishers, 1985: 115–131.
11. Bakris GL, Williams M, Dworkin L, et al. Preserving renal function in adults with hypertension and diabetes: a consensus approach. Am J Kidney Dis 2000;36: 646–661.
12. Hyman DJ, Pavlik VN. Characteristics of patients with uncontrolled hypertension in the United States. N Eng J Med 2001;345:479–486.
13. Coresh J, Wei GL, McQuillan G, et al. Prevalence of high blood pressure and elevated serum creatinine level in the United States: findings from the Third National Health and Nutrition Examination Survey (1988–1994). Arch Intern Med 2001;161:1207.
14. Hebert LA, Wilmer WA, Falkenhain ME, et al. Renoprotection: one or many therapies? Kidney Int 2001;59:1211–1226.
15. Taal MW, Brenner BM. Renoprotective benefits of RAS inhibition: from ACEI to angiotensin II antagonists. Kidney Intl 2000;57:1803–1817.
16. Toto R. Angiotensin II subtype 1 receptor blockers and renal function. Arch Intern Med 2001;161:1492–1499.
17. Brenner BM. Hemodynamically mediated glomerular injury and the progressive nature of kidney disease [clinical conference]. Kidney Int 1983;23(4):647–655.
18. Bennett PH, Haffner S, Kasiske BL, et al. Diabetic renal disease recommendations. Screening and management of microalbuminuria in patients with diabetes mellitus: recommendations to the scientific advisory board of the National Kidney Foundation from an ad hoc committee of the council on diabetes mellitus of the National Kidney Foundation. Am J Kid Dis 1995;25:107–112.
19. Mogensen CE, Keane WF, Bennett PH, et al. Prevention of diabetic renal disease with special reference to microalbuminuria. Lancet 1995;346(8982):1080–1084.
20. Andersen S, Tarnow L, Rossing P, Hansen BV, Parving HH. Renoprotective effects of angiotensin II receptor blockade in type 1 diabetic patients with diabetic nephropathy. Kidney Int 2000 Feb;57(2):601–606.
21. Nelson RG, Tan M, Beck GJ, et al. Changing glomerular filtration with progression from impaired glucose tolerance to type II diabetes mellitus. Diabetologia 1999;42(1):90–93.

22. Nelson RG, Meyer TW, Myers BD, Bennett PH. Course of renal disease in Pima Indians with non-insulin-dependent diabetes mellitus. Kidney Int Suppl 1997; 63:S45–S48.
23. Blouch K, Deen WM, Fauvel JP, Bialek J, Derby G, Myers BD. Molecular configuration and glomerular size selectivity in healthy and nephrotic humans. Am J Physiol 1997;273(3 Pt 2):F430–F437.
24. Lemley KV, Blouch K, Abdullah I, et al. Glomerular permselectivity at the onset of nephropathy in Type 2 diabetes mellitus. J Am Soc Nephrol 2000;11:2095–2105.
25. Nelson RG, Bennett PH, Beck GJ, et al. for the Diabetic Renal Disease Study Group. Development and progression of renal disease in Pima Indians with non- insulin-dependent diabetes mellitus. N Engl J Med 1996;335(22):1636–1642.
26. Hunsicker LG, Adler S, Caggiula A, et al. Predictors of the progression of renal disease in the Modification of Diet in Renal Disease Study. Kidney Int 1997; 51(6):1908–1919.
27. Klahr S, Schreiner G, Ichikawa I. The progression of renal disease. N Engl Med 1988;318:1657–1666.
28. Klahr S. Low protein diets and angiotensin-converting enzyme inhibition in progressive renal failure. Am J Kid Dis 1993;22(1):114–119.
29. Klahr S, Levey A, Beck G, et al. The effects of dietary protein restriction and blood pressure control on the progression of chronic renal disease. N Engl JMed 1994;330:877–884.
30. Peterson JC, Adler S, Burkart JM, et al. For the Modification of Diet in Renal Disease Study. Blood pressure control, proteinuria, and the progression of renal disease. Ann Intern Med 1995;123(10):754–762.
31. Klahr S, Breyer JA, Beck GJ, et al. for the Modification of Diet in Renal Disease Study Group Dietary protein restriction, blood pressure control, and the progression of polycystic kidney disease. [published erratum appears in J Am Soc Nephrol 1995 Oct;6(4):1318]. J Am Soc Nephrol 1995;5(12):2037–2047.
32. Klahr S. Role of dietary protein and blood pressure in the progression of renal disease. Kidney Int 1996;49(6):1783–1786.
33. Benigni A, Remuzzi G. How renal cytokines and growth factors contribute to renal disease progression. Am J Kidney Dis 2001;37:S21–S24.
34. Ruggenenti P, Perna A, Benini R, Remuzzi G. for the Gruppo Italiano di Studi Epidemiologici in Nefrologia (GISEN). Effects of dihydropyridine calcium channel blockers, angiotensin-converting enzyme inhibition, and blood pressure control on chronic, nondiabetic nephropathies. J Am Soc Nephrol 1998;9(11):2096–2101.
35. Ruggenenti P, Perna A, Gherardi G, Benini R, Remuzzi G. Chronic proteinuric nephropathies: outcomes and response to treatment in a prospective cohort of 352 patients with different patterns of renal injury. Am J Kidney Dis 2000;35(6): 1155–1165.
36. Ruggenenti P, Perna A, Benini R, et al. for the Gruppo Italiano Studi Epidemiologici in Nefrologia (GISEN). In chronic nephropathies prolonged ACE inhibition can induce remission: dynamics of time-dependent changes in GFR. J Am Soc Nephrol 1999;10(5):997–1006.
37. Ruggenenti P, Perna A, Gherardi G, Gaspari F, Benini R, Remuzzi G. for the Gruppo Italiano di Studi Epidemiologici in Nefrologia (GISEN). Renal function and requirement for dialysis in chronic nephropathy patients on long-term ramipril: REIN follow-up trial. Ramipril Efficacy in Nephropathy [see comments]. Lancet 1998;352(9136):1252–1256.

38. Ruggenenti P, Perna A, Mosconi L, et al. for the Gruppo Italiano di Studi Epidemiologici in Nefrologia (GISEN). Proteinuria predicts end-stage renal failure in non-diabetic chronic nephropathies. Kidney Int Suppl 1997;63:S54–S57.
39. Remuzzi G, Bertani T. Pathophysiology of progressive nephropathies. N Engl J Med 1998;339(20):1448–1456.
40. Ecder T, Chapman AB, Brosnahan GM, Edelstein CL, Johnson AM, Schrier RW. Effect of antihypertensive therapy on renal function and urinary albumin excretion in hypertensive patients with autosomal dominant polycystic kidney disease [see comments]. Am J Kidney Dis 2000;35(3):427–432.
41. Plum J, Bunten B, Nemeth R, Grabensee B. Effects of the angiotensin II antagonist valsartan on blood pressure, proteinuria, and renal hemodynamics in patients with chronic renal failure and hypertension.
42. Myers BD, Nelson RG, Tan M, et al. Progression of overt nephropathy in non-insulin-dependent diabetes. Kidney Int 1995;47(6):1781–1789.
43. Austin SM, Lieberman JS, Newton LD, Mejia M, Peters WA, Myers BD. Slope of serial glomerular filtration rate and the progression of diabetic glomerular disease. J Am Soc Nephrol 1993;3(7):1358–1370.
44. The HOPE Trial (Heart Outcomes Prevention Evaluation Study) Investigators. Effects of ramipril on cardiovascular and microvascular outcomes in people with diabetes mellitus: results of the HOPE study and MICRO-HOPE substudy. Heart Outcomes Prevention Evaluation Study Investigators [see comments]. Lancet 2000;355(9200):253–259.
45. Toto RD, Adams-Huet B, Fenves AZ, Mitchell HC, Mulcahy W, Smith RD. Effect of ramipril on blood pressure and protein excretion rate in normotensive nondiabetic patients with proteinuria. Am J Kidney Dis 1996;28(6):832–840.
46. Bakris GL, Weir MR, DeQuattro V, McMahon FG. Effects of an ACE inhibitor/ calcium antagonist combination on proteinuria in diabetic nephropathy. Kidney Int 1998;54(4):1283–1289.
47. Bakris GL, Griffin KA, Picken MM, Bidani AK. Combined effects of an angiotensin converting enzyme inhibitor and a calcium antagonist on renal injury. J Hypertens 1997;15(10):1181–1185.
48. Hannedouche T, Landais P, Goldfarb B, et al. Randomised controlled trial of enalapril and beta blockers in non- diabetic chronic renal failure. Br Med J 1994;309(6958):833–837.
49. Ihle BU, Whitworth JA, Shahinfar S, Cnaan A, Kincaid-Smith PS, Becker GJ. Angiotensin-converting enzyme inhibition in nondiabetic progressive renal insufficiency: a controlled double-blind trial. Am J Kidney Dis 1996;27(4):489–495.
50. Ravid M, Savin H, Jutrin I, Bental T, Katz B, Lishner M. Long-term stabilizing effect of angiotensin-converting enzyme inhibition on plasma creatinine and on proteinuria in normotensive type II diabetic patients. Ann Intern Med 1993; 118(8):577–581.
51. Jafar TH, Schmid CH, Landa M, et al. Angiotensin-converting enzyme inhibitors and progression of nondiabetic renal disease: a meta-analysis of patient-level data. Ann Intern Med 2001;135:73–87.
52. MaGee JH, Unger AM, Richardson DW. Changes in renal function associated with drug or placebo therapy of human hypertension. Am J Med 1964;36:795–804.
53. Moyer JH, Heider C, Pevey K, Ford RV. The effect of treatment on the vascular deterioration associated with hypertension, with particular emphasis on renal function. Am J Med 1958;24:177–192.
54. Peterson JC, Adler S, Burkart JM, et al. for the Modification of Diet in Renal Disease Study. Blood pressure control, proteinuria, and the progression of renal disease. Ann Intern Med 1995;123(10):754–762.

55. Viberti G, Morgensen GCE, Groop LC, Pauls JF. Effect of captopril on progression to clinical proteinuria in patients with insulin-dependent diabetes mellitius and microalbuminuria. J Am Med Assoc 1994;271:275–279.
56. Hebert LA, Bain RP, Verme D, et al. Remission of nephrotic reange proteinuria in Type 1 diabetes. Kidney Int 1994;46:1688–1693. Au Term ok?
57. Bakris GL, Copley JB, Vicknair N, Sadler R, Leurgans S. Calcium channel blockers versus other antihypertensive therapies on progression of NIDDM associated nephropathy. Kidney Int 1996;50(5):1641–1650.
58. Smith AC, Toto R, Bakris GL. Differential effects of calcium channel blockers on size selectivity of proteinuria in diabetic glomerulopathy. Kidney Int 1998; 54(3):889–896.
59. GISEN. Randomised placebo-controlled trial of effect of ramipril on decline in glomerular filtration rate and risk of terminal renal failure in proteinuric, non-diabetic nephropathy. [see comments]. Lancet 1997;349(9069):1857–1863.
60. Maschio G, Alberti D, Janin G, et al. for the Angiotensin-Converting- Enzyme Inhibition in Progressive Renal Insufficiency Study Group. Effect of the angiotensin-converting-enzyme inhibitor benazepril on the progression of chronic renal insufficiency. N Engl J Med 1996;334(15):939–945.
61. Toto RD, Mitchell HC, Smith RD, Lee HC, McIntire D, Pettinger WA. "Strict" blood pressure control and progression of renal disease in hypertensive nephrosclerosis. Kidney Int 1995;48(3):851–859.
62. Agodoa LY, Appel L, Bakris GL, et al. Effect of ramipril vs amlodipine on renal outcomes in hypertensives: a randomized controlled trial. JAMA 2001; 285(2719):2728.
63. Should all patients with type 1 diabetes mellitus and microalbuminuria receive angiotensin-converting enzyme inhibitors? A meta-analysis of individual patient data. Ann Intern Med. 2001;134(5):370–379.
64. Lewis E, Hunsicker LG, Bain RP, Rohde RD, the Collaborative Study Group. The effect of angiotensin-converting enzyme inhibition on diabetic nephropathy. N Engl Med 1993;329:1456–1462.
65. Parving H-H, Lehnert H, Brochner-Mortensen J, Gomis R, Andersen S, Arner P, the Irbesartan in Patients with Type 2 Diabetes and Microalbuminuria Study Group. The Effect of Irbesartan on the Development of Diabetic Nephropathy in Patients with type 2 Diabetes. N Engl J Med 2001;345:870–878.
66. Brenner BM, Cooper ME, de Zeeuw D, et al. Effects of losartan on renal and cardiovascular outcomes in patients with Type 2 diabetes and nephropathy. The RENAAL Study Investigators N Engl J Med 2001;345:861–869.
67. Lewis EJ, Hunsicker LG, Clarke WR, et al. Renoprotective effect of the angiotensin-receptor antagonist irbesartan in patients with nephropathy due to Type 2 diabetes. The Collaborative Study Group. N Engl J Med 2001;345:851–860.
68. UK Prospective Diabetes Study Group. Tight blood pressure control and risk of macrovascular and microvascular complications in Type 2 diabetes: UKPDS 38. [see comments] [published erratum appears in Br Med J 1999;318(7175):29]. Br Med J 1998;317(7160):703–713.
69. Smith AC, Toto RD, Bakris GL. Differential effects of calcium channel blockers on size selectivity of proteinuria in diabetic glomerulopathy. Kidney Intl 1998;54:889–896.
70. Ruggenenti P, Perna A, Benini R, Remuzzi G for the Gruppo Italiano di Studi Epidemiologici in Nefrologia (GISEN). Effects of dihydropyridine calcium channel blockers, angiotensin-converting enzyme inhibition, and blood pressure control on chronic, nondiabetic nephropathies. J Am Soc Nephrol 1998;9:2096–2101.

71. Hostetter TH, Rosenberg ME, Ibrahim HN, Juknevicius I. Aldosterone in renal disease. Curr Opin Nephrol Hypertens 2001;10:105–110
72. Chrysostomou A, Becker G. Spironolactone in addition to ACE inhibition to reduce proteinuria in patients with chronic renal disease. N Engl J Med , 2001;345: 925–926.

# 4 Diagnostic Evaluation for Patients With Renovascular Hypertension

*Sumeska Thavarajah,* MD
*and William B. White,* MD

*Contents*



## INTRODUCTION

The overall prevalence of renovascular hypertension is low, accounting for only 5% of all hypertensive patients in the general population and between 10 and 45% of those in a hypertension subspecialty practice *(1,2)*. Thus, routine screening is neither cost effective nor efficient; screening should be performed only on those patients with historical and physical findings, which raise suspicion for renovascular disease. Additionally, renal artery stenosis in not synonymous with renovascular hypertension, as illustrated by multiple autopsy series *(3–5)*. In a series of 154 randomly selected autopsies, Schwartz and White showed a strong association between renal artery stenosis and advancing age but no correlation between stenosis and increased diastolic blood pressure (DBP) *(4)*. Similarly, Holley and coworkers *(3)* found that 49% of normoten-

From: *Secondary Hypertension: Clinical Presentation, Diagnosis, and Treatment*
Edited by: G. A. Mansoor © Humana Press Inc., Totowa, NJ

sive and 77% of hypertensive patients have evidence of moderate to severe renal artery stenosis.

Renal artery stenosis is typically defined as narrowing of the luminal diameter of a large renal artery by at least 50–75% whereas renovascular hypertension is stenosis coupled with renin-dependent hypertension in unilateral disease or combined with hypervolemia in bilateral arterial disease. Left untreated, renal artery stenosis may progress and cause renal dysfunction. The progression of arterial luminal narrowing and the associated decline in renal function is demonstrated by a series of 1189 patients who underwent serial angiograms for the workup of cardiac ischemia *(6)*. Stenotic renal lesions noted on the first study were reassessed at the time of a followup angiogram. There was progression in the severity of stenosis in 11.1% of the patients and associated decline in renal function. The workup of a patient with suspected renovascular hypertension should be designed to identify those lesions that cause pathophysiological changes associated with hypertension and renin dependency as well as ultimately providing anatomic data to guide management.

## ASSESSMENT AND SCREENING OF THE PATIENT POPULATION

Because of the low prevalence of renovascular hypertension in the general population, routine screening is neither cost effective nor high yield. Additionally, the predictive value of screening tests for the identification of renal artery stenosis and the response to revascularization is limited in a population with low prevalence of renovascular hypertension. Screening should be limited to those with clinical features that raise suspicion for renovascular disease.

Clinical features suggestive of renovascular disease were identified in a retrospective analysis of patients who underwent surgical intervention for renovascular disease and now are used to stratify patients by risk prior to screening *(1,6,7–11)*. Data collected from the Cooperative Study of Renovascular Hypertension on 339 essential hypertensives and 175 patients with renovascular disease demonstrated an association between renovascular disease and advancing age, sudden onset of hypertension, accelerated hypertension, and coexisting vascular disease (Table 1) *(7)*. Essential hypertension tends to have a more variable onset, to present in middle age, and to occur in those patients with a family history of hypertension. In contrast, renovascular hypertension tends to occur in the extremes of age, attributable more often to fibromuscular disease in younger patients and atheromatous disease in older patients. In those individuals presenting with hypertension after age 60, there is a 10%

Table 1
Features Suggestive of Renovascular Hypertension

- Age of onset <30 or >55
- Accelerated hypertension
- Resistant to therapy despite ≥3 drugs
- Unexplained renal dysfunction
- Azotemia after ACEI or ARB administration
- Abdominal bruit
- Coexistant vascular disease: coronary artery disease, cerebrovascular disease, peripheral vascular disease
- Recurrent pulmonary edema

ACEI, angiotension-converting enzyme inhibitor; ARB angiotension receptor blocker.

chance of an etiology of renovascular hypertension *(12)*. Renovascular hypertension is more likely to be accelerated and refractory to treatment, with many patients presenting with grade III or IV retinopathy and severe diastolic hypertension at the time of diagnosis, as well as requiring multiple antihypertensive agents *(1,2,6,9)*. For example, a series of 52 patients with renovascular hypertension were found to have resistant hypertension with a mean systolic blood pressure of 208 mmHg and DBP of 106 mmHg, renal insufficiency (mean serum creatinine of 1.7 mg/dL), an average regimen of 2.8 antihypertensive agents, and symptoms of recurrent pulmonary edema *(13)*.

Atheromatous disease is a major risk factor for renovascular hypertension; 40% of patients with renal artery stenosis have bruits in major vessels and up to 30% have concomitant coronary artery disease or peripheral vascular disease *(1,5,14)*. Historical factors such as claudication, previous myocardial infarction, cerebrovascular accidents, hyperlipidemia, and smoking are associated with increased risk. For example, Nicholson et al. *(15)* demonstrated that smokers comprised 88% of the population with renovascular disease but just 42% of the patient population with essential hypertension.

In renal artery stenosis, the kidney supplied by the stenotic vessel develops tubular atrophy and interstitial fibrosis secondary to hypoperfusion while the contralateral kidney, exposed to higher pressures, develops glomerulosclerosis resulting in proteinuria and ultimate decline in renal function. The blood flow distal to the stenosis is dependent in part on angiotensin II (Ang II) driven vasoconstriction in the efferent arteriolar circulation. The rise in serum creatinine and decline in glomerular filtration rate (GFR) seen with use of an angiotensin-converting enzyme inhibitor (ACEI) or an angiotensin II receptor blocker (ARB) is caused by removal of Ang II-mediated renal efferent arteriolar vasoconstriction. Unexplained renal insufficiency and azotemia following ACEI or ARB challenge are both factors that should raise suspicion for the presence of renovascular disease.

## SCREENING TESTS

Because not all stenotic lesions of the renal arteries have functional significance, any screening workup should obtain both anatomic and functional data. The conventional angiogram is the gold standard for diagnosis, combining visualization of lesions, determination of hemodynamic significance, and possible therapeutic intervention, but the procedure has a variety of associated risks. The diagnostic goal is to minimize the number of patients exposed to these procedural risks by using other noninvasive screening tests. Several anatomic and functional screening tests have been developed that accurately identify renal artery stenosis and predict prognostic outcome following revascularization.

### *Functional Tests*

The functional tests to screen for renovascular hypertension are shown in Table 2. These tests generally include biochemical parameters coupled with stimulation or imaging studies using agents that block the renin-angiotensin system to provide information about the functional significance of the stenosis and aid in predicting the benefits of revascularization with regard to blood pressure (BP) control and renal function.

#### Plasma Renin Levels/ Stimulated Plasma Renin Levels

The most general screening test is the sampling of peripheral plasma renin activity (PRA). In response to diminished renal perfusion, the kidney supplied by the stenotic artery secretes excess renin. However, an elevated systemic plasma renin level is not very specific for renovascular hypertension given the overlap for elevated PRA levels in essential hypertension and potential for normal levels of PRA in renovascular hypertension: 50–80% of renovascular hypertensive patients have elevated PRA levels, whereas 15–20% of essential hypertensive patients have elevated levels *(16)*. The predictive value of the systemic PRA levels is enhanced by measuring the response in renin levels after administration of an ACEI (usually oral captopril or parenteral enalaprilat), based on the finding that the affected kidney will have exaggerated renin release caused by both the fall in arterial pressure and the removal of the effects of Ang II on the efferent arterioles in the nephron. Early studies examined the predictive value of the stimulated plasma renin tests in

Table 2
Functional Tests for Renovascular Hypertension

| *Diagnostic test* | *Diagnostic criteria* | *Advantages* | *Disadvantages* |
|---|---|---|---|
| Stimulated PRA | PRA > 12 ng/mL/hr<br>↑ of > 10 ng/mL/hr<br>↑ of ≥ 150% | Noninvasive, inexpensive | Affected by many antihypertensives<br>Cannot differentiate between bilateral and unilateral disease |
| Renal vein renin ratio | Lateralization >1.5<br><br>Invasive<br>Contralateral <1.0 | Lateralization can be determined | Technically difficult<br>Ipsilateral >1.5 |
| Renal scintigraphy | Changes in renogram<br>Pre/post ACEI administration | Noninvasive<br>No radio-contrast<br>Can distinguish bilateral vs unilateral | Expensive<br>Affected by other kidney disorders |

PRA, plasmas renin activity; ACEI, angiotension-converting enzyme inhibitor.

those patients diagnosed with renovascular hypertension by conventional angiography. A series by Haward and colleagues of 12 patients demonstrated a sensitivity of 89% and specificity of 100% for stimulated plasma renin levels for identifying those patients who would respond to revascularization *(13)*.

The limitations of the captopril renin test are primarily related to the effects of various antihypertensive therapies. Because most antihypertensive agents can affect the level of renin, all antihypertensive agents with a potential effect on the PRA should be discontinued for 2 to 4 weeks before testing. Calcium channel blockers (CCBs) have often been used for hypertension management until the biochemical testing has been completed. Plasma renin levels are drawn before and 1 hour after dosing with a short-acting ACEI, and BP measurements are completed at baseline and at 15-minute intervals throughout the testing.

In a retrospective analysis of 246 patients with renovascular hypertension, Muller and colleagues*(17)* defined the three criteria for a positive stimulated renin test:

1. stimulated plasma renin level of greater than 12 ng/mL/hour
2. an absolute increase in plasma renin activity of greater than 10 ng/mL/hour.
3. a greater than 150% increase in PRA or greater than 400% increase in PRA if the baseline PRA was less than 3 ng/mL/hour.

Although neither that sensitive nor specific in patients with renal insufficiency or bilateral disease, when applied to those with preserved renal function these criteria for the captopril test are 100% sensitive and specific for diagnosis of renal artery stenosis but not necessarily renovascular hypertension. Attempts to reproduce Muller's results in prospective studies have failed to achieve similar accuracy for the captopril test with sensitivity ranging from 34 to 95% and specificity ranging from 66 to 93% *(18–22)*. The largest series involved 485 patients with hypertension using the three criteria for plasma renin levels and had a sensitivity of 79% and specificity of 89% *(19)*. Accuracy for the captopril test has been shown to be lower in younger patients, African-Americans, patients on diuretics, and patients with renal insufficiency (serum creatinine >1.7 mg/dL). Davidson et al. *(23)* attempted to redefine the diagnostic cut-off criteria in an effort to improve the predictive value of the test, designating a plasma renin level of greater than 5.7ng/mL/hr as a positive test in the evaluation of 36 patients with renovascular hypertension. Of these 36 patients, 69.4% had been cured (BP < 140/90 mmHg on no medication) or improved (DBP decreased by 10–15% and less medication) by surgical revascularization. The stimulated plasma renin test was positive in 24 of the 25 patients who responded to intervention

(96% sensitivity) and negative in 6 of the 11 nonresponders (54.5% specificity). Applying Muller's criteria to this same group improves specificity to 63% but decreases the sensitivity to 83%.

The lack of reproducible results and confounding factors of renal insufficiency, volume depletion, smoking, and autonomic dysfunction have markedly limited the utility of this test. It is inconvenient and potentially unsafe for patients with stage II and III hypertension to be taken off of most antihypertensive agents for several weeks. Another major limitation is the lack of any anatomic data and inability to differentiate unilateral vs bilateral disease. Given its limited utility and the inaccurate results in a low- to moderate-risk population, this test is no longer typically used in the evaluation for renovascular disease.

### Renal Vein Renin Sampling

In contrast to the stimulated plasma renin test, renal vein renin testing provides information about the renin production of each kidney. Given the invasive nature of the test, however, it has not been used as a first-line screening test in patients at low risk for renovascular disease. Renin samples are obtained via selective catheterization of the renal veins under fluoroscopic guidance. The affected kidney will typically have elevated renin secretion and thus an increased renal vein renin to vena caval renin ratio while the contralateral kidney will show suppressed renin secretion. A renal vein to vena caval renin ratio of more 1.5 is predictive of a beneficial BP response to treatment in 90% of the patients with unilateral stenosis *(24)*. The normal renal vein to vena caval renin ratio is 1.24 with only 10% of normotensive patients having a ratio of more than 1.5. The kidney contralateral to the stenotic artery has a suppressed renal vein renin to vena caval renin ratio of less than 1.0 with less than 20% of renovascular hypertensive patients having suppressed ratios.

Multiple studies have demonstrated that a ratio of more than 1.5 as a criterion for diagnosis of renovascular hypertension has an 80% sensitivity and a 62% specificity but does not always predict response to intervention *(13,25,26)*. In those patients with renovascular hypertension undergoing surgical revascularization *(25)*, 45 of 50 of those cured and 26 of the 34 improved by surgery demonstrated lateralization of the renin levels (cut-off ratio was >1.4). Although lateralization was predictive of beneficial response to surgical intervention, the failure to lateralize did not predict failure since 7 of 14 patients with a ratio less than 1.4, showed improvement after surgery highlighting the fact that a patient cannot be excluded from renal revascularization based on the split renal vein renin sampling. Up to 30% of patients who fail to lateralize have a beneficial response to surgery *(27)*. There is the potential for many technical errors to account for the number of false-negative results, such as sampling from the wrong branch of the renal vein, improper collection and processing of samples, and stimulation of renin secretion by dye injection. The technical errors in combination with the multiple inherent risks of the test, including intravenous catheterization and nephrotoxicity from the dye load, have steered many away from using split renal vein renin sampling as part of a diagnostic workup.

### Renal Scintigraphy

Radionuclide scintigraphy has become a primary method for screening patients with normal renal function for renovascular hypertension by assessing renal perfusion, renal size, and excretory capacity. The renogram consists of three phases: (a) the rapid upslope or uptake of tracer in the first minute, the tubular phase or the time to peak of the clearance curve (about 3 to 5 minutes and a correlate of renal plasma flow) and (b) the secretory phase associated with a gradual decline in tracer over the next 30 minutes (a correlate of urinary flow). The administration of a short-acting ACEI enhances the functional differences between the kidneys in patients with renovascular hypertension. Those patients on ACEIs or ARBs should hold therapy for at least 48 hours before to the renal scan. Changes in the baseline renogram between the kidneys and changes between pre- and post-ACE inhibition are then assessed (Fig. 1). Asymmetry in uptake of radionuclide 1.5 to 2.5 minutes after injection defined as less than 40% uptake on the affected side and more than 60% on the unaffected side, in excretion, time to peak activity, or the percentage of peak activity 15–20 minutes postinjection, are indicative of renal artery stenosis *(16,28)*. Using these criteria, the renogram has been reported to have a sensitivity of 85–90% (range 45–94%) and a specificity of 93–98% (range of 81–100%) *(29–31)*.

The choice of the radiolabeled agents also may affect the precision of renal scintigraphy. $I^{131}$- I orthoiodohippuric acid (OIH) is a marker of renal plasma flow, taken up and retained in tubular cells because of the inability to be washed out when the GFR is reduced. The OIH renograms are characterized by prolongation of cortical transit time and cortical retention in the affected kidney. The sensitivity and specificity of OIH renograms are equivalent to detection of renal artery stenosis by intravenous pyelography *(2)*. Other radiotracers have far better resolution and pick up more of the branch arteries *(30)*. Technetium-99 diethylenetriamine pentaacetic acid (DTPA) is a pure glomerular agent with limited protein binding that is eliminated by glomerular filtration and therefore has decreased intensity with declining GFR. DTPA–captopril renograms have been reported to have a sensitivity of 91% and a specificity of 94% for greater than 50% of patients with renal artery

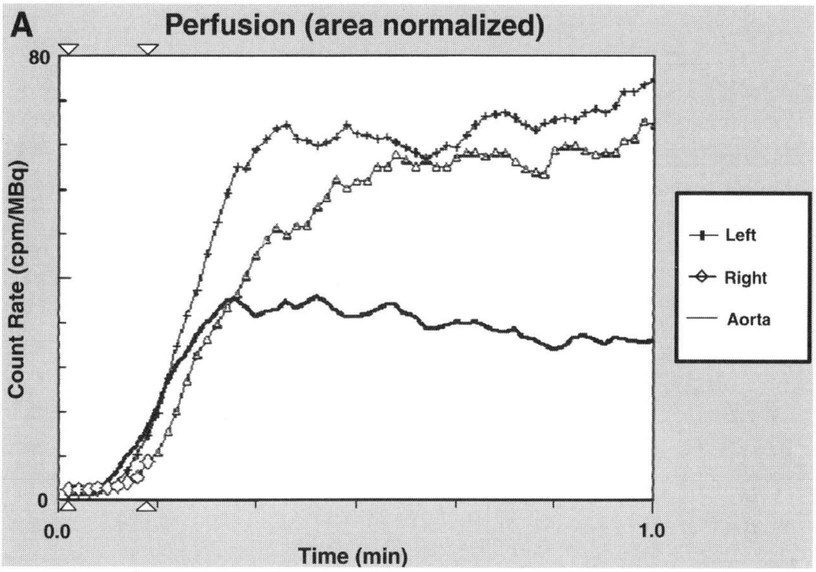


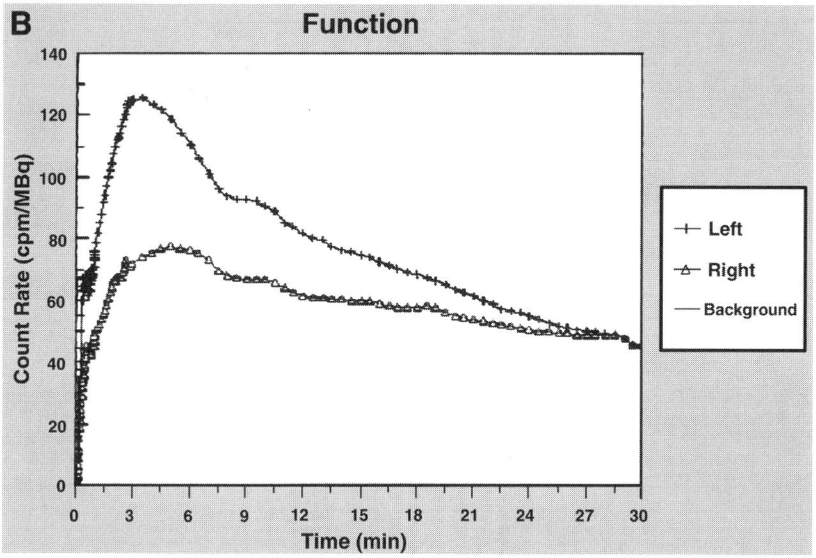


**Fig. 1.** Two-part renogram of a 61-year-old female on ACEI with 3.2mCi of Technetium-99m MAG3.

(A) Baseline perfusion study.

(B) Baseline function. During peak concentration the left kidney contributes 65% of the renal funtion. Half-time emptying for the left kidney in 17 minutes, not reached in the right kidney (normal 5 to 7 minutes).

(C) Perfusion study after 2 mg of intravenous enalaprilat.

(D) Functional study after 2 mg enalaprilat. In comparison to baseline renogram, high probability of right renal artery stenosis. (Fig. 1C & D, *next page*.)

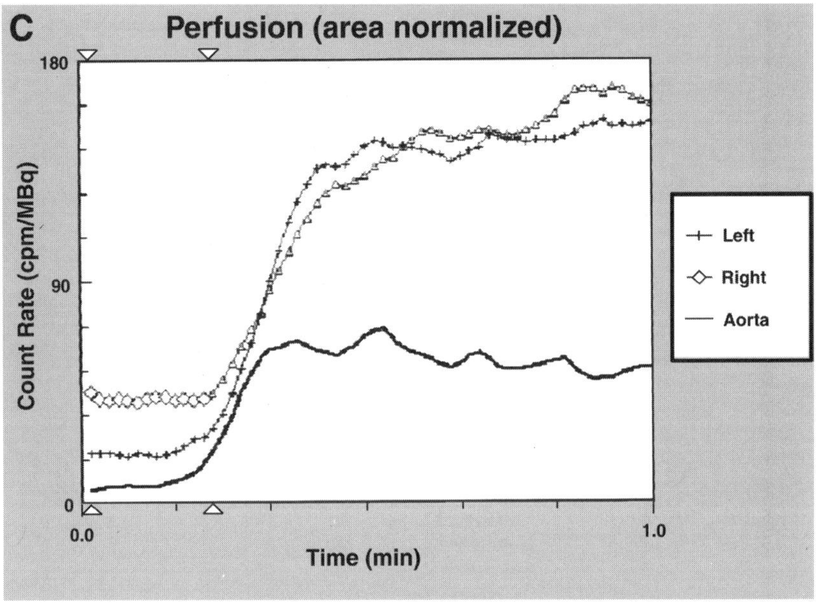


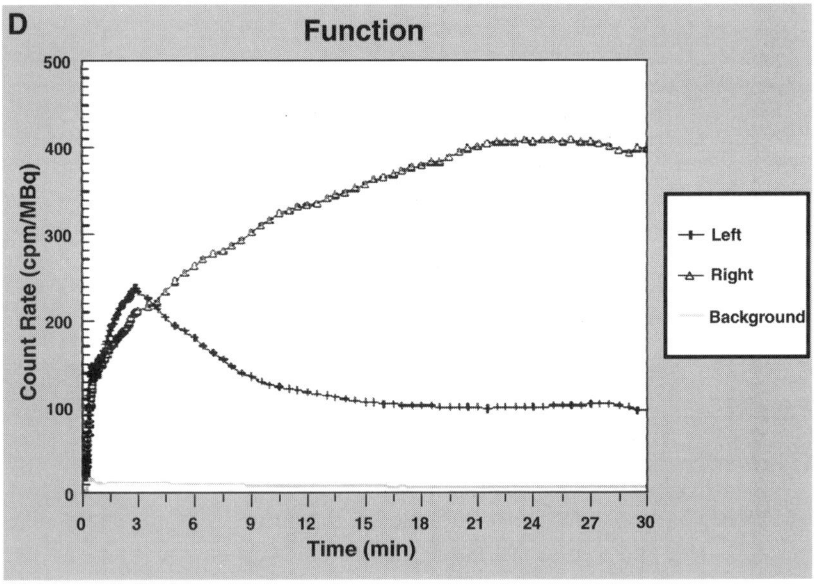


stenosis *(32)*. In addition to detection, there was a high concordance for predicting response to revascularization in those patients with positive captopril scans.

In the setting of impaired renal function (serum creatinine > 1.4), the accuracy of DTPA renograms is compromised *(33,34)*. Technetium-99 mercaptoacetyltriglycine (MAG3) is another agent secreted by the tubules, which visualizes the collecting system and cortex. It has become the radionuclide of choice for the assessment of renovascular hypertension. It is effective in those patients with renal insufficiency because it provides more distinct images and exposes the patient to a lower radiation dose *(16)*. In a series of 84 patients, 51 of whom were evaluated by captopril renal scintigraphy (using either DTPA or MAG3 as the contrast agent) in addition to conventional angiography, there was a positive predictive value of 97% and a negative predictive value of 72% for beneficial response to treatment, highlighting the significant predictive value of renal scintigraphy for response to intervention *(28)*. This again is demonstrated in the review of data on the use of renal scintigraphy over 15 years by van Jaarsveld *(35)*. Using renal scintigraphy with a sensitivity of 68% and a specificity of 90% in a population with 3% prevalence of renovascular disease, it was demonstrated that in order to detect 20 cases of renovascular hypertension, 117 patients would require angiography *(35)*. In contrast, without using renal scintigraphy as a screening test, 667 patients with hypertension would undergo angiography to detect 20 cases of renovascular hypertension.

## EVALUATION OF RENAL ARTERY ANATOMY

In addition to identifying the presence of renovascular hypertension, another important goal is to define the responsible stenotic lesion and assess whether it is amenable to treatment with either percutaneous angioplasty or bypass surgery (Table 3). Prior to revascularization, every patient will undergo conventional angiography. The goal would be to determine whether kidney function is salvageable and thereby prevent those who would not benefit from intervention from proceeding with unnecessary angiography.

### Intravenous Pyelography

In the past, intravenous pyelography (IVP) was a common screening test used to detect the ischemic changes in the kidney ipsilateral to the stenosis. Diagnostic criteria included a disparity in renal length of at least 1.5 cm and a greater than 1-minute delay in calyceal appearance time *(16)*. Compared to arteriography, this modality had a sensitivity of 74.5% and specificity of 86.2% *(16)*. However, there are a high number of false negatives attributed to bilateral or segmental renal artery disease. More significant was the poor predictive value for response to intervention. In reviewing results of the pyelography, only 60 to 73% of the patients with abnormal pyelograms had a beneficial response to surgical revascularization, whereas 40–85% of those with normal

**Table 3**
**Anatomic Tests for Renovascular Hypertension**

| *Test* | *Diagnostic criteria* | *Advantages* | *Disadvantages* |
|---|---|---|---|
| IV Pyelogram | Diff between kidneys<br>> 1.5 cm<br>> 1 min calyceal appearance after dye injection | Easy to perform<br>Can continue medications | Dye load<br>Poor predictive value |
| Duplex Doppler Ultrasound | Kidney size<br>Peak flow >180 cm/s<br>Ratio R/A >3.5 | Noninvasive<br>Can be used in all patients and continue medications | Time consuming<br>Operator dependent |
| CT Angiogram | Visualization of Stenotic vessels | Good visualization of main and accessory vessels | Dye load |
| MRA | Visualization of stenotic vessels | Good visualization of lesions in main renal arteries | Misses accessory vessels<br>Over/underestimates degree of stenosis |

pyelograms had a beneficial response to surgery *(16,24)*. This poor sensitivity and specificity, as well as poor predictive value, and the risks of large amounts of contrast dye and radiation exposure have virtually eliminated the use of IVP as a screening test.

#### Duplex Doppler Ultrasonography

Duplex doppler ultrasonography is a unique modality that provides both anatomic and some functional data. Renal size assessment and visualization of renal arteries is performed via B-mode imaging. As the lumen of a vessel narrows, the velocity of blood flow increases and the severity of stenosis can be determined by comparing the systolic flow velocity through the renal artery compared with that through the aorta using a color Doppler unit *(16,34)*. Compared to conventional angiography, Doppler ultrasound has a sensitivity of 88–95% and specificity of 90–99% with positive and negative predictive values of 99% and 97%, respectively *(24,36,37)*.

In a series of 98 patients evaluated with both duplex ultrasound and radionuclide scintigraphy, Johansson and colleagues *(38)* showed that the kidney ipsilateral to the stenosis was smaller ($10.1 \pm 0.2$ cm) than in the contralateral unaffected kidney ($11.4 \pm 0.1$ cm ($p < 0.01$). The duplex ultrasound allows for assessment of renal size and asymmetry between kidneys, ureteral abnormalities, vascular abnormalities, and identification of stenotic vessels.

Classically stenotic lesions have been defined ultrasonographically by a peak flow velocity of more than 180cm/second through the vessel and a ratio of renal arterial flow velocity to aortic flow velocity of more than 3.5 *(37)*. In an effort to improve sensitivity and specificity, Hoffman et al redefined the criteria of stenosis as a combination of three factors: delayed time to early systolic peak velocity (acceleration time), decreased acceleration within segmental hilar arteries (acceleration index), and loss of the normal early systolic compliance peak with a resultant sensitivity of 95% and specificity of 97%.

Other radiologists using duplex ultrasonography as a screening method have tried to define more objective measurements that have a greater predictive value for prognosis and intervention. In a series of 5950 hypertensive patients screened with Doppler ultrasonography, Radermacher et al. evaluated the utility of the resistance index (RI) as a predictor of successful intervention *(39)*.

$$\text{Resistance Index (RI)} = (1 - \text{End diastolic velocity/max systolic Velocity}) \times 100$$

Of the 35 patients with a resistance index greater than 80, 34 failed to have a beneficial response in blood pressure postrevascularization and 28 of these patients had a decline in renal function, whereas of the 96 patients with a resistance index of less than 80, only 6% failed to have some improvement in blood pressure and 3 % had a decline in renal function. In another series of 214 hypertensive patients involving 53 subjects with renal artery stenosis, the resistance index had a 92% sensitivity and 96% specificity for detection of greater than 70% stenosis *(40–42)*. Another measure of arterial flow is the pulsatility index (PI):

PI = (Peak systolic velocity - End diastolic velocity)/Mean velocity

All these measurements have comparable sensitivity and specificity for detection of stenosis but are useful in making the diagnosis of renal artery stenosis less subject to observer bias.

The main advantage of ultrasonography is that it is a modality that can be used in almost every patient becaue the results are not affected by use of antihypertensives or underlying renal insufficiency. It is noninvasive with no exposure to irradiation or contrast dye. Its main drawback is that it is a time-consuming procedure and highly operator dependent for accuracy. Unless an institution has extensive experience with dedicated ultrasonography technicians or radiologists, the accuracy of this test does not approach that of other screening modalities.

### Spiral Computed Tomography Angiography

Spiral computed tomography (CT) angiography provides another modality to image the renal arteries noninvasively with the accuracy of conventional angiography. In a group of 50 patients undergoing both spiral CT angiography and intra-arterial digital subtraction arteriography (DSA), spiral CT angiography detected 126 of 127 renal arteries and 27 of 28 of the accessory renal arteries detected by DSA (96% detection rate) *(43)*. In this study, spiral CT angiography had four false-negatives, two false-positives, two underestimations of stenosis, and one overestimation of stenosis, all involving accessory renal arteries. For a greater than 50% stenosis, in any renal artery, spiral CT angiography had a sensitivity of 90% and a specificity of 97%; when only the main renal arteries were evaluated, the sensitivity and specificity improved to 100% and 97%, respectively. These results were corroborated in studies by Elkohen et al. *(44)* where spiral CT angiography had a sensitivity of 87.5% and specificity of 98% in detecting 14 of 16 significant stenotic lesions with the missed lesions in only branch arteries. Beregi et al. *(45)* demonstrated a sensitivity of 88% and specificity of 98% for detection of renal artery stenosis and 100% sensitivity and 98% specificity when evaluating only main renal arteries.

A significant disadvantage of this screening modality is the use of contrast and the risk of nephrotoxicity. A spiral CT angiogram usually requires 150–200 cc of noniodinated contrast and thus limits its use to patients with normal renal function. The accuracy of this study is limited in those patients with impaired renal function; Olbricht et al. *(46)* studied 62 patients evaluated with spiral CT angiography and conventional arteriography. Evaluation by spiral CT angiography had a sensitivity of 98% and specificity of 94%, which fell to a 93% sensitivity and 81% specificity in those patients with serum creatinine levels of greater than 1.7 mg/dL *(46)*.

### Magnetic Resonance Angiography

Magnetic resonance angiography (MRA) provides a noninvasive, nonnephrotoxicalternative to conventional angiography. Images are derived from signals originating from moving and fixed protons. There are three protocols used to reconstruct the renal arteries: two-dimensional time of flight (2DTOF), three-dimensional time of flight (3DTOF), and three-dimensional phase contrast (3DPC). 2DTOF images detect slow-flowing vessels. 3DTOF images have better spatial resolution and can visualize perinephric tissue well. 3DPC images allow for subtraction of background tissue, thus highlighting the area of interest. Kim et al. *(47)* evaluated 25 patients with 2DTOF with a specificity of 92% and sensitivity of 100% for detection of stenosis, but there was an overestimation and underestimation of stenosis severity *(46)*. Yucel et al. applied all three modalities in evaluating 16 patients with a 100% sensitivity and 93% specificity *(48)*.

When compared to contrast arteriography, MRA had a sensitivity of 91% and overall accuracy of 81% when evaluating 32 renal arteries *(49)*. Although MRA has equivalent accuracy to conventional arteriography for main arterial lesions, it fails to detect lesions in many accessory renal arteries. In a series of 37 patients with hypertension evaluated with MRA and intra-arterial DSA, MRA had a sensitivity of 100% and specificity of 96% for detecting stenotic lesions in main renal arteries but missed 9 of 12 of the lesions in accessory renal arteries.

MRA is being used more frequently as a noninvasive method for visualizing vessels and the kidneys in those patients with significant renal impairment. Its accuracy is comparable to conventional angiography for proximal or main renal arteries but is less accurate for the detection of accessory vessels. Grading the severity of the lesions is subject to observer error, leading to overestimation and underestimation of the degree of luminal narrowing.

### Contrast Angiography

Contrast angiography remains the gold standard for assessment of renal artery stenosis. Via a major artery, the renal arteries are catheterized and visualized with injections of contrast. In addition to identifying the location of stenosis, the severity and the hemodynamic significance may be determined by measuring the gradient across stenotic lesions. Contrast angiography evaluates the kidney size quite precisely because a kidney at least 9 cm in length with evidence of retrograde filling of distal renal arteries should have the best outcome with regard to renal function *(49,50)*. Unlike other screening tests, this is the only modality that is diagnostic and can become potentially therapeutic Fig. 2.

Contrast angiography is not without risks because it exposes patients to the risks of arterial catheterization, contrast dye, irradiation, cholesterol emboli, and aortic dissection. In patients with renal insufficiency, there is a 10–15% risk of contrast-induced nephropathy *(50)*.

A few protocols have been developed in an attempt to approximate the accuracy of conventional angiography with less risk of complications. One protocol is intravenous digital subtraction angiography (intravenous DSA). This method does not require hospitalization or arterial catheterization. It is especially useful in patients with severe atherosclerotic disease, thus minimizing cholesterol embolization risk. A review of 13 studies reveals a sensitivity of 87.6 % and specificity of 89.5% for detection of renal artery stenosis *(50)*. However, the images do not have the resolution of conventional angiography and expose patients to a dye load. Additionally, images of vessels can be obscured by overlying mesenteric vessels. Intra-arterial DSA is another protocol, that uses intra-arterial injections of contrast material but in combination with computer technology to enhance images to minimize the amount of dye used. This modality provides an equivalent level of accuracy as seen with conventional angiography. Recently, the use of carbon dioxide ($CO_2$) as a contrast agent to eliminate the risk of renal toxicity has gained popularity for evaluating both renal and peripheral vascular disease. $CO_2$ is used as the contrast agent and the images are then enhanced with DSA. This combination of $CO_2$ and DSA provides images of the vessels with a high percentage of diagnostic agreement with conventional angiography. $CO_2$ angiography can visualize second and third branches of renal arteries accurately. Beyond this requires about a 10 cc injection of contrast; this small amount poses little nephrotoxic risk. Since this agent is a gas, bowel gas can interfere with adequate visualization. This is often minimized by the use of glucagon.

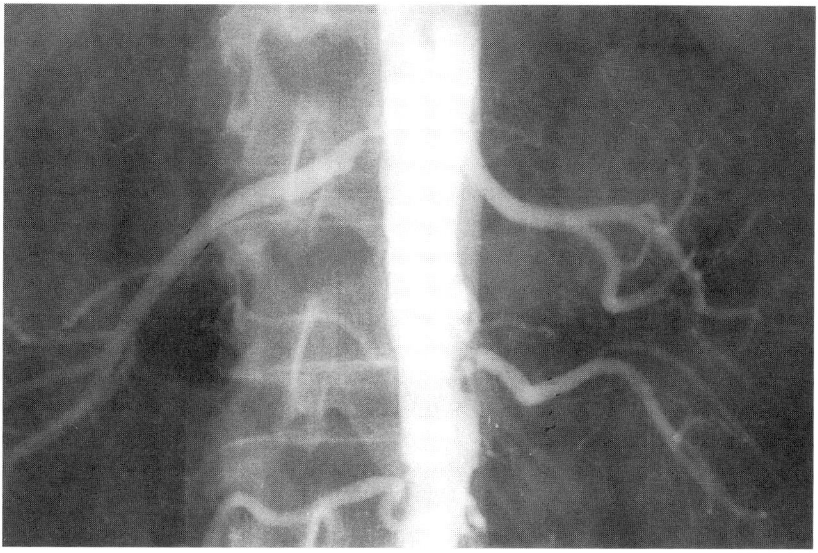

**Fig. 2.** Contrast angiography demonstrating renal artery stenosis.

## CONCLUSION

It is not feasible to develop a single algorithm for the diagnosis of renovascular hypertension; rather, the choice of screening tests is tailored to the level of clinical suspicion and the individual's clinical characteristics. While conventional angiography is superior diagnostically and has potential therapeutically, it has too many risks to use as a routine procedure. The diagnostic assessment needs to provide enough anatomic and functional data to warrant proceeding to angiography and potential intervention with angioplasty. Many of the early tests such as plasma renin levels, renal vein renins, and intravenous pyelography do not have acceptable levels of accuracy and have been eliminated in most workups (Table 4). Captopril renal scintigraphy has come to the forefront as an initial screening test in those patients with historical and physical findings suggestive of renovascular hypertension. Those with positive renal scans could proceed directly to angiography. Those with equivocal or negative scans, but highly suspicious clinical features, could be further evaluated with MRA and, based on those findings, proceed to conventional angiography. Another modality that can be used as a initial screening test is duplex Doppler ultrasonography. The reliability of this modality depends on an institution's experience and the presence of a

Table 4
Overview of the Predictive Value of Diagnostic Tests

| *Test* | *Sensitivity (%)* | *Specificity (%)* |
|---|---|---|
| Renal scintigraphy | 85–90 | 93–98 |
| Duplex Doppler ultrasonography | 88–95 | 90–99 |
| Spiral CT angiography | 90–98 | 94–98 |
| MR angiography | 91–100 | 76–92 |

well-trained technician. It is an attractive alternative because it provides both anatomic and functional information and is not affected by renal function or antihypertensive agents. It does not expose patients to risks of contrast dye or irradiation, and is relatively inexpensive. Whatever modalities are used in the initial screening, however, the final diagnosis is virtually always made with angiography.

## REFERENCES


1. Conlon PJ, O'Riordan E, Kalra PA. New insights into the epidemologic and clinical manifestations of atherosclerotic renovascular disease. Am J Kid Dis 2000; 35(4):573–87.
2. Nally JV, Barton DP. Contemporary Approach to Diagnosis and Evaluation of Renovascular Hypertension. Urologic Clinics of North America. 2001;28(4):781–91.
3. Holley KE, Hunt JC, Brown AL, Kincaid OW, Sheps SG. Renal artery stenosis: a clinical-pathological study in normotensive and hypertensive patients. Am J Med 1964;37:14–22.
4. Schwartz CJ, White TA.Stenosis of the renal artery: an unselected necropsy study. Br Med J 1964;2:1415–1421.
5. Olin JW, Melia M, Young JR, Graor RA, Risius B. Prevalence of atherosclerotic renal artery stenosis in patients with atherosclerosis elsewhere. Am J Med 1990;88:46N–51N.
6. Crowley JJ, Santos RM, Peter RH, et al. Progression of renal artery stenosis in patients undergoing cardiac catherization. Am Heart J 1998;136(5):913–8.
7. Maxwell MH, Bleifer KH, Franklin SS, Varady PD.Cooperative study of renovascular hypertension: demographic analysis of the study. JAMA. 1972;220: 1195–1204.
8. Harding MB, Smith LR, Himmelstein SI, et al. Renal artery stenosis: prevalence and associated risk factors in patients undergoing routine cardiac catheterization. J Am Soc Nephrol 1992;2:1608–1616.
9. Davis BA, Crook JE, Vestal RE, Oakes JA.Prevalence of renovascular hypertension in patients with grade III or IV retinopathy. N Engl J Med 1979;301:1273–1276.
10. Working Group on Renovascular Hypertension. Detection, evaluation, and treatment of renovascular hypertension. Final report. Arch Intern Med 1987;147: 820–829.

11. Kalra PA, MacDowall P, O'Donoghue P, et al. Analysis of vascular comorbidity in patients with atheromatous renovascular disease. J Am Soc Nephrol 1996;7:1390A.
12. Anderson GH Jr, Blakeman N, Streeten DHP. Prediction of renovascular hypertension: comparison of clinical diagnostic indices. Am J Hyperten 1988;1:301–304.
13. Harward TRS, Poindextor B, Huber TS, Carlton LM, Flynn TC, Seeger JM. Selection of patients for renal artery repair using captopril testing. American J Surg 1995;170(2):183–187.
14. Vetrovec GW, Landweher DM, Edwards VL.Incidence of renal artery stenosis in hypertensive patients undergoing coronary angiography. J Intervent Cardiol 1989;2:69–76.
15. Nicholson JP, Teichman SL, Alderman MH, Sos TA, Pickering TG, Laragh JH.Cigarette smoking and renovascular hypertension. Lancet 1983;2(8353):765–6.
16. Mann SJ, Pickering TG.Detection of Renovascular Hypertension—State of the art: 1992. Ann Intern Med 1992;117:845–853.
17. Muller FB, Sealey JE, Case DB, et al. The captopril test of identifying renovascular disease in hypertensive patients. Am J Med 1986;80:633–44.
18. Nally JV, Chen C, Fine E, et al. Diagnositic criteria of renovascular hypertension with captopril renography: a consensus statement. Am J Hyperten 1991;4: 749S–752S.
19. Lenz T, Kia T, Rupprecht G, et al. Captopril test: time over? J Hum Hyperten 1999;13:431–435.
20. Svetkey LP, Mimmelstein SI, Dunnick NR. Prospective analysis strategies for diagnosing renovascular hypertension: Hypertension. 1989;14:247–257.
21. Hansen PB, Garsdal P, Fruergaard P. The captopril test for identification of renovascular hypertension: value and immediate adverse effects. J Intern Med 1990; 228:159–163.
22. Postma CT, van der Steen PHM, Hoegnagels HL, et al. The captopril test in detection of renovascular disease in hypertensive patients. Arch Intern Med 1990; 150:625–28.
23. Davidson R, Barri Y, Wilcox C. The simplified captopril test: an effective tool to diagnose renovascular Hypertension. Am J Kidney Dis 1994;24:660–664.
24. Canzanello VJ, Textor SC.Noninvasive Diagnosis of Renovascular Disease. Mayo Clinic Proc 1994;69:1172–81.
25. Stanley JG, Gewertz BL, Fry WJ. Renal system renin indices and renal vein renin ratios as prognostic indicators in remediable renovascular hypertension. J Surg Res 1976;20:149–155.
26. Couch NP, Sullivan J, Crane C. The predictive accuracy of renal vein renin activity in the surgery of renovascular hypertension. Surgery 1976;79:70–6.
27. Dean RH, Rhamy RK. Split renal function studies in renovascular hypertension. Renovascular Hypertens 1984:135–145.
28. Dondi M, Fanti S, DeFabritis A, et al. Prognostic value of captopril renal scintigraphy in renovascular hypertension. J Nucl Med 1992;33:2040–2044.
29. Geyskes GG, Oei HY, Puylaert GBAJ, et al. Renography with captopril: Changes in a patient with hypertension and unilateral renal artery stenosis. Arch Intern Med 1986;146:1705–08.
30. Sfakianakis G, Sfakianaki E, Bourgoigne J. Renal scintigraphy following angiotensin converting enzyme inhibition in diagnosis of renovascular hypertension (captopril scintigraphy). Nucl Med Annual 1998:125–68.
31. Svetkey LP, Wilkinson R Jr, Dunnick NR, et al. Captopril renography in the diagnosis of renovascular disease. Am J Hypertens. 1991;4:711S–715S.

32. Humke U, Uder M.Renovascular hypertension: the diagnosis and management of renal ischaemia. BJU Int. 1999;84:555–569.
33. Scoble JE, McClean A, Stansby G, Hamilton G, Sweny P, Hilson AJW. The use of captopril DTPA scanning in the diagnosis of atherosclerotic renal artery stenosis in patients with impaired renal function. Am J Hypertens. 1991;4:721S–723S.
34. Textor SC. Renovascular hypertension. Endocrinol Metab Clin North Am 1994;23(2):235–53.
35. van Jaarsveld BC, Krijnen P, Derkx FHM, Oei HY, Postma CT, Schalekamp MADH. The place of renal Scintigraphy in the diagnosis of renal artery stenosis: fifteen years of clinical experience. Arch Intern Med 1997;157(11):1226–34.
36. Hansen KJ, Tribble RW, Reavis SW, et al. Renal duplex sonography: evaluation of clinical utility. J Vasc Surg. 1990;2:227–236.
37. Hoffmann U, Edwards JM, Carter S, et al. Role of duplex scanning for detection of atherosclerotic renal artery disease. Kidney Int 1991;39:1232–1239.
38. Johansson M, Jensen G, Aurell M, et al. Evaluation of duplex ultrasound and captopril renography for detection of renovascular hypertension. Kidney Int 2000;58:774–782.
39. Rademacher J, Chavan A, Block J, et al. Use of Doppler ultrasonography to predict the outcome of therapy for renal artery stenosis. N Engl J Med 2001;344:410–7.
40. Riehl J, Schmitt H, Bongartz D, Bergmann D, Sieberth HG. Renal artery stenosis: evaluation with colour duplex ultrasonograph. Nephrol Dial Transplant. 1997;12: 1608–1614.
41. Krumme B, Blum U, Schwertfeger E,et al. Diagnosis of renovascular disease by intra- and extrarenal Doppler scanning. Kidney Int. 1996;50:1288–1292.
42. Edwards JM, Zaccardi JM, Strandness DE. A preliminary study of the role of duplex scanning in defining adequacy of treatment of patients with renal artery fibromuscular dysplasia. J Vasc Surg. 1992;15:604–609.
43. Kim TS, Chung JW, Park JH, Kim SH, Yeon KM, Chung M. Renal artery evaluation: comparison of spiral CT angiography to intraarterial DSA. J Vasc Interventional Rad 1998;9:553–559.
44. Elkohen M, Beregi JP, Deklunder G, et al. A prospective study of helical computed tomography angiography vs. angiography for detection of renal artery stenosis in hypertensive patients. J Hypertens 1996;14:525.
45. Beregi JP, Elkohen M, Deklunder G, Artaud D, Coullet JM, Wattianne L.Helical CT angiography compared with arteriography in detection of renal artery stenosis. Am J Roentgenol 1996;167:495–501.
46. Olbricht CJ, Paul K, Prokop M, et al. Minimally invasive diagnosis of renal artery stenosis by spiral computed tomography angiography. Kidney Int 1995;48:1332.
47. Kim D, Edelman R, Kent K, Porter D, Skillmann JJ. Abdominal aorta and renal artery stenosis: vvaluation with MR angiography. Radiology. 1990;174:727–731.
48. Yucel EK, Kaufman JA, Prince M, Bazari H, Fang LS, Waltman AC. Time of flight renal MR angiography: utility in patients with renal insufficiency. Magn Reson Imaging. 1993;11:925–930.
49. Hertz SM, Holland GA, Baum RA, Haskal ZJ, Carpenter JP.Evaluation of renal artery stenosis by magnetic resonance angiography. Am J Surg. 1994;168(2):140–143.
50. Khauli RB. Defining the Role of Renal angiography in the diagnosis of renal artery disease. A J Kid Dis 1994;24:679–684.

# 5 Interventional Treatments for Renal Artery Stenosis

*George A. Mansoor,* MD, FRCP (EDIN)

*CONTENTS*



## INTRODUCTION

Hemodynamically significant renal artery stenosis may cause hypertension *(1)*, chronic renal failure *(2)*, and recurrent congestive heart failure *(3)*. Anatomically, there are two main types of renal artery stenosis, fibromuscular dysplasia (FMD) and atherosclerotic renal artery stenosis (ARAS). Physiologically, when the lesions are hemodynamically significant, they have similar effects in generating and maintaining hypertension, but there is a greater tendency for ARAS to be associated with chronic renal insufficiency. The appearance of hypertension in a young person, typically female, usually leads to the discovery of FMD. The person with ARAS, however, is usually older and male and has

From: *Secondary Hypertension: Clinical Presentation, Diagnosis, and Treatment*
Edited by: G. A. Mansoor © Humana Press Inc., Totowa, NJ

concurrent cardiovascular risk factors in the setting of hypertension and/or chronic renal disease. Less commonly, ARAS may be considered after repeated unexplained episodes of congestive heart failure (CHF) and when revascularization appears to improve symptoms *(3,4)*. Although the discovery of FMD of the renal artery in the setting of significant hypertension usually leads to intervention with angioplasty, ARAS is usually approached much more cautiously with regard to intervention.

## FIBROMUSCULAR DYSPLASIA OF THE RENAL ARTERY

FMD is a disturbance of the arterial wall structure involving small to medium-sized arteries *(5)*. The lesions are not associated with inflammation and may afflict any vascular territory; however, the renal arteries are affected in about 75% of cases. In about one quarter of patients, two vascular areas may be simultaneously or sequentially affected by this disorder *(5)*. The lesions of FMD tend to be multiple and are likely to affect distal portions of the renal arteries. Genetics and possibly hormonal factors play a role in the appearance of FMD because of the reported familial occurrence and female predominance.

Histologically, several types of arterial wall involvement have been described, with the media being almost universally affected and another layer in about two-thirds of cases *(6,7)*. Hypertension is typically the presenting feature of FMD and, although progression of the lesions may occur, this rarely leads to total occlusion. Luckily, if the main renal artery is affected, expert angioplasty is relatively safe, is usually technically successful, and provides good short-and long-term results. Furthermore, restenosis rates are generally less than 25%. *Consensus and extended followup of cohorts of patients indicate that angioplasty without stenting provides good results for FMD lesions of the renal artery.*

In the setting of renovascular hypertension, angioplasty of an FMD lesion leads to significant improvement or cure in the majority of patients *(8–10)*. In one of the early case series of angioplasty in FMD of the renal artery, 93% of patients with FMD had either improved or were cured of hypertension at the time of followup *(10)*. However, only some 50% of patients are cured *(11)*. In one study examining predictive factors for cure of hypertension at 6 months, younger age, lower preintervention systolic blood pressure (BP), and shorter duration of hypertension emerged as significant predictors *(12)*. Apart from immediate technical complications that are relatively infrequent, restenosis may occur in as many as 8–25% of patients over an extended period of followup. Surgical intervention may become necessary especially for more distal lesions or for complicated presentations.

In general, therefore, management of FMD of the renal artery in patients with hypertension can be done medically if BP is easily controlled or by angioplasty if BP cannot be controlled. Local expertise, patient demographics, and preference may make one management strategy more suitable for a particular patient.

No large trials have examined medical versus interventional management of FMD when it is discovered in the setting of hypertension.

## ATHEROSCLEROTIC RENAL ARTERY STENOSIS

The patient with ARAS is typically older and presents with new or worsening hypertension that may be associated with chronic renal dysfunction. The majority of these patients will have other cardiovascular risk factors such as smoking, hyperlipidemia, or vascular disease *(13)*. Less commonly, the presentation of ARAS may be dominated by recurrent episodes of congestive heart failure or unstable angina *(3,4)*. The lesions of ARAS tend to be ostial more often than those of FMD and may be unilateral or bilateral. There may also be associated disease of the aorta and its branches.

Interventional therapies for ARAS may include angioplasty, angioplasty and stenting, and/or open surgical intervention. There is, however, considerable uncertainty regarding the outcome of each method of treatment and its relative value compared to medical management. Although a few clinical trials have compared medical management to interventional treatments, no clear consensus has evolved to manage unilateral or bilateral ARAS.

## ANGIOGRAPHIC CONSIDERATIONS IN RENAL ARTERY STENOSIS

Despite advances in magnetic resonance and other imaging methods, catheter-based angiography remains the method of choice for diagnosing hemodynamically significant renal artery stenosis. However, several criteria must be fulfilled during angiography to ensure optimal evaluation. Preangiography preparation is needed to minimize contrast renal injury *(14)*, and risks of intervention such as contrast renal dysfunction and cholesterol embolism must be communicated to the patient. As discussed in one guideline regarding renal artery revascularization *(15)*, several angulated views of the patient may be needed to avoid false negative assessments of ARAS lesions. Most operators perform angiography of the abdominal aorta first to exclude the presence of an aortic aneurysm and to visualize the main renal arteries. Most hemodynamically significant lesions (>70%) will be evident either at this stage or after branch-selective injection of contrast. To estimate the severity, the operator measures the diameter of the narrowest diseased section and compares it to the normal proximal or distal segments of the artery. In cases where there is uncertainty regarding the significance of a lesion (50–70%), pressure gradients may be helpful, and a gradient of greater than 10% or a change of greater than 20 mmHg but preferably greater than 40 mmHg *(16)* or more in systolic BP may be used as an indicator of hemodynamic significance. Routine revascularization for incidentally discovered renal artery stenosis—for example, at coronary angiography—should not be performed *(17)*.

The operator has several options if a hemodynamically significant lesion is found and anticipated benefit from revascularization outweighs the risks. Primary angioplasty may be performed and, if a good result is obtained, especially in the case of FMD of the renal artery, no further intervention is needed. If primary angioplasty fails or is complicated, stent placement becomes necessary in FMD. Restenosis lesions may be dealt with by angioplasty alone or by stenting in FMD. Primary stent placement is increasingly being used in ARAS; a stent is placed without prior dilation. For ostial ARAS lesions, stent placement is the procedure of choice and confers higher patency rates at 6 months (75% vs 29%) and similar clinical outcomes than angioplasty alone *(18)*. At the end of the procedure, angiography is repeated to ascertain the final result, and gradients may also be repeated. A desired result is one that is uncomplicated and has resulted in a residual diameter of less than 30%. Stents should be placed to completely cover the offending lesion and, in the case of ostial lesions, the stent may be left minimally protruding into the aorta *(15)*. Despite widespread use of stenting for ARAS, there is still about a 20% restenosis rate, which appears to affect mainly vessels less than 4.5 mm in diameter *(19)*.

Several serious and nonserious complications may occur during angioplasty and stent placement. The rate of complications varies widely and ranges from 12 to 36%. The most common are related to the puncture site and include groin hematoma and puncture-site trauma. These include but are not limited to stent arterial dissection, malposition, stent nondeployment, and vascular complications requiring immediate surgery. Postprocedure complications may include arterial thrombosis, contrast renal injury, cholesterol embolism, and restenosis. Surgical salvage is needed in less than 3% of cases. With modern methods and appropriate experience, the complication rate should be around 14%, of which the majority are not life jeopardizing. Cholesterol embolism, for which only supportive care is available, may be seen several days after intervention and may affect the kidneys' viscera, peripheries, or central organs.

## SURGICAL OPTIONS IN RENAL ARTERY STENOSIS

Surgical intervention is used much less often today because percutaneous interventions have matured and become widely available *(20)*. Several surgical procedures have been used to treat both FMD and ARAS. These include a variety of bypass procedures, reimplantation methods, and nephrectomy. Surgery is used mainly for complicated aortorenal lesions. In one small randomized trial comparing angioplasty and surgical reconstruction in unilateral ARAS, technical success was higher for surgery, as were primary patency rates and secondary patency rates. Clinical results were similar in the two groups *(21)*.

## CLINICAL TRIALS COMPARING MEDICAL MANAGEMENT WITH INTERVENTIONAL MANAGEMENT

No large defining randomized trial has been performed in ARAS. Only three randomized trials have directly compared medical therapy to revascularization. These studies suffer from design flaws and small numbers of enrolled patients *(22–24)*. In total, they enrolled 210 patients (106 patients to angioplasty and 104 to medical therapy), and therefore both individually and when taken together have very limited power. All studies looked at the endpoints of BP and renal function but with very limited followup of 3 months and 6 months. The majority of patients in the interventional arms received angioplasty, and stenting was not used routinely.

In the trial by Webster *(22)*, a randomized comparison was made of percutaneous angioplasty and medical therapy in ARAS. Many eligible patients were not randomized, which limits the applicability of this study, and only patients with bilateral disease appeared to benefit from angioplasty in terms of a significant lowering of BP. No benefit was seen for unilateral disease or in serum creatinine, and procedure-related complications were relatively frequent. Similarly, in a randomized trial *(24)* comparing medical treatment ($n = 26$) with angioplasty ($n = 23$) in unilateral ARAS, there was benefit in terms of lowering medication requirements but no change in calculated creatinine clearance *(24)*. Similar to the study by Webster et al. *(22)*, a high rate of procedural complications was seen. BP also declined more in the angioplasty group in a randomized trial of angioplasty (*n* = 56) compared to medical therapy (*n* = 50) in ARAS *(23)*. This last study, however, was difficult to interpret because of a high cross-over rate from medical to angioplasty groups.

In another randomized trial *(25)*, the aim was to examine surgical revascularization and medical treatment in patients with the entire renal mass at risk. These patients included bilateral ARAS, a stenosis to a solitary kidney, or a unilateral stenosis with elevated creatinine (>1.5 mg/dL). Hence, 27 patients were randomized to medical management and 25 to surgical management. A variety of surgical procedures were done, but the aim was surgical revascularization in the surgical group. Followup was 74 months on average. No differences were seen in BP control, death-free survival, or dialysis-free survival. Larger, more definitive studies are needed in this subgroup of patients with ARAS.

Because of the small numbers in these trials, two meta-analyses *(26, 27)* have been performed that included 210 patients in three trials. Theses studies concluded that caution and larger studies were needed to be certain of the effects of revascularization compared to medical therapy. Both found that balloon angioplasty is modestly more effective than medical therapy in reducing both systolic and diastolic BP. However, although the reduction is modest, it could potentially convey significant cardiovascular benefits. Little effect was shown on renal function in either meta-analysis. We await randomized trials examining modern percutaneous intervention using stenting with its excellent primary patency rate as a primary procedure vs medical treatment in ARAS.

## CLINICAL TRIALS COMPARING ANGIOPLASTY TO SURGICAL RECONSTRUCTION

One randomized trial compared renal angioplasty to surgical treatment *(21)*. The authors recruited hypertensive nondiabetic subjects who had unilateral ARAS and serum creatinine less than 3.4 mg/dL. If both surgery and angioplasty were deemed possible, the patient was randomized. In this manner, 29 were randomized to angioplasty and 29 to surgery. Surgery was technically superior to angioplasty, with a patency rate of 97% vs 83% for the angioplasty group. By the end of 24 months, there were six restenoses in the angioplasty group and one restenosis in the surgical group. No difference was seen in BP control in the two groups. Major and minor complications related to intervention were not different.

## CONCLUSIONS

Renal artery stenosis that is physiologically important may present with a variety of clinical syndromes: hypertension, renal dysfunction, and unexplained CHF. In the case of FMD of the renal artery, expert angioplasty is usually successful if BP cannot be controlled or if a decision is made to intervene. In the case of ARAS, stenting leads to superior patency rates compared to angioplasty alone. However, the few randomized clinical trials comparing revascularization to medical therapy are too small for a meaningful conclusion regarding their relative utility to be made. There is a need for large multicenter studies that compare a conservative approach to a revascularization approach in a variety of subtypes with ARAS. It is likely that some subgroups with ARAS will derive more benefit from revascularization.

## REFERENCES

1. Granger JP, Schnackenberg CG. Renal mechanisms of angiotensin II-induced hypertension. Semin Nephrol 2000;20:417–425.
2. Textor SC. Pathophysiology of renal failure in renovascular disease. Am J Kidney Dis 1994;24:642–651.
3. Pickering TG, Herman L, Devereux RB, et al. Recurrent pulmonary oedema in hypertension due to bilateral renal artery stenosis: treatment by angioplasty or surgical intervention. Lancet 1988; 2:551–552.
4. Gray BH, Olin JW, Childs MB, Sullivan TM, Bacharach JM. Clinical benefit of renal artery angioplasty with stenting for the control of recurrent and refractory congestive heart failure. Vasc Med 2002;7:275–279.
5. Begelman SM, Olin JW. Fibromuscular dysplasia. Curr Opin Rheumatol 2000;12:41–47.
6. Harrison EG Jr, McCormack LJ. Pathologic classification of renal arterial disease in renovascular hypertension. Mayo Clin Proc 1971;46:161–167.
7. Alimi Y, Mercier C, Pellissier JF, Piquet P, Tournigand P. Fibromuscular disease of the renal artery: a new histopathologic classification. Ann Vasc Surg 1992;6:220–224.
8. Tegtmeyer CJ, Selby JB, Hartwell GD, Ayers C, Tegtmeyer V. Results and complications of angioplasty in fibromuscular disease. Circulation 1991;83:I155–I161.
9. Birrer M, Do DD, Mahler F, Triller J, Baumgartner I. Treatment of renal artery fibromuscular dysplasia with balloon angioplasty: a prospective follow-up study. Eur J Vasc Endovasc Surg 2002;23:146–152.
10. Sos TA, Pickering TG, Sniderman K, et al. Percutaneous transluminal renal angioplasty in renovascular hypertension due to atheroma or fibromuscular dysplasia. N Engl J Med 1983;4;309:274–279.
11. Ramsay LE, Waller PC. Blood pressure response to percutaneous transluminal angioplasty for renovascular hypertension: an overview of published series. Br Med J 1990;300:569–752.
12. Davidson RA, Barri Y, Wilcox CS. Predictors of cure of hypertension in fibromuscular renovascular disease. Am J Kidney Dis 1996;28:334–338.

13. Conlon PJ, O'Riordan E, Kalra PA. New insights into the epidemiologic and clinical manifestations of atherosclerotic renovascular disease. Am J Kidney Dis 2000; 35:573–587.
14. Lindholt JS. Radiocontrast induced nephropathy. Eur J Vasc Endovasc Surg 2003;25:296–304.
15. Rundback JH, Sacks D, Kent KC, et al for the American Heart Association. Guidelines for the reporting of renal artery revascularization in clinical trials. Circulation 2002;106:1572–1585.
16. Messerli FH, Genest J, Nowaczynski W, et al. Hypertension with renal arterial stenosis: humoral, hemodynamic and histopathologic factors. Am J Cardiol 1975;36:702–707.
17. Textor SC. Progressive hypertension in a patient with "incidental" renal artery stenosis. Hypertension 2002;40:595–600.
18. van de Ven PJ, Kaatee R, Beutler JJ, et al. Arterial stenting and balloon angioplasty in ostial atherosclerotic renovascular disease: a randomised trial. Lancet 1999; 353:282–286.
19. Lederman RJ, Mendelsohn FO, Santos R, Phillips HR, Stack RS, Crowley JJ. Primary renal artery stenting: characteristics and outcomes after 363 procedures. Am Heart J 2001;142:314–323.
20. Mackrell PJ, Langan EM 3rd, Sullivan TM, et al. Management of renal artery stenosis: effects of a shift from surgical to percutaneous therapy on indications and outcomes. Ann Vasc Surg 2003;17:54–59.
21. Weibull H, Bergqvist D, Bergentz SE, Jonsson K, Hulthen L, Manhem P. Percutaneous transluminal renal angioplasty versus surgical reconstruction of atherosclerotic renal artery stenosis: a prospective randomized study. J Vasc Surg 1993; 18:841–850.
22. Webster J, Marshall F, Abdalla M, et al for the Scottish and Newcastle Renal Artery Stenosis Collaborative Group. Randomised comparison of percutaneous angioplasty vs continued medical therapy for hypertensive patients with atheromatous renal artery stenosis. J Hum Hypertens 1998;12:329–335.
23. van Jaarsveld BC, Krijnen P, Pieterman H, et al for the Dutch Renal Artery Stenosis Intervention Cooperative Study Group. The effect of balloon angioplasty on hypertension in atherosclerotic renal-artery stenosis. N Engl J Med 2000;6;342:1007–1014.
24. Plouin PF, Chatellier G, Darne B, Raynaud A for the Essai Multicentrique Medicaments vs Angioplastie (EMMA) Study Group. Blood pressure outcome of angioplasty in atherosclerotic renal artery stenosis: a randomized trial. Hypertension 1998;31:823–829.
25. Uzzo RG, Novick AC, Goormastic M, Mascha E, Pohl M. Medical versus surgical management of atherosclerotic renal artery stenosis. Transplant Proc 2002;34: 723–725.
26. Ives NJ, Wheatley K, Stowe RL, et al. Continuing uncertainty about the value of percutaneous revascularization in atherosclerotic renovascular disease: a meta-analysis of randomized trials. Nephrol Dial Transplant 2003;18:298–304.
27. Nordmann AJ, Woo K, Parkes R, Logan AG. Balloon angioplasty or medical therapy for hypertensive patients with atherosclerotic renal artery stenosis? a meta-analysis of randomized controlled trials. Am J Med 2003;114:44–50.

# 6 Medical Management of Renovascular Hypertension

*Vincent J. Canzanello, MD*

*CONTENTS*



## INTRODUCTION

All patients with renovascular hypertension will require treatment with antihypertensive drugs during some stage of their disease. The duration, intensity, and complexity of treatment can vary widely. In a young woman with the abrupt onset of hypertension and an abdominal bruit, an astute clinician will suspect renovascular hypertension caused by fibromuscular dysplasia (FMD). With early diagnosis, the course of

From: *Secondary Hypertension: Clinical Presentation, Diagnosis, and Treatment*
Edited by: G. A. Mansoor © Humana Press Inc., Totowa, NJ

drug therapy is often short (weeks to months) and followed by curative revascularization *(1,2)*. In the case of hypertension associated with atherosclerotic renovascular disease (ARVD), essential hypertension is usually present before ARVD is diagnosed, and most patients receive treatment with one or more antihypertensive drugs for several years before worsening control of blood pressure (BP) or unexplained deterioration of renal function leads to the discovery of underlying renovascular disease. Unlike patients with FMD, most patients with ARVD continue to require antihypertensive drug therapy despite successful renal revascularization, and, not infrequently, the dose and number of drugs before and after the intervention are similar *(3)*. Several of the retrospective and prospective studies reviewed below have demonstrated that many patients with ARVD, with or without renal insufficiency, can be successfully managed medically for years. For these reasons, the clinician should be familiar with the benefits and risks of the drugs, treatment regimens, and monitoring approaches used for this challenging population of patients.

## CHOOSING THE BEST CANDIDATE FOR MEDICAL THERAPY

Perhaps the most difficult aspect of managing a patient with hypertension who has renovascular disease is the decision of whether to treat medically or to proceed with revascularization, either surgically or with balloon angioplasty (with or without stent placement). At one end of the spectrum, the decision is not difficult. For example, for a young woman with FMD, medical treatment may mean a lifetime of taking several antihypertensive drugs, but revascularization offers the likelihood of cure or improvement in hypertension. Clearly, the latter option is preferable in this case. At the other end of the spectrum is an elderly patient with hypertension who has extensive ARVD, multiple comorbid conditions, and advanced renal insufficiency (e.g., a serum level of creatinine of 3 mg/dL or higher). For this patient, revascularization poses a significant risk and the patient is less likely to have improvement in BP control and renal function *(4)*. Few would argue that without revascularization, this elderly patient has a very high risk of subsequent cardiovascular morbidity and mortality *(5)*. However, there are little data in support of this risk being substantially reduced by revascularization even if BP control is improved *(6,7)*. Although the underlying renal disease may progress, most patients die of complications from atherosclerotic involvement of other vascular beds, such as the coronary, cerebrovascu-

Table 1
Clinical Characteristics Associated With Unfavorable BP or Renal Function Outcome Following Renal Revascularization

| |
|---|
| Advanced age *(3,12)* |
| Advanced renal insufficiency (serum creatinine ≥ 3.0 mg/dL) *(4,6,13)* |
| Atherosclerotic as opposed to fibromuscular dysplastic cause *(14,15)* |
| Renal resistance index by Doppler ultrasonography ≥ 80 *(16)* |
| Decreased kidney size (< 9 cm on radiographs or ultrasonograms) *(17)* |

lar, and peripheral circulations. Indeed, according to a recent study from the Mayo Clinic on elderly patients with extensive ARVD, medical management generally was able to achieve adequate control of BP; also, the condition of the patients rarely progressed to end-stage renal disease caused by ischemic nephropathy, and their survival rate was similar to that of patients who had revascularization *(8)*. However, most patients are somewhere in between the patients at these two extremes of the spectrum. The majority of patients are older than 60 years, have renovascular disease caused by atherosclerosis, and have various degrees of mild to moderate renal insufficiency. This is the group of patients that is the focus of this chapter. This is also the group of patients for which several prospective randomized studies have suggested that, with equivalent degrees of BP control, revascularization has little benefit compared with medical therapy *(9–11)*. Several clinical characteristics of these patients that are associated with an unfavorable outcome after renal revascularization are listed in Table 1.

## PROGRESSION OF ATHEROSCLEROTIC RENOVASCULAR DISEASE

The concept of the progression of ARVD continues to evolve. The results of several studies in which this issue was considered are shown in Table 2. In the retrospective study by Schreiber et al. *(18)* at the Cleveland Clinic, progression of ARVD was assessed in 85 patients (126 renal arteries) who underwent two or more renal angiographic studies between 1960 and 1979. Progressive vascular obstruction was demonstrated in 37 patients (44%) over a mean followup of 52 months. This included 14 patients (16%) who had progression to total arterial occlusion, most within a mean angiographic followup of 13 months. As might be expected, the patients whose lesions were most stenotic at baseline had the greatest risk of progression. The majority of patients with progressive unilateral lesions demonstrated almost no development of *de novo*

Table 2
**Studies on Progression of Atherosclerotic Renovascular Disease**

| *Study* | *Design* | *No. of patients/ No. of arteries* | *Mean followup, mo* | *Outcome* |
|---|---|---|---|---|
| Schreiber et al. *(18)* | Retrospective review of renal arteriograms | 85/126 | 52 | Overall progression in 44%<br>Progression to occlusion in 16%<br>Average monthly progression rate of 1.6% |
| Zierler et al. *(19)* | Prospective using renal artery duplex ultrasonography | 76/132 | 32 | Cumulative incidence of progression from < 60% to > 60% stenosis was 48% by 3 yr<br>Cumulative incidence of progression from > 60% to occlusion was 7% at 3 yr<br>Average monthly progression rate of 7%<br>Trend toward association of progression with poor BP control |
| Caps et al. *(20)* | Prospective using renal artery duplex ultrasonography | 122/204 | 33 | Cumulative incidence of renal atrophy (decrease in renal length > 1 cm) was 11.7% and 20.8% in patients with < 60% and > 60%, respectively, baseline renal artery stenosis<br>Systolic BP and increasing serum creatinine correlated positively with these changes |

lesions in the contralateral renal artery. Progression of ARVD was associated with a progressive increase in creatinine serum levels and a decrease in renal size, whereas the degree of BP control was similar in patients whether or not the lesions progressed. Although more recent prospective studies with serial renal artery duplex ultrasonography generally have demonstrated a similar overall rate of progression *(19,20)* (Table 2), the cumulative incidence of progression of high-grade lesions (i.e., 60% stenosis or greater) to occlusion was less than one half (7 vs 16%) of that in the retrospective study of Schreiber et al. *(18)* and occurred over 36 months vs 13 months. This discrepancy may be related in part to better BP control and attendance to other risk factors such as treatment of dyslipidemia. Also, because the study of Schreiber et al. *(18)* was retrospective, repeat renal angiography may have been applied more selectively to patients who had worsening BP control or decreasing renal function (or both), thus enriching the study population with patients who had more aggressive ARVD.

Currently, prospective renal artery duplex ultrasonographic studies provide the best estimates for both the overall progression of ARVD and, more important, the risk of progression to arterial occlusion. Current estimates suggest that there may be a reasonable window of opportunity to assess the response to aggressive medical management with antihypertensive therapy and control of other atherosclerotic risk factors such as dyslipidemia, cigarette smoking, and diabetes mellitus.

## EVOLUTION OF MEDICAL THERAPY FOR THE TREATMENT OF RENOVASCULAR HYPERTENSION

### *The Era Before Angiotensin-Converting Enzyme Inhibitors (ACEIs)*

One of the first reports of the medical treatment of renovascular hypertension was published in 1963 by Dustan et al. *(21)*. In this study of 32 patients, treatment with a combination of hydralazine, guanethidine, and a thiazide diuretic achieved control or substantial improvement of hypertension in 41% of patients. Through the 1970s, treatment with this combination of drugs and other combinations, including propranolol and methyldopa, produced control or improvement rates that averaged about 40 to 50% *(22)*.

### *The Era of ACEIs*

In the early 1980s, the introduction of ACEIs into clinical practice led to marked improvement in the management of hypertension associated with renovascular disease. One of the first and largest studies of the use of ACEIs in the treatment of renovascular hypertension was reported by Hollenberg *(23)* (Table 3). This study included 269 patients (mean age, 50 years) who had predominantly ARVD; 56% of the patients had bilateral renal artery stenoses or stenosis of the renal artery of a solitary functioning kidney. In 41% of the patients, the baseline creatinine serum level was 1.5 mg/dL or higher. The BP of most patients had not been controlled with a regimen of three or more traditional antihypertensive drugs such as diuretics, sympatholytics, and vasodilators. These patients were hospitalized, and the multidrug therapy was replaced with captopril, starting at 25 mg/day and titrating upward to a regimen of three doses daily, culminating in an average daily dose of almost 400 mg. Diuretics, followed by β-blockers, were used as second- and third-line agents. At the end of 3 months of followup, the overall rate of BP control (defined as diastolic BP <95 mmHg) was 74%. Another 8% of patients had a partial response. Captopril therapy was discontinued for 13% of patients, mainly because of rash, dysgeusia, or proteinuria, which might be expected with the high dose of medication. Unexpectedly, relatively small changes occurred in renal function, with the mean serum creatinine level increasing by 0.6 and 0.3 mg/dL in patients with baseline azotemia and normal renal function, respectively. Acute renal failure developed within the first month of treatment, requiring captopril to be stopped or the dose decreased, in eight patients, all of whom had bilateral renal artery stenoses or stenosis of the renal artery to a solitary functioning kidney. The changes in renal function were reversible in all but one patient, who required dialysis.

The next largest study of medical therapy with ACEIs was that of Franklin and Smith *(24)*. This prospective randomized double-blind study of 75 patients with renovascular hypertension compared the efficacy of enalapril (5 to 40 mg/day) and hydrochlorothiazide with a combination of timolol (10 mg), hydralazine (50 mg twice daily), and hydrochlorothiazide. Of these patients, 81% had ARVD and 44% had bilateral renal artery stenoses. At baseline, the mean BP was 172/102 mmHg and the serum creatinine level was 1.4 mg/dL. Over the course of the 8-week study, systolic BP decreased 32 and 20 mmHg in the enalapril and control groups, respectively, and diastolic BP decreased 20 and 18 mmHg, respectively. A "good response," defined as diastolic BP of 90 mmHg or less, was achieved in 94% of the patients in the enalapril group and in 82% of those in the control group. With respect to renal function, 20% of the patients in the enalapril group and 3% in the control group had a 0.3 mg/dL or greater increase in the serum creatinine level.

Table 3
Prospective Medical Treatment Trials of Renovascular Hypertension

| *Author/year (reference)* | *No. patients (age, y)* | *Duration of study, mo* | *Drug regimen* | *Baseline BP, mmHg* | *Final BP, mmHg* | *Outcome* |
|---|---|---|---|---|---|---|
| Hollenberg 1983 *(23)* | 236 (50) | 3 | Captopril ± diuretic ± β-blocker | DBP > 110 | NA | 74% achieved DBP < 95 mmHg |
| Franklin and Smith 1985 *(24)* | 75 (60) | 2 | Enalapril + diuretic | 172/102 | 140/82 | 94% achieved DBP ≤ 90 mmHg |
| Plouin et al. 1998 *(9)* | 49 (59) | 6 | Nifedipine ± clonidine ± prazosin ± enalapril ± atenolol | 149/89* | 141/84* | 7/26 crossed over to angioplasty for refractory hypertension |
| Webster et al. 1998 *(10)* | 55 (61) | 12 | Atenolol + diuretic + calcium channel blocker ± methyldopa ± prazosin | Unilateral stenosis—171/09<br>Bilateral stenoses—179/93 | 168/91<br>171/91 | SBP improved in group with bilateral stenoses treated with angioplasty |
| van Jaarsveld et al. 2000 *(11)* | 106 (60) | 12 | Amlodipine + atenolol or enalapril + diuretic | 180/103 | 163/96 | 23/50 crossed over to angioplasty for refractory hypertension |

*Average 24-hour BP by ambulatory monitoring.
BP, blood pressure; DBP, diastolic blood pressure; SBP, systolic blood pressure.

Of note, no episode of acute oliguric renal failure occurred, even among the 18 patients in the enalapril group who had bilateral renal artery stenoses, although the largest increase in the creatinine serum level was in patients who, at baseline, had renal insufficiency and the most severe degree of bilateral renal artery stenoses.

Three other studies by Plouin et al. *(9)*, Webster et al. *(10)*, and van Jaarsveld et al. *(11)* have further explored the role of medical therapy in the management of hypertension associated with renovascular disease (Table 2). All these studies were randomized trials that compared medical therapy with percutaneous transluminal balloon angioplasty (PTA). They focused on patients who had ARVD and normal or near-normal renal function.

The study of Plouin et al. *(9)* was limited to patients who had unilateral renal artery stenosis. Initially, the diastolic BP of all the subjects was stabilized at less than 110 mmHg by using slow-release nifedipine with add-on therapy consisting of clonidine and prazosin. Atenolol, furosemide, or enalapril (or a combination of these) was added to the baseline regimen of the 26 patients who were randomly assigned to medical therapy to achieve a diastolic BP of less than 95 mmHg. Of these 26 patients, 7 (27%) eventually required PTA to control BP. At the end of the 6-month study, the BP of those still in the medical treatment group was no different from that of those in the PTA group (141/84 vs 140/81 mmHg); however, patients in the medical treatment group were taking at least three antihypertensive drugs. No patient in the medical treatment group developed clinically important renal insufficiency.

The study of Webster et al. *(10)*, unlike that of Plouin et al. *(9)*, contained about an equal number of patients who had unilateral renal artery stenosis (27 patients) and bilateral renal artery stenoses (28 patients). All patients were required to have a baseline diastolic BP of 95 mmHg or greater with at least two antihypertensive drugs. Before being randomly assigned to medical therapy or PTA, all participants had a 4-week run-in period with a regimen that included atenolol, a thiazide diuretic, or a calcium channel blocker (CCB) (or a combination of these). Of note, ACEIs were not permitted during this study. After randomization, additional drug choices included furosemide, methyldopa, and prazosin. The medical treatment and PTA groups were each divided into bilateral stenoses and unilateral stenosis groups. Of the patients with unilateral stenosis, those in the medical treatment group had an unimpressive change in BP from 171/90 mmHg at the end of the run-in period to 168/91 mmHg; importantly, this was not different from that of those in the PTA group. Of the patients with bilateral stenoses, those in the medically treated group fared similarly to patients with unilateral stenosis, whereas patients in the PTA group had a significant decrease in systolic BP from 185/95 to 152/83 mmHg. No significant differences in the serum creatinine level were detected throughout the study in any of the groups. Webster et al. *(10)* concluded that for patients with bilateral renal artery stenoses, PTA can result in modest improvement in systolic BP compared with medical therapy. In fact, one could conclude from the data that neither therapy led to satisfactory control of BP. From a clinician's viewpoint, this study had several limitations: ACEIs were proscribed (the use of these drugs almost certainly would have improved BP control in the medically treated group), and stenting of the renal arteries was not performed (stenting may have improved the outcome in the PTA group).

In the largest of the three studies comparing medical therapy and PTA, van Jaarsveld et al. *(11)* randomly assigned 50 patients to medical therapy and 56 to PTA. Approximately 20% of the patients in each group had bilateral renal artery stenoses. The medical regimen consisted of stepped dosing of either amlodipine plus atenolol or enalapril plus hydrochlorothiazide, with the addition of other unspecified drugs as needed to achieve a diastolic BP less than 95 mmHg. By 3 months, 22 patients (44%) in the medical therapy group either had not reached the BP goal or had developed progressive renal insufficiency (≥ 0.2 mg/dL increase in the serum level of creatinine) and had PTA, which resulted in good BP control and renal outcome. It was not stated whether medical therapy was more likely to fail in patients with bilateral disease. The BP of patients who were still in the medical treatment group at 12 months of followup was similar to that of patients in the PTA group, 159/91 vs 160/93 mmHg; patients in the medical treatment group were taking a mean of 2.4 antihypertensive drugs compared with 1.9 for those in the PTA group. Renal function was similar in both groups.

In summary, the studies discussed here demonstrated that, in a majority of patients, ARVD can be managed safely and effectively with medical therapy, at least compared with balloon angioplasty. In at least two of these studies, ACEIs were included in the drug regimen and were apparently well tolerated.

A recent report from Mayo Clinic, as mentioned previously, also suggested that, in older patients with extensive ARVD, BP can be well controlled and renal function maintained with medical therapy alone *(8)*. In this retrospective study, 68 patients (mean age, 72 years; 31% with bilateral renal artery stenoses or stenosis of the artery to a solitary functioning kidney) did not initially have revascularization for various reasons. The clinical data were assessed an average of 39 months after the initial renal arteriographic study. The average BP was 157/83 mmHg at the beginning of this interval and 155/79 mmHg at the end. BP less than 140/90 mmHg was achieved in one-third of the patients and BP less than 160/95 mmHg, in almost two-thirds of the entire group. The average number of drugs required per patient increased from 1.6 to 1.9. Of note, almost one-third of the patients received treatment with ACEIs. During followup, the mean creatinine serum level for the group increased from 1.4 to 2.0 mg/dL, with an increase greater than 50% above the baseline value in 15% of patients. Two patients had revascularization during followup: one for refractory hypertension and the other for progressive renal insufficiency. The condition of only one patient reached end-stage renal disease due to ischemic nephropathy. The overall survival of the entire cohort was similar to the reported 4-year survival of a similar cohort managed with balloon angioplasty and stenting of the renal arteries *(6)*.

## CONCERNS ABOUT MEDICAL THERAPY

### *Acute Renal Failure*

Acute or subacute renal failure following the initiation of ACEI therapy in patients with renovascular hypertension was first reported in the early 1980s *(25,26)*. This phenomenon was limited almost entirely to patients who had either bilateral renal artery stenoses or stenosis of the artery to a solitary functioning kidney, and it initially was estimated to occur in 23 to 38% of these patients *(27,28)*. Many other studies, however, have demonstrated that clinically important changes in renal function are uncommon in patients with unilateral renal artery stenosis who receive treatment with ACEIs *(14)*. To complicate the issue further, acute renal failure after the initiation of ACEI therapy has been reported for patients in whom no significant renal artery stenoses were documented *(29–31)*, an observation that has limited the diagnostic usefulness of acute renal failures in identifying renovascular disease.

In one of the largest and best-conceived studies, van de Ven et al. *(32)* were able to provoke a 20% increase in the serum creatinine level in all 52 patients with severe bilateral renal artery stenoses who received ACEI treatment (with or without a loop diuretic) for 4 to 14 days. A similar increase in the creatinine level also occurred in 37% of patients with unilateral renal artery stenosis and in 13% of those with normal renal arteries. No patient had acute renal failure, and all changes in renal function were reversed after treatment with either the loop diuretic or ACEI was discontinued. In the studies of Hollenberg *(23)* and Franklin and Smith *(24)* on ACEIs in ARVD, discussed above, acute renal dysfunction was rarely encountered, despite the inclusion of a large proportion of patients who had extensive occlusive disease.

### *Progressive Renal Ischemia*

This is one of the most important concerns of a clinician caring for a patient who has renovascular disease. Clearly, ARVD is a progressive disorder, as mentioned above. As discussed here, prospective studies conducted in the early 1990s *(19,20)* have demonstrated that the rate of progression in medically treated patients is less than that suggested by earlier retrospective analyses *(18)*. Still, these lesions can progress and lead to advanced renal insufficiency and end-stage renal disease despite successful revascularization *(4,14)*. It is reassuring that, as shown by the randomized trials of medical therapy vs PTA discussed above *(9–11)*, the renal outcome was not different for the two treatments. Because the optimal management of hypertension in most cases requires ACEI therapy, concern has been expressed that ACEIs may hasten progressive renal ischemia by decreasing blood flow distal to a stenosis of the renal artery. There have been isolated clinical reports of renal artery thrombosis in patients with unilateral atherosclerotic renal artery stenosis treated with ACEIs *(33)*; however, in most instances, it is difficult to determine whether the medical therapy or the progression of the underlying stenotic lesion was the cause *(28)*. Recent large-scale clinical trials of patients with heart failure have provided indirect evidence that progressive ischemic nephropathy is rare during ACEI therapy *(14)*. These trials included a large proportion of patients who had ischemic cardiomyopathy, and because up to 20% of patients with coronary artery disease also have previously unrecognized renovascular disease *(34,35)*, progressive renal insufficiency might be postulated in this subpopulation (but it was not observed). Transient increases in the serum creatinine level usually responded to a decrease in the dose of the diuretic and continuation of ACEI therapy. Also, ACEIs *(36–38)* and, more recently, angiotensin receptor blockers (ARBs) *(39,40)* have shown important benefits in decreasing cardiovascular morbidity and mortality and limiting the progression of both diabetic and nondiabetic renal disease, comorbid conditions in most patients who have ARVD. Therefore, it is likely that most patients with medically managed renovascular disease will be taking ACEIs or at least have other clinically important indications for their use.

It is important, however, to avoid precipitous decreases in systemic BP that may predispose to acute renal failure or occlusion of the renal artery. Methods to avoid this situation include the temporary discontinuation of diuretic therapy during the initiation of ACEI treatment (to reduce the risk of volume depletion) and the slow addition and titration of other antihypertensive drugs. Recommendations for monitoring renal function during medical therapy are discussed here.

### *Hyperkalemia*

An increase in the serum level of potassium of 0.5 mEq/L or greater has been reported in 0.4 to 5% of patients receiving ACEI therapy *(41)*. Risk factors for hyperkalemia include baseline renal dysfunction, diabetes mellitus, congestive heart failure, and the concomitant use of potassium supplements or other drugs known to impair the renal excretion of potassium—for example, potassium-sparing diuretics. Clinically important hyperkalemia was rare in the clinical trials discussed above and should be preventable if appropriate attention is given to patients at high risk. The serum level of potassium should be measured regularly, usually within 1 week after the initiation of ACEI therapy and then every 3 to 6 months, depending on the level of risk. If the serum level of potassium is greater than 5.5 mEq/L, a nonpotassium-sparing diuretic should be added to the regimen. Replacement of a thiazide diuretic with a loop diuretic is usually successful and should allow continued treatment with an ACEI. Another approach may be the substitution of an ARB for the ACEI. In a recent crossover study by Bakris et al. *(42)*, of a group of patients with a glomerular filtration rate (GFR) of 60 mL/min per 1.73 $m^2$ or less and normal baseline serum levels of potassium, treatment with lisinopril produced a significantly greater increase in the potassium concentration than did the ARB valsartan, 0.28 and 0.12 mEq/L, respectively.

## A PERSONAL APPROACH TO THE MEDICAL MANAGEMENT OF HYPERTENSION ASSOCIATED WITH RENOVASCULAR DISEASE

There are no set guidelines for the medical management of hypertension associated with renovascular disease. It is important to avoid the use of nonsteroidal anti-inflammatory drugs, which can exacerbate both hypertension and renal dysfunction. It is equally important to attend to factors that contribute to the progression of atherosclerosis, such as dyslipidemia, cigarette smoking, and diabetes mellitus. Usually, it is the inability to control BP despite treatment with two or three drugs that leads to the initial evaluation culminating in the diagnosis of renovascular disease. In the author's experience, most of the patients who come for evaluation of uncontrolled BP are already taking a CCB and a variable number are taking a β-blocker or other sympatholytic agent. Many are also taking a thiazide diuretic, which has limited effectiveness in patients with renal insufficiency (e.g., a serum creatinine level above 1.5 mg/dL). A sizeable proportion of patients had previously received treatment with an ACEI or ARB, which may have been discontinued because of either the precipitation of acute renal insufficiency or, more likely, reluctance of the clinician to continue the treatment (for the reasons discussed above) after renovascular disease was diagnosed.

Because of the success of ACEI treatment demonstrated in the clinical trials discussed here, this drug class usually should be included in the medical regimen. A prudent approach is to withhold diuretic therapy for several days and then begin treatment with a low dose of an ACEI (e.g., lisinopril, 2.5 mg/d). Serum electrolytes, blood urea nitrogen, and creatinine levels should be checked within 1 week after the start of treatment. If renal function is stable, the dose can be increased and, depending on BP response, diuretic therapy can be reintroduced. It is not clear from review of the current literature at what baseline level of renal dysfunction ACEIs or ARBs should be avoided; however, these drugs have been used safely in many diabetic and nondiabetic patients with serum creatinine levels as high as 4 mg/dL *(39,43)*.

For patients whose BP does not respond to a regimen that includes a diuretic, ACEI or ARB, CCB, and β-blocker, other options exist. The author's preference is the addition of a vasodilator, typically minoxidil, starting at 2.5 mg/day for males and hydralazine starting at 25 mg twice daily for females (to avoid hirsutism). Treatment with these vasodilators often allows the patient to stop taking the CCB, a considerable cost savings. Because most patients are already taking a β-blocker, reflex tachycardia usually is not an issue. Clonidine can be prescribed for patients for whom β-blocker therapy is contraindicated. Fluid retention associated with vasodilator therapy can be minimized by paying careful attention to weight and adjusting the dose of the loop diuretic accordingly. Because of a relatively short duration of action, furosemide should be taken twice daily, with the second dose taken in the late afternoon—not the evening—to avoid nocturia. The starting dose usually prescribed by the author is 20 mg twice daily. For patients who complain of urinary urgency while taking furosemide, replacement with torsemide, a loop diuretic with a more gradual onset of action and prolonged effect, may be helpful and allow once-daily dosing. The usual starting dose is 5 mg once daily.

For monitoring patients during the titration phase of treatment with these drugs, it is prudent to encourage the use of out-of-office BP measurements with an accurate device and to monitor renal function approximately every 2 weeks. Once the patient's BP is stabilized, there is no clear-cut consensus on the best method of followup. Some authors have recommended that BP and the serum creatinine level be measured every 3 months and noninvasive renal imaging (e.g., renal artery duplex scanning) be performed every 6 to 12 months to assess kidney size and progression of stenotic lesions *(44)*. Others have recommended periodic nuclear imaging studies, which estimate the blood flow and GFR for each kidney *(2)*. Nuclear imaging studies or measurements of GFR by creatinine or iothalamate clearance may be particularly helpful in patients who have normal baseline renal function, in which the serum creatinine level alone may be an insensitive indicator of progressive renovascular disease. All of these recommendations are probably reasonable with two caveats. One, for patients with FMD, BP monitoring and annual renal function tests may be adequate because the disease typically is not progressive and the lesions are often difficult to assess noninvasively. Two, for patients with advanced ARVD and who were originally considered poor candidates for revascularization, the need for routine follow-up imaging studies might be questioned because the results are unlikely to prompt subsequent intervention.

## MANAGEMENT OPTIONS FOR THE PATIENT IN WHOM MEDICAL THERAPY IS FAILING

Failure to achieve satisfactory BP control is less common than previously because of the large number of potent antihypertensive drugs that are available. If the patient has a lesion of the renal artery considered to be amenable to revascularization, balloon angioplasty or surgery should be considered. Not infrequently, however, refractory hypertension is related to a severely ischemic atrophic kidney that is not amenable to revascularization. The kidney of a patient with FMD usually is not atrophic, but it may not be amenable to revascularization because of the location or complexity of the stenotic lesions. The mechanism of hypertension in patients with such extensive or complex FMD almost certainly is caused by continued renin secretion from the affected kidney, and the hypertension would be expected to respond to high doses of ACEIs. Possibly, however, the degree of converting enzyme inhibition is incomplete or angiotensin II is being produced by alternative pathways *(45)*. Because of this possibility, the author has occasionally used the combination of an ACEI and an ARB in this setting and has had good results. The therapeutic benefit of this combination has been demonstrated recently in patients with heart failure *(46)* or proteinuric renal disease *(47)*. If the combination of an ACEI and ARB cannot be prescribed or is not effective, the remaining option is nephrectomy. Recently, Mayo Clinic experience with 63 patients who had refractory hypertension and nephrectomy of an atrophic nonfunctioning kidney was reviewed *(48)*. After a mean followup of 2.9 years, BP control was improved significantly in 78% of patients and no significant decrease in renal function was detected during the first year after nephrectomy. The widening availability of laparoscopic nephrectomy no doubt will increase the attractiveness of this therapeutic option *(49)*.

## REFERENCES

1. Aurell M, Jensen G. Treatment of renovascular hypertension. Nephron 1997;75: 373–378.
2. Safian RD, Textor SC. Renal-artery stenosis. N Engl J Med 2001;344:431–442.
3. Xue F, Bettmann MA, Langdon DR, Wivell WA. Outcome and cost comparison of percutaneous transluminal renal angioplasty, renal arterial stent placement, and renal arterial bypass grafting. Radiology 1999;212:378–384.
4. Hallett JW Jr, Textor SC, Kos PB, et al. Advanced renovascular hypertension and renal insufficiency: trends in medical comorbidity and surgical approach from 1970 to 1993. J Vasc Surg 1995;21:750–759.
5. Conlon PJ, Athirakul K, Kovalik E, et al. Survival in renal vascular disease. J Am Soc Nephrol 1998;9:252–256.
6. Dorros G, Jaff M, Mathiak L, et al. Four-year follow-up of Palmaz-Schatz stent revascularization as treatment for atherosclerotic renal artery stenosis. Circulation 1998;98:642–647.
7. Butterly DW, Schwab SJ. Renal artery stenosis: the case for conservative management. Mayo Clin Proc 2000;75:435–436.
8. Chabova V, Schirger A, Stanson AW, McKusick MA, Textor SC. Outcomes of atherosclerotic renal artery stenosis managed without revascularization. Mayo Clin Proc 2000;75:437–444.
9. Plouin PF, Chatellier G, Darne B, Raynaud A for the Essai Multicentrique Medicaments vs Angioplastie (EMMA) Study Group. Blood pressure outcome of angioplasty in atherosclerotic renal artery stenosis: a randomized trial. Hypertension 1998;31:823–829.
10. Webster J, Marshall F, Abdalla M, et al. for the Scottish and Newcastle Renal Artery Stenosis Collaborative Group. Randomised comparison of percutaneous angioplasty vs continued medical therapy for hypertensive patients with atheromatous renal artery stenosis. J Hum Hypertens 1998;12:329–335.
11. van Jaarsveld BC, Krijnen P, Pieterman H, et al. for the Dutch Renal Artery Stenosis Intervention Cooperative Study Group. The effect of balloon angioplasty on hypertension in atherosclerotic renal-artery stenosis. N Engl J Med 2000;342: 1007–1014.
12. Helin KH, Lepantalo M, Edgren J, Liewendahl K, Tikkanen T, Tikkanen I. Predicting the outcome of invasive treatment of renal artery disease. J Intern Med 2000;247:105–110.
13. Paulsen D, Klow NE, Rogstad B, et al. Preservation of renal function by percutaneous transluminal angioplasty in ischaemic renal disease. Nephrol Dial Transplant 1999;14:1454–1461.

14. Textor SC. Revascularization in atherosclerotic renal artery disease. Kidney Int 1998;53:799–811.
15. Giroux MF, Soulez G, Therasse E, et al. Percutaneous revascularization of the renal arteries: predictors of outcome. J Vasc Interv Radiol 2000;11:713–720.
16. Radermacher J, Chavan A, Bleck J, et al. Use of Doppler ultrasonography to predict the outcome of therapy for renal-artery stenosis. N Engl J Med 2001;344:410–417.
17. Jacobson HR. Ischemic renal disease: an overlooked clinical entity? Kidney Int 1988;34:729–743.
18. Schreiber MJ, Pohl MA, Novick AC. The natural history of atherosclerotic and fibrous renal artery disease. Urol Clin North Am 1984;11:383–392.
19. Zierler RE, Bergelin RO, Davidson RC, Cantwell-Gab K, Polissar NL, Strandness DE Jr. A prospective study of disease progression in patients with atherosclerotic renal artery stenosis. Am J Hypertens 1996;9:1055–1061.
20. Caps MT, Zierler RE, Polissar NL, et al. Risk of atrophy in kidneys with atherosclerotic renal artery stenosis. Kidney Int 1998;53:735–742.
21. Dustan HP, Page IH, Poutasse EF, Wilson L. An evaluation of treatment of hypertension associated with occlusive renal arterial disease. Circulation 1963;27:1018–1027.
22. Hollenberg NK. Medical therapy for renovascular hypertension: a review. Am J Hypertens 1988;1:338S–343S.
23. Hollenberg NK. Medical therapy of renovascular hypertension: efficacy and safety of captopril in 269 patients. Cardiovasc Rev Rep 1983;4:852–875.
24. Franklin SS, Smith RD. Comparison of effects of enalapril plus hydrochlorothiazide versus standard triple therapy on renal function in renovascular hypertension. Am J Med 1985;79:14–23.
25. Hricik DE, Browing PJ, Kopelman R, Goorno WE, Madias NE, Dzau VJ. Captopril-induced functional renal insufficiency in patients with bilateral renal-artery stenoses or renal-artery stenosis in a solitary kidney. N Engl J Med 1983;308:373–376.
26. Curtis JJ, Luke RG, Welchel JD, Diethelm AG, Jones P, Dustan HP. Inhibition of angiotensin-converting enzyme in renal-transplant recipients with hypertension. N Engl J Med 1983;308:377–381.
27. Jackson B, Matthews PG, McGrath BP, Johnston CI. Angiotensin converting enzyme inhibition in renovascular hypertension: frequency of reversible renal failure. Lancet 1984;1:225–226.
28. Hricik DE, Dunn MJ. Angiotensin-converting enzyme inhibitor-induced renal failure: causes, consequences, and diagnostic uses. J Am Soc Nephrol 1990;1:845–858.
29. Thind GS. Renal insufficiency during angiotensin-converting enzyme inhibitor therapy in hypertensive patients with no renal artery stenosis. J Clin Hypertens 1985;1:337–343.
30. Toto RD, Mitchell HC, Lee HC, Milam C, Pettinger WA. Reversible renal insufficiency due to angiotensin converting enzyme inhibitors in hypertensive nephrosclerosis. Ann Intern Med 1991;115:513–519.
31. Bridoux F, Hazzan M, Pallot JL, et al. Acute renal failure after the use of angiotensin-converting-enzyme inhibitors in patients without renal artery stenosis. Nephrol Dial Transplant 1992;7:100–104.
32. van de Ven PJ, Beutler JJ, Kaatee R, Beek FJ, Mali WP, Koomans HA. Angiotensin converting enzyme inhibitor-induced renal dysfunction in atherosclerotic renovascular disease. Kidney Int 1998;53:986–993.
33. Hoefnagels WH, Thien T. Renal artery occlusion in patients with renovascular hypertension treated with captopril. Br Med J (Clin Res Ed) 1986;292:24–25.

34. Vetrovec GW, Landwehr DM, Edwards VL. Incidence of renal artery stenosis in hypertensive patients undergoing coronary angiography. J Interv Cardiol 1989; 2:69–76.
35. Harding MB, Smith LR, Himmelstein SI, et al. Renal artery stenosis: prevalence and associated risk factors in patients undergoing routine cardiac catheterization. J Am Soc Nephrol 1992;2:1608–1616.
36. Lewis EJ, Hunsicker LG, Bain RP, Rohde RD for the Collaborative Study Group. The effect of angiotensin-converting-enzyme inhibition on diabetic nephropathy. N Engl J Med 1993;329:1456–1462.
37. Maschio G, Alberti D, Janin G, et al. for the Angiotensin-Converting-Enzyme Inhibition in Progressive Renal Insufficiency Study Group. Effect of the angiotensin-converting-enzyme inhibitor benazepril on the progression of chronic renal insufficiency. N Engl J Med 1996;334:939–945.
38. Yusuf S, Sleight P, Pogue J, Bosch J, Davies R, Dagenais G for the Heart Outcomes Prevention Evaluation Study Investigators. Effects of an angiotensin-converting-enzyme inhibitor, ramipril, on cardiovascular events in high-risk patients. N Engl J Med 2000;342:145–153.
39. Lewis EJ, Hunsicker LG, Clarke WR, et al. Renoprotective effect of the angiotensin-receptor antagonist irbesartan in patients with nephropathy due to type 2 diabetes. N Engl J Med 2001;345:851–860.
40. Brenner BM, Cooper ME, de Zeeuw D, et al. Effects of losartan on renal and cardiovascular outcomes in patients with type 2 diabetes and nephropathy. N Engl J Med 2001;345:861–869.
41. Drug Facts & Comparisons 2002: Pocket Version, 6th ed. St. Louis, Mo: Facts and Comparisons, 2001.
42. Bakris GL, Siomos M, Richardson D, et al. for the VAL-K Study Group. ACE inhibition or angiotensin receptor blockade: impact on potassium in renal failure. Kidney Int 2000;58:2084–2092.
43. Giatras I, Lau J, Levey AS for the Angiotensin-Converting-Enzyme Inhibition and Progressive Renal Disease Study Group. Effect of angiotensin-converting enzyme inhibitors on the progression of nondiabetic renal disease: a meta-analysis of randomized trials. Ann Intern Med 1997;127:337–345.
44. Plouin PF, Rossignol P, Bobrie G. Atherosclerotic renal artery stenosis: to treat conservatively, to dilate, to stent, or to operate? J Am Soc Nephrol 2001;12: 2190–2196.
45. McLaughlin K, Jardine AG. Angiotensin converting enzyme inhibitors and angiotensin receptor (AT1) antagonists: either or both for primary renal disease? Nephrol Dial Transplant 1999;14:25–28.
46. Hamroff G, Katz SD, Mancini D, et al. Addition of angiotensin II receptor blockade to maximal angiotensin-converting enzyme inhibition improves exercise capacity in patients with severe congestive heart failure. Circulation 1999;99:990–992.
47. Russo D, Pisani A, Balletta MM, et al. Additive antiproteinuric effect of converting enzyme inhibitor and losartan in normotensive patients with IgA nephropathy. Am J Kidney Dis 1999;33:851–856.
48. Kane GC, Textor SC, Schirger A, Garovic VD. The role of nephrectomy in refractory hypertension and atherosclerotic renal artery occlusion. Circulation 2001;104 Suppl:II-501–II-502.
49. Janetschek G, Marberger M. Laparoscopic surgery in urology. Curr Opin Urol 2000;10:351–357.

# 7 Primary Reninism or Renin-Secreting Tumors

*Timothy L. Reudelhuber,* PhD

CONTENTS



## THE RENIN-ANGIOTENSIN SYSTEM AND PHYSIOLOGICAL CONTROL OF RENIN SECRETION

The renin-angiotensin system (RAS) is a major regulator of salt and fluid balance in mammals. Within the circulation, angiotensinogen derived from the liver is cleaved by active renin, which comes primarily from the juxtaglomerular (JG) cells of the renal afferent arteriole, to release the decapeptide angiotensin I (Ang I). Ang I is in turn cleaved by endothelial cell-bound angiotensin-converting enzyme (ACE) to produce the vasoactive peptide angiotensin II (Ang II). Ang II exerts its actions by binding to two types of receptors; the angiotensin type 2 receptor (AT2), whose function remains a bit of a mystery, and the angiotensin type 1 receptor (AT1), which is responsible for most of the known cardiovascular effects of Ang II and is the target for the class of drugs referred to as angiotensin receptor blockers (ARBs). By acting through the AT1 receptor, Ang II modulates vasoconstriction, stimu-

From: *Secondary Hypertension: Clinical Presentation, Diagnosis, and Treatment*
Edited by: G. A. Mansoor © Humana Press Inc., Totowa, NJ

lates aldosterone release from the adrenal gland, and promotes sodium retention in the kidney.

The cleavage of angiotensinogen by renin represents the rate-limiting step in the circulating RAS, and changes in the levels of either of these components will result in increases in production of Ang II. Nevertheless, angiotensinogen levels respond rather slowly to physiological signals, whereas active renin levels can change rapidly in response to a number of stimuli. In general terms, renin secretion is suppressed by increases in distal tubular sodium content as sensed by the macula densa or by increases in blood pressure (BP), interstitial pressure, or circulating Ang II levels as sensed by the JG cells of the afferent arteriole. Conversely, renin secretion is increased by decreases in BP, decreased distal tubular sodium, decreased Ang II feedback on JG cells, and rapid increases in sympathetic nerve activity.

## PATHOPHYSIOLOGICAL STATES OF EXCESS RENIN SECRETION

Excess secretion of renin results primarily from a disruption of the normal physiological control mechanisms of renin regulation. Perhaps the most common cause of hyperreninemia is renal ischemia secondary to renal artery stenosis. The resulting renovascular hypertension is a direct effect of an increase in renin release and will be treated in other chapters of the current text. Hypersecretion of renin also occurs with pharmacologic blockade of the RAS with either ACE inhibition or use of ARBs because both classes of drugs block the repressive action of Ang II on the renin-secreting JG cells. Finally, unregulated secretion of renin occurs in renin-producing tumors that have escaped the hemodynamic and hormonal control of the normal environment of the afferent arteriole. Distinction between these causes remains crucial in determining the course of treatment.

## HYPERRENINISM CAUSED BY A RENIN-SECRETING TUMOR

Renin-secreting tumors can be divided roughly into renal and nonrenal tumors. A surprisingly wide variety of nonrenal tumors have on occasion been found to secrete renin and to be associated with hypertension including lung cancers *(1)*, hepatoblastomas *(2)*, paragangliomas *(3,4)*, pancreatic carcinomas *(5)*, adenocarcinoma of the colon *(6)*, adrenal carcinomas *(7)*, and various types of ovarian *(8,9)* and fallopian tube *(10)* tumors. It is important to note that production of renin by these tumor types is rare and unexpected and likely to be caused by the particular chromosomal mutations or rearrangements undergone by the cancer cells. Treatment of hypertension in these cases has focused on the use of RAS inhibitors and tumor ablation, although hypertension is likely to reappear with new tumor growth or metastasis *(3)*.

In the kidney, hypersecretion of renin is infrequently associated with renal carcinomas and quite frequently (>50% of cases) with Wilms' tumors *(11)*. Although renal masses can cause compression-induced hypertrophy of the JG apparatus leading to increased renin secretion *(12)*, it is now clear that Wilms' tumor cells themselves secrete renin *(11–13)*. Another exceedingly rare type of tumor associated with renin-dependent hypertension is the JG cell tumor, sometimes referred to as reninomas. These tumors are benign neoplasms that are most often clinically detected as causes of hypertension associated with severe hypokalemia in very young patients. The first report of such a tumor occurred only in 1967 and to date the English literature contains less than 100 reports of such tumors. Two very thorough and informative reviews on the subject of JG cell tumors have been published in recent years *(14,15)*, and, because of the rarity of these cases, they will likely remain excellent sources in the foreseeable future of information and of reference to primary cases for the interested reader.

## *Diagnosis*

Patients with renin-producing tumors are invariably hyperreninemic, resulting in hyperaldosteronemia and hypokalemia upon initial examination. However, increased plasma renin activity (PRA) is not always apparent in these patients *(15)*. Diagnosis by PRA is also complicated in patients being treated for hypertension with medications that lead to increased renin secretion such as ARBs and ACE inhibitors (ACEIs). In addition, increased circulating renin is also seen in other conditions including renovascular hypertension and renal failure, making the evidence of increased PRA more equivocal. Perhaps the best evidence in the diagnosis of a JG cell reninoma is the appearance of significant hypertension associated with hypokalemia (perhaps the most significant finding in these patients) in relatively young patients without other apparent risk factors *(15)*. In analyzing previously reported cases in the medical literature, Martin et al *(14)* noted that the mean age at diagnosis for these cases was 26.8 years, with less than one-quarter of patients being diagnosed after 40 years of age. Although not as diagnostic, many of the patients display hypertension that becomes increasingly difficult to control with standard therapy over time. If left untreated, patients may present with complaints commonly associated with severe hypertension including headache, vomiting, polyuria, nocturia, and dizziness.

Three clinical tests have been used with limited success to provide support for the diagnosis of a reninoma. First, treatment with an ACEI or ARB, which normally results in a rise in renin secretion in patients with essential hypertension, will sometimes fail to elicit increased renin secretion in a patient with a reninoma, because the tumor cells may have escaped the normal feedback regulation on renin secretion *(15)*. However, the hormonal response of these tumors is not uniform or entirely predictable *(15)*. It may also be impractical to administer such tests because most suspect cases will already be dependent on RAS-targeted antihypertensive therapy to control their BP. Second, renal vein PRA measurements have been used to test for lateralization of renin secretion from the tumor-bearing kidney because the healthy kidney suppresses renin secretion in response to the hypertension. However, renin secretion from the tumor-bearing kidney is not always increased *(16,17)*, perhaps because of either alternate vascularization of the tumor or direct generation of the vasoactive peptide Ang II within some of the tumors. It should also be noted that patients with unilateral artery stenosis may lateralize renin secretion to the ischemic kidney, making this symptom equivocal in the diagnosis. Finally, renal arteriograms may be used to detect larger tumors and in some cases to rule out stenosis as a cause of the hyperreninism. However, most reninomas are less than 4 cm in diameter *(14,15)* and may not appear on an arteriogram. Ultimately, a careful analysis of a computed tomograhy (CT) scan of the kidneys will be the best adjunct when a reninoma is suspected because it should have the necessary resolution to detect even small tumors, which can be clinically significant even at sizes under 1 cm in diameter. Importantly, there is no obvious correlation between the severity of hypertension and the size of the responsible reninoma *(14)*.

## *Histopathology*

The histo- and molecular pathology of Wilm's tumors has been described elsewhere and will not be dealt with further in this chapter. However, in cases where these tumors have contributed to renin-dependent hypertension, some cells within the tumors invariably stain with antirenin or antiprorenin antibody *(18,19)*, although this analysis is unlikely to determine the course of treatment of these patients.

In contrast, diagnosis of a JG cell reninoma provides an opportunity for curative treatment of hypertension in affected patients. Gross examination of these tumors at surgery reveals a well-delimited and encap-

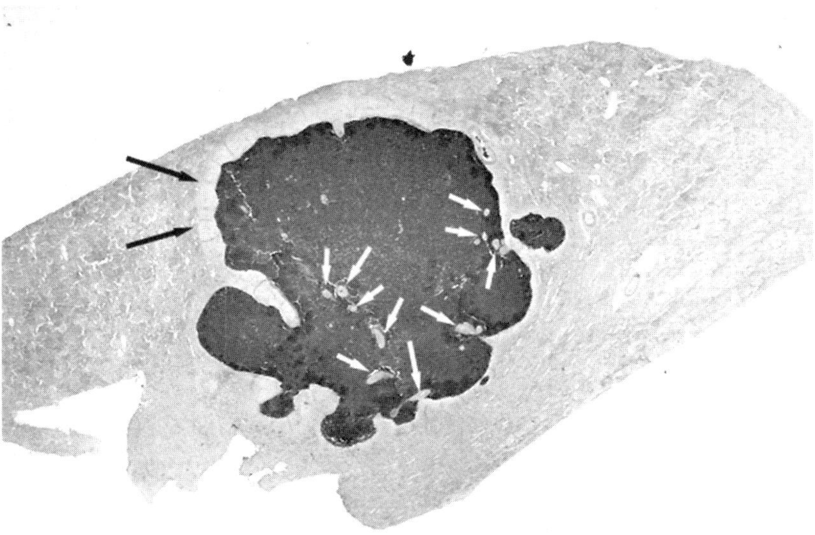

**Fig. 1.** Renin staining of a juxtaglomerular (JG) cell tumor. Paraffin sections of a JG cell tumor resected from the left kidney of a 10-year-old male were stained with antihuman renin antibody. Note the uneven distribution of the dark renin staining, the enclosure of the tumor in a thick fibrous capsule (black arrows), and the heavy vascularization (white arrows). Average tumor diameter was 1.2 cm. Original magnification ×5.5.

sulated cortical mass (Fig. 1). Intratumoral hemorrhage is also a common finding because these tumors are commonly heavily vascularized. Other frequently described characteristics of reninomas are entrapment of renal tubules, cyst formation, and focal necrosis. Histologic examination reveals a well-circumscribed and heavily vascularized uniform mass covered by a thick fibrous capsule (Fig. 1). The tumor cells vary in size and contain an eosinophylic cytoplasm and oval irregularly shaped nuclei.

Immunohistochemistry provides the best confirmation of a reninoma. As expected, tumor cells stain positive for renin (Fig. 1) but do not always stain uniformly *(19)*. Most likely because of the smooth-muscle origin of JG cells, these tumors also stain for smooth muscle α actin *(14)*. Although the wider application of their finding needs to be confirmed, Martin et al. *(14)* recently reported that four out of four reninomas examined are positive for CD34 staining, and, like others, they found them to be negative for cytokeratin, chromogranin, synaptophysin, HMB-45, S-100, c-kit, CD31, factor VIII, and desmin.

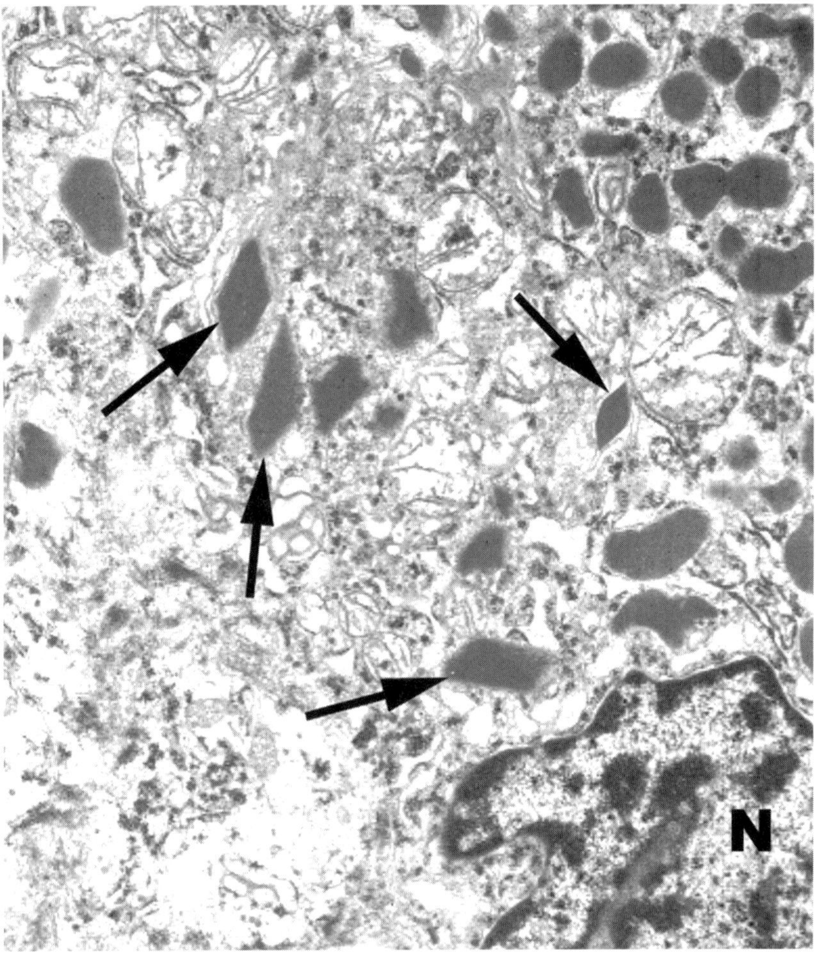


Fig. 2. Electron micrograph of a reninoma cell. Tumor cells from the reninoma shown in Fig. 1 were stained with uranyl-acetate and observed in the electron microscope. Note the diamond-shaped granules present in the cytoplasm of tumor cells (black arrows) and the irregular shape of the nucleus (N). Original magnification x10,000.

Ultrastructural examination reveals another clear diagnostic characteristic of reninomas; the cytoplasm contains rhomboid-shaped granular inclusions highly characteristic of renin-producing cells (Fig. 2). This characteristic clearly distinguishes a reninoma from other tumors with similar clinical or pathological presentation including glomus tumors, hemangiopericytomas, angiomyolipomas, and renal cell carcinomas *(14)*.

## TREATMENT

Treatment of hypertension associated with an uncorrected renin-secreting tumor of any sort consists of RAS-targeted antihypertensive therapy and may become more difficult with time as the tumor grows or metastasizes *(3)*. There is no doubt, however, that the ultimate correction of this problem is by ablation of the tumor. Patients harboring a JG cell reninoma have a particularly good prognosis in this regard. In more than 90% of cases, reninoma-associated hypertension is smoothly and completely reversed by surgical resection of the tumor. In most of the remaining cases, only mild hypertension persists, perhaps because of secondary organ damage, and can be managed by standard therapy *(15)*. Because JG cell tumors are benign, there have been no reported cases of metastases or recurrence after surgery.

## CONCLUSIONS

The diagnosis of a renin-secreting tumor is a challenge because of the paucity of clinically distinguishing characteristics. To date, the most common findings are hypertension associated with hypokalemia in a young individual without any compelling risk factors. Diagnosis of a reninoma of JG origin is strongly aided by CT scan of the kidney, and surgical ablation of this type of tumor can lead to a correction of the associated hypertension and an excellent prognosis for the patient.

## REFERENCES


1. Genest J, Rojo-Ortega JM, Kuchel O, et al. Malignant hypertension with hypokalemia in a patient with renin-producing pulmonary carcinoma. Trans Assoc Am Physicians 1975;88:192–201.
2. Moritake H, Taketomi A, Kamimura S, et al. Renin-producing hepatoblastoma. J Pediatr Hematol Oncol 2000;22:78–80.
3. Arver S, Jacobsson H, Cedermark B, et al. Malignant human renin producing paraganglionoma-localization with 123I-MIBG and treatment with 131I-MIBG. Clin Endocrinol (Oxf) 1999;51:631–635.
4. Andiran N, Koseoglu V, Andiran F, Buyukpamukcu N, Kutluk T, Buyukpamukcu M. Malignant hypertension and paraganglioma in a 14-year-old girl. Pediatr Hematol Oncol 1999;16:67–70.
5. Langer P, Bartsch D, Gerdes B, et al. Renin producing neuroendocrine pancreatic carcinoma: a case report and review of the literature. Exp Clin Endocrinol Diabetes 2002;110:43–49.
6. Ringrose TR, Phillips PA, Lindop GB. Renin-secreting adenocarcinoma of the colon. Ann Intern Med 1999;131:794–795.
7. Yamanaka K, Iitaka M, Inaba M, Morita T, Sasano H, Katayama S. A case of renin-producing adrenocortical cancer. Endocr J 2000;47:119–125.

8. Iwamoto H, Hirata S, Honda T, Fukasawa H, Kimura N, Hoshi K. Renin-producing serous cystoadenocarcinoma of the ovary: a case report. Eur J Gynaecol Oncol 2002;23:183–186.
9. Stephen MR, Lindop GB. A renin secreting ovarian steroid cell tumour associated with secondary polycythaemia. J Clin Pathol 1998;51:75–77.
10. Zabernigg A, Muller-Holzner E, Gasc JM, Gattringer C. An unusual case of a renin-producing tumour of the fallopian tube. Eur J Cancer 1997;33:1709.
11. McKenzie KJ, Ferrier RK, Howatson AG, Lindop GB. Demonstration of renin gene expression in nephroblastoma by in situ hybridization. J Pathol 1996;180:71–73.
12. Yokomori K, Hori T, Takemura T, Tsuchida Y. Demonstration of both primary and secondary reninism in renal tumors in children. J Pediatr Surg 1988;23:403–409.
13. Lindop GB, Lever AF. Anatomy of the renin-angiotensin system in the normal and pathological kidney. Histopathology 1986;10:335–362.
14. Martin SA, Mynderse LA, Lager DJ, Cheville JC. Juxtaglomerular cell tumor: a clinicopathologic study of four cases and review of the literature. Am J Clin Pathol 2001;116:854–863.
15. Corvol P, Pinet F, Plouin PF, Bruneval P, Menard J. Renin-secreting tumors. Endocrinol Metab Clin North Am 1994;23:255–270.
16. Koriyama N, Kakei M, Yaekura K, et al. A case of renal juxtaglomerular cell tumor: usefulness of segmental sampling to prove autonomic secretion of the tumor. Am J Med Sci 1999;318:194–197.
17. Kashiwabara H, Inaba M, Itabashi A, Ishii J, Katayama S. A case of renin-producing juxtaglomerular tumor: effect of ACE inhibitor or angiotensin II receptor antagonist. Blood Press 1997;6:147–153.
18. Tomita T, Poisner A, Inagami T. Immunohistochemical localization of renin in renal tumors. Am J Pathol 1987;126:73–80.
19. Lindop GB, Millan DW, Murray D, Gibson AA, McIntyre GD, Leckie BJ. Immunocytochemistry of renin in renal tumours. Clin Exp Hypertens A 1987;9:1305–1323.

# III Adrenal Cortex and Hypertension

# 8 Primary Aldosteronism

*Diagnosis*

*William F. Young, Jr.*, MD

*Contents*



## INTRODUCTION

The syndrome of primary aldosteronism was first described by Conn in 1955 *(1)* and is characterized by hypertension, suppressed plasma renin activity (PRA), increased plasma aldosterone concentration (PAC), and unsuppressible aldosterone levels in the blood or urine. Prevalence estimates for primary aldosteronism when hypokalemia was one of the diagnostic criteria varied from 0.05 to 2% of the population with hypertension. However, with the recognition that most patients who have primary aldosteronism are normokalemic and with improved screening methods, it appears that primary aldosteronism is the most common form of secondary hypertension, affecting 5 to 12% of patients with presumed essential hypertension *(2–6)* and 23 to 26% of patients with resistant hypertension *(7)*.

Distinguishing the subtype of primary aldosteronism is critical to appropriate therapy (Table 1). Conn's first case was a 34-year-old woman with a 4 cm unilateral aldosterone-producing adenoma (APA); hypertension was cured with unilateral adrenalectomy *(1)*. A more common subtype of primary aldosteronism is idiopathic hyperaldosteronism (IHA) caused by bilateral zona glomerulosa hyperplasia; this form of

From: *Secondary Hypertension: Clinical Presentation, Diagnosis, and Treatment*
Edited by: G. A. Mansoor © Humana Press Inc., Totowa, NJ

Table 1
Subtypes of Primary Aldosteronism

| | |
|---|---|
| May be treated surgically for cure | |
| | Aldosterone-producing adenoma (APA) |
| | Primary (unilateral) adrenal hyperplasia (PAH) |
| | Aldosterone-producing adrenocortical carcinoma |
| Should be treated medically | |
| | Idiopathic hyperaldosteronism (IHA) |
| | Glucocorticoid-remediable aldosteronism (GRA) |

primary aldosteronism is rarely cured with adrenal surgery *(8–10)*. Primary adrenal hyperplasia (PAH) or unilateral adrenal hyperplasia is an uncommon subtype. A hyperplastic adrenal gland that morphologically resembles that in IHA but mimics the APA response to physiological maneuvers and unilateral or subtotal adrenalectomy characterizes PAH *(9,11)*. Glucocorticoid-remediable aldosteronism (GRA) is autosomal dominant in inheritance and associated with variable degrees of hyperaldosteronism, high levels of hybrid steroids (e.g., 18-hydroxycortisol), and suppression with exogenous glucocorticoid *(12,13)*.

Unilateral adrenalectomy cures hypokalemia in all patients and improves or cures hypertension in most patients who have APA and PAH, but surgery is not as effective for patients with IHA and GRA. The key management issues addressed in this chapter are screening, confirmatory testing, and subtype evaluation.

## DIAGNOSIS

The diagnosis of primary aldosteronism is usually made in patients who are in the third to sixth decades. Few symptoms are specific to the syndrome. Patients with marked hypokalemia may have muscle weakness, cramping, headaches, palpitations, polydipsia, polyuria, or nocturia, or a combination of these. There are no specific physical findings. The degree of hypertension is usually moderate to severe and may be resistant to the usual pharmacological treatments *(9,10)*. Hypokalemia is frequently absent; thus, all patients with hypertension are candidates for this disorder. Several studies have shown that patients with primary aldosteronism may be at higher risk than other patients with hypertension for target organ damage of the heart and kidney *(14–25)*. Hypokalemia reduces the secretion of aldosterone, and it is optimal to restore the serum level of potassium to normal before performing diagnostic studies.

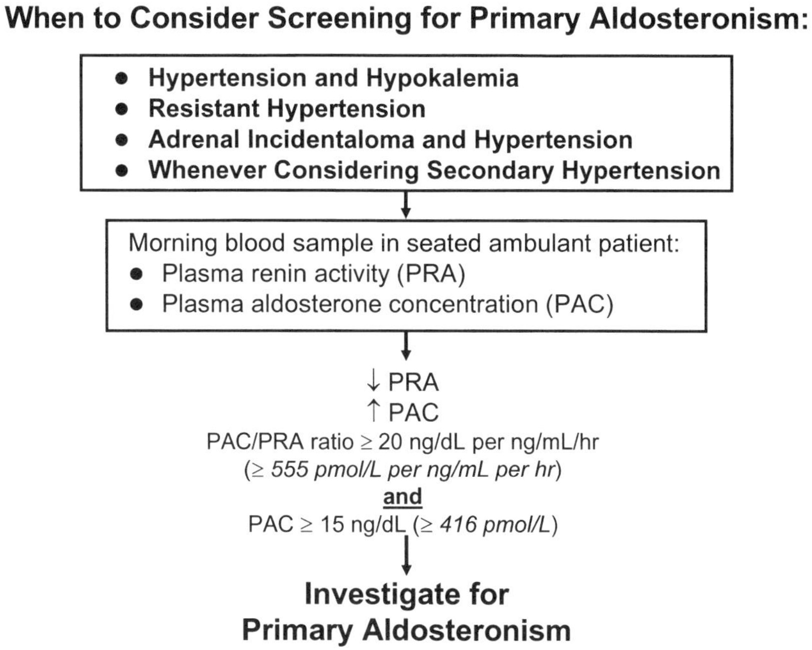


**Fig. 1.** Use of plasma aldosterone concentration (PAC)-to-plasma renin activity (PRA) ratio to screen for primary aldosteronism.

## *Screening Tests*

Spontaneous hypokalemia is uncommon in patients with uncomplicated hypertension and, when present, strongly suggests associated mineralocorticoid excess. However, normokalemia does not exclude primary aldosteronism. Several studies have shown that most patients with primary aldosteronism have baseline serum levels of potassium in the normal range *(2,26,27)*. Therefore, hypokalemia is not required to make the diagnosis of primary aldosteronism. Patients with hypertension and hypokalemia, regardless of presumed cause (e.g., diuretic treatment), and most patients with treatment-resistant hypertension should undergo screening for primary aldosteronism (Fig. 1).

In patients with suspected primary aldosteronism, screening can be accomplished by measuring a morning (preferably 8 a.m.) ambulatory paired random PAC and PRA (Fig. 1). This test may be performed while the patient is taking antihypertensive medications and without posture stimulation *(7,28)*. Spironolactone is the only medication that will uniformly interfere with interpretation of the ratio. Angiotensin-converting enzyme inhibitors (ACEIs) have the potential to "falsely elevate" PRA.

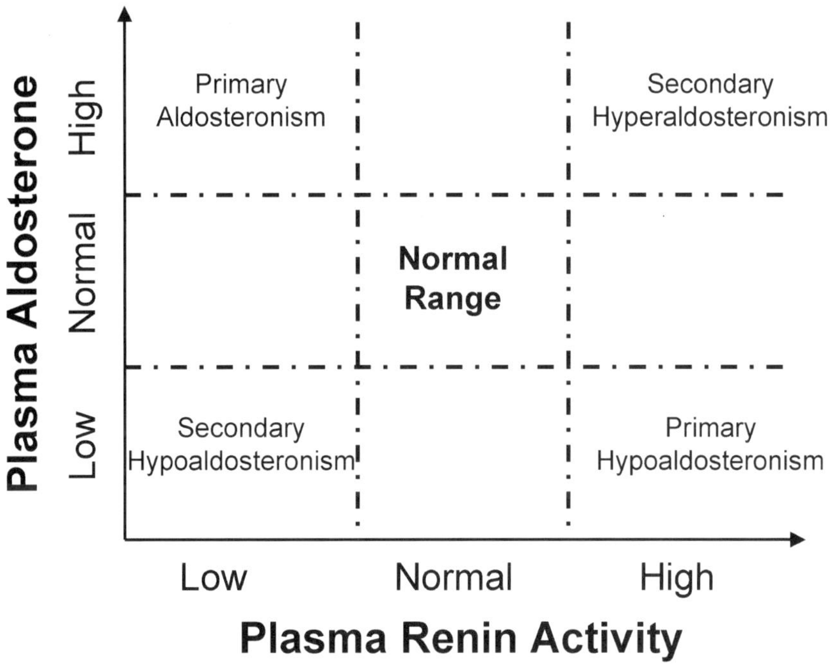


**Fig. 2.** Paired hormone measurements help to distinguish among different types of hyperfunction and hypofunction of the renin-angiotensin-aldosterone axis. PAC, plasma aldosterone concentration; PRA, plasma renin activity.

Therefore, in a patient treated with an ACEI, the findings of a detectable PRA level or a low PAC/PRA ratio do not exclude the diagnosis of primary aldosteronism. Additionally, a strong predictor for primary aldosteronism is a PRA level undetectably low in a patient taking an ACEI.

The PAC/PRA ratio, first proposed as a screening test for primary aldosteronism in 1981 *(29)*, is based on the concept of paired hormone measurements *(30)* (Fig. 2). For example, in a hypertensive hypokalemic patient, (a) secondary hyperaldosteronism should be considered when both PRA and PAC are increased and the PAC/PRA ratio is less than 10 (e.g., renovascular disease),( b) an alternate source of mineralocorticoid receptor agonism should be considered when both PRA and PAC are suppressed (e.g., hypercortisolism), and (c) primary aldosteronism should be suspected when PRA is suppressed and PAC is increased (Fig. 3). Fifteen prospective studies have been published on the use of the PAC/PRA ratio in screening for primary aldosteronism *(2,3,28,29,31-41)*. Although there is some uncertainty about test charac-

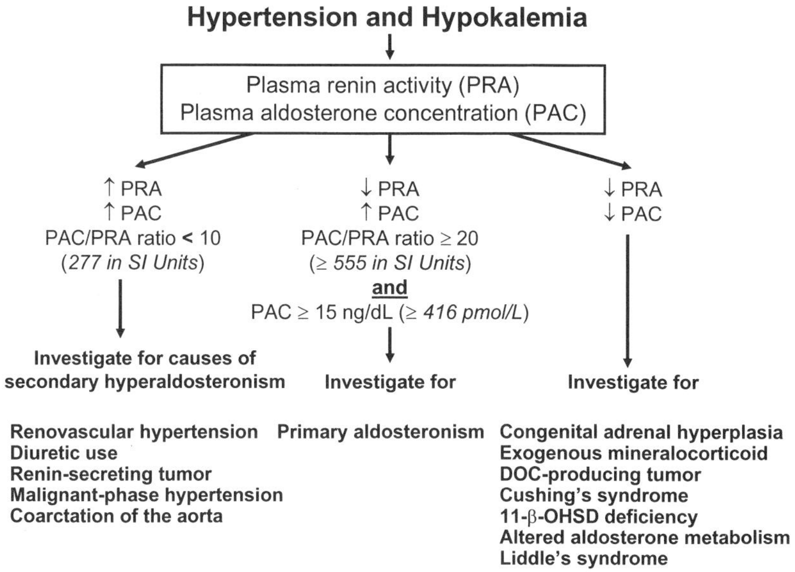


**Fig. 3.** Use of plasma aldosterone concentration (PAC)-to-plasma renin activity (PRA) ratio to distinguish among different causes of hypertension and hypokalemia. DOC, deoxycorticosterone; OHSD, hydroxysteroid dehydrogenase. (Adapted from ref. *9*.)

teristics and lack of standardization *(42)*, the PAC/PRA ratio is widely accepted as the screening test of choice for primary aldosteronism *(43,44)*. It has been suggested erroneously that the PAC/PRA ratio is not useful because it does not provide a renin-independent measure of circulating aldosterone suitable for determining whether PAC is increased relative to PRA *(45)*. However, the diagnostic value of the PAC/PRA ratio is that it is denominator-dependent (Fig. 2) and not an independent "index." A suppressed level of PRA is critical to the diagnosis of primary aldosteronism—just as a suppressed level of thyroid-stimulating hormone is a key finding in hyperthyroidism. Increasingly, the PAC/PRA ratio is being used to screen for primary aldosteronism (Fig. 4). The increased use of the PAC/PRA has resulted in a 10-fold increased annual detection rate of primary aldosteronism *(4,5)*.

Assays of plasma renin concentration are being offered by some laboratories. However, few studies have examined the diagnostic efficacy of a PAC/renin concentration ratio as a screening test for primary aldosteronism. In one study, a PAC/renin concentration ratio greater than 50 (pg/mL per pg/mL) was 89% sensitive and 96% specific for primary aldosteronism *(46)*. Until additional studies demonstrate simi-

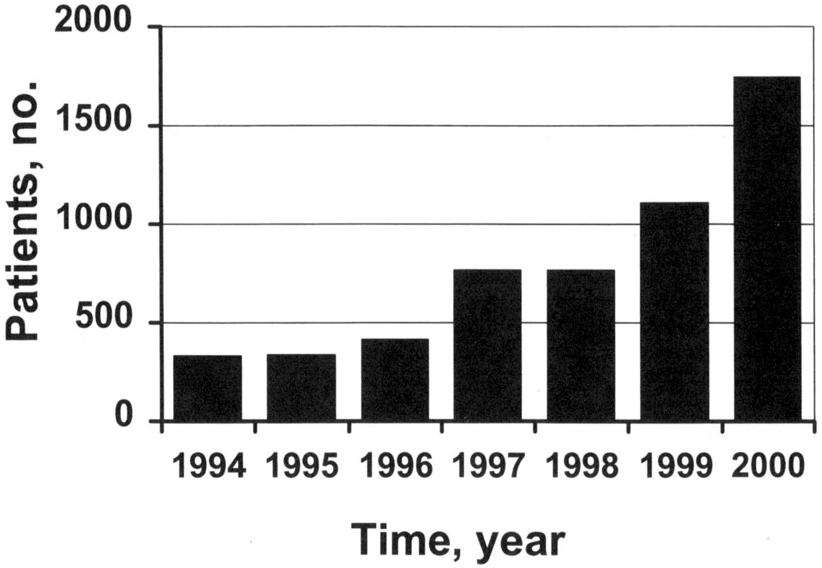


**Fig. 4.** Number of patients screened annually at Mayo Clinic for primary aldosteronism with the plasma aldosterone concentration (PAC)/ plasma renin activity (PRA) ratio. The increased frequency of screening has led to a 10-fold increase in the annual detection rate of primary aldosteronism.

lar test characteristics in larger patient cohorts, the plasma renin concentration should not replace the plasma renin activity assay in screening for primary aldosteronism.

It is important to understand that the lower limit of detection varies among different PRA assays and can have a dramatic effect on the PAC/PRA ratio *(4,5,47)*. As an example, a very different ratio is obtained if the lower limit of detection for PRA is 0.6 ng/mL per hour rather than 0.1 ng/mL per hour; for a PAC of 16 ng/dL, the PAC/PRA ratio would be 27 and 160, respectively. Thus, the cutoff for a "high" PAC/PRA ratio depends on the laboratory and, more specifically, on the PRA assay. Weinberger et al. *(48)* found that the combination of a PAC/PRA ratio greater than 30 and PAC greater than 20 ng/dL had a sensitivity of 90% and a specificity of 91% for APAs. Hirohira et al. *(45)* found that a PAC/PRA ratio greater than 32 had a sensitivity of 100% and a specificity of 61% for APA. At the Mayo Clinic, a PAC (in ng/dL)/PRA (in ng/mL per hour) ratio greater than or equal to 20 *and* PAC greater than or equal to 15 is used to indicate probable primary aldosteronism. Also, the combination of a PAC/PRA ratio greater than or equal to 20 and a PAC greater than or equal to 15 has been found in more than 90% of

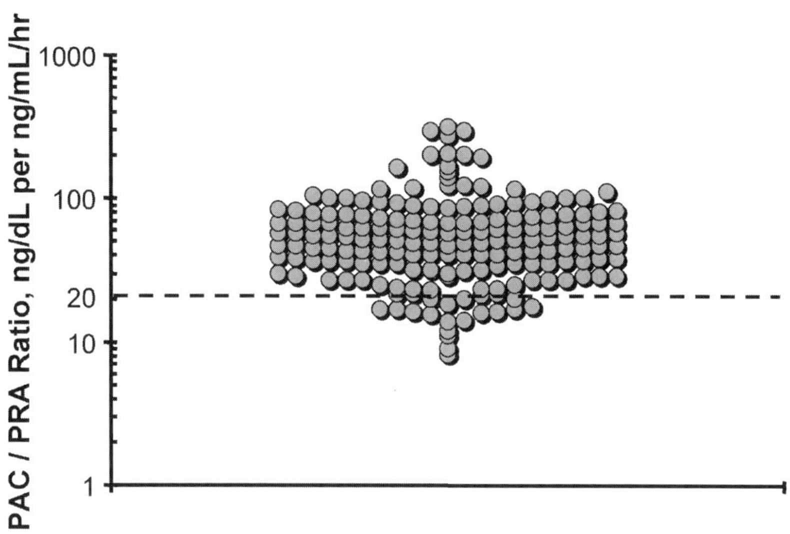


**Fig. 5.** Plasma aldosterone concentration (PAC)/plasma renin activity (PRA) ratios in 184 patients with surgically confirmed aldosterone-producing adenomas; 91.3% had a PAC/PRA ratio ≥ 20.

patients with surgically confirmed APA (Fig. 5). In patients without primary aldosteronism, most of the variation occurs within the normal range (Fig. 6). A high PAC/PRA ratio is a positive screening test result, a finding that warrants further testing.

## *Confirmatory Tests*

An increased PAC/PRA ratio is not diagnostic by itself, and primary aldosteronism must be confirmed by demonstrating inappropriate aldosterone secretion. The list of drugs and hormones capable of affecting the renin-angiotensin-aldosterone axis is extensive, and frequently in patients with severe hypertension, a "medication-contaminated" evaluation is unavoidable. Calcium channel blockers (CCBs), $\alpha_1$-adrenergic receptor blockers (ARBs), and β-adrenergic blocks do not affect the diagnostic accuracy in most cases *(8)*. It is impossible to interpret data obtained from patients receiving treatment with spironolactone. Therefore, spironolactone treatment should not be initiated until the evaluation has been completed and the final decisions about treatment have been made. If primary aldosteronism is suspected in a patient receiving treatment with spironolactone, the treatment should be discontinued for at least 6 weeks.

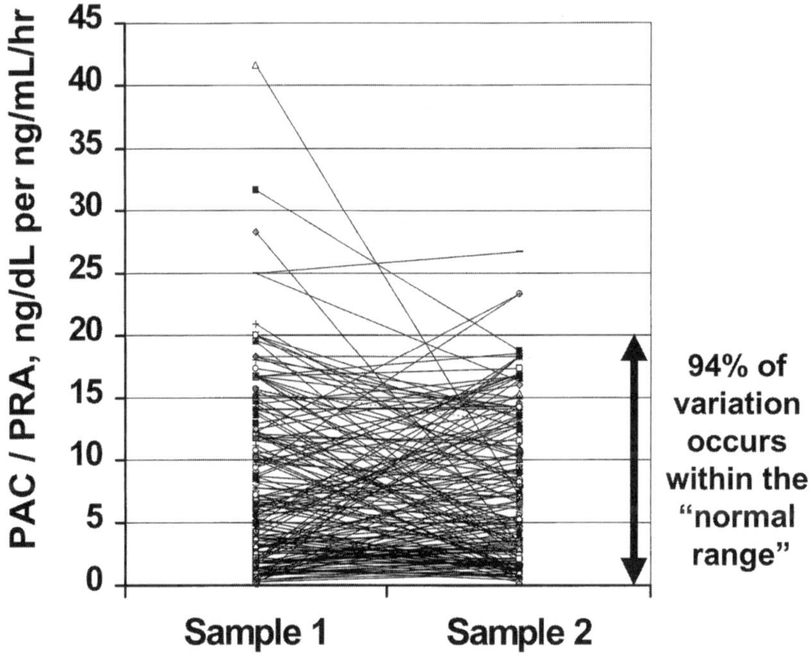


**Fig. 6.** The variation in repeat plasma aldosterone concentration (PAC)/plasma renin activity (PRA) ratios in 174 patients without primary aldosteronism. Only 6% of patients had one PAC/PRA ratio greater than 20. The mean interval between the ratios was 60.4 weeks. Most of the variation (94%) occurred within the normal range.

Aldosterone suppression testing can be performed with orally administered sodium chloride and measurement of urinary aldosterone *(8)* or with intravenous sodium chloride loading and measurement of PAC *(26,49)*. Our practice has been oral salt loading over 3 days. After hypertension and hypokalemia are controlled, patients should receive a high-sodium diet (supplemented with sodium chloride tablets if needed) for 3 days. The risk of increasing dietary sodium in patients with severe hypertension must be assessed in each case. Because the high-salt diet can increase kaliuresis and hypokalemia, vigorous replacement of potassium chloride may be needed and the serum level of potassium should be monitored daily. On day 3 of the high-sodium diet, a 24-hour urine specimen is collected for measurement of aldosterone, sodium, and potassium. To document adequate sodium repletion, the 24-hour urinary sodium excretion should exceed 200 mEq. Urinary aldosterone excretion greater than 12 μg/24 hours in this setting is consistent with autonomous aldosterone secretion *(50)*.

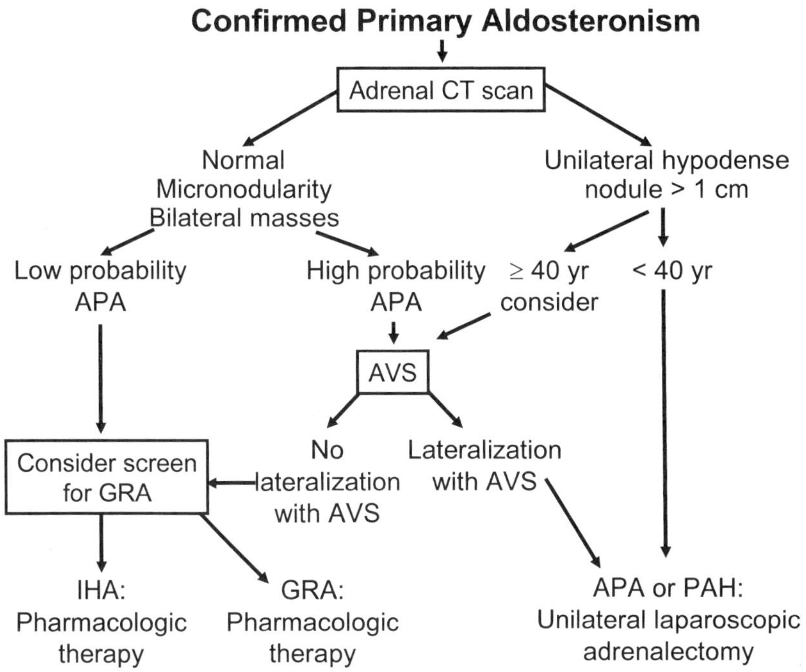


**Fig. 7.** Subtype evaluation of primary aldosteronism. The details are discussed in the text. APA, aldosterone-producing adenoma; AVS, adrenal venous sampling; CT, computed tomography; GRA, glucocorticoid-remediable aldosteronism; IHA, idiopathic hyperaldosteronism; PAH, primary adrenal hyperplasia. (Adapted from ref. *9*.)

## *Subtype Studies*

Following screening and confirmatory testing, the third management issue guides the therapeutic approach by distinguishing APA and PAH from IHA and GRA. Unilateral adrenalectomy in patients with APA or PAH results in normalization of hypokalemia in all; hypertension is improved in all and is cured in approximately 30 to 60% of these patients *(51)*. In IHA and GRA, unilateral or bilateral adrenalectomy seldom corrects the hypertension *(8)*. Although hypertension is frequently cured with unilateral adrenalectomy in patients with APA and PAH, the average cure rate for IHA is only 19% after unilateral or bilateral adrenalectomy *(8)*. IHA and GRA should be treated medically.

### Computed Tomography

Primary aldosteronism subtype evaluation may require one or more tests, the first of which is imaging the adrenal glands with computed tomography (CT) (Fig. 7). In 143 surgically treated APAs at the author's

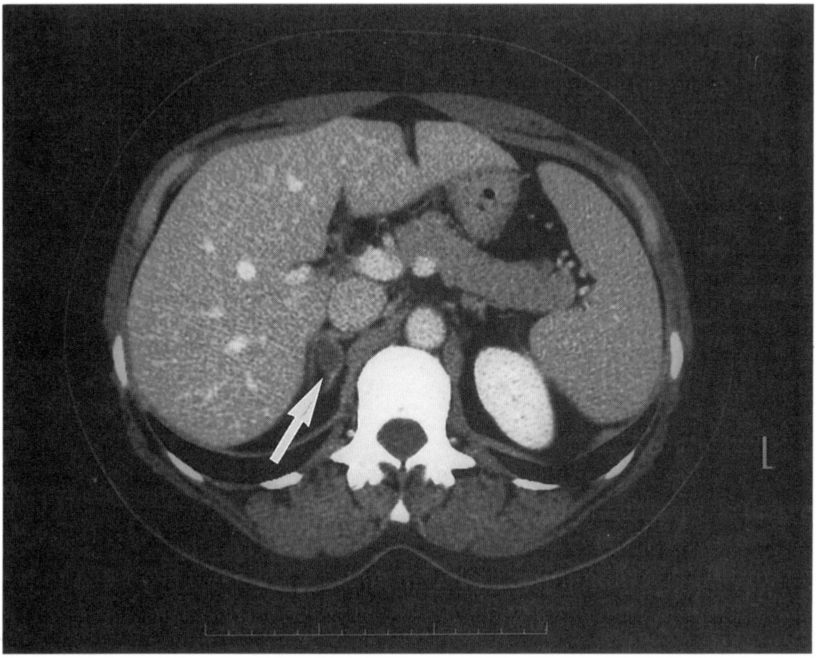


**Fig. 8.** Appearance of a 0.8 × 1.2 cm aldosterone-producing adrenal cortical adenoma (arrow) on contrast-enhanced computed tomography in a 36-year-old woman. The patient had been hypertensive for 10 years, with poor control for the last 3 years; her antihypertensive medication program included an ACEI , a CCB, and a β-adrenergic blocker. The screening test for primary aldosteronism was positive, with a normal range PAC of 17 ng/dL and low PRA at less than 0.6 ng/mL/hr (PAC/PRA ratio > 28). The 24-hour urinary excretion of aldosterone was increased at 16 μg (urinary sodium = 215 mEq/24 h). CT showed a clear hypodense right adrenal gland nodule. However, some mild thickening of the left adrenal gland necessitated adrenal venous sampling, which lateralized the tumor to the right adrenal gland. She underwent laparoscopic right adrenalectomy and a 1.7 × 1.0 × 1.0 cortical adenoma was found. The postoperative PAC was 2.5 ng/dL. Five years later, she was normotensive without the aid of antihypertensive agents.

institution, the mean diameter of the adenoma was 1.8 cm, although in nearly one-fifth (19%) it was less than 1 cm *(8)*. When a solitary unilateral macroadenoma (> 1 cm) and normal contralateral adrenal morphology are found on CT in a young patient (< 40 years) with primary aldosteronism, unilateral adrenalectomy is a reasonable therapeutic option (Fig. 8). However, in many cases, CT may show normal-appearing adrenals, minimal unilateral adrenal limb thickening, unilateral microadenomas (≤ 1 cm), or bilateral macroadenomas. In these cases, additional testing is required to determine the source of excess aldosterone secretion. Small APAs may be labeled incorrectly as IHA on the basis of CT findings of bilateral nodularity or normal-appearing adrenals. Also, apparent adrenal microadenomas may represent areas of hyperplasia, and unilateral adrenalectomy would be inappropriate. Additionally, nonfunctioning unilateral adrenal macroadenomas are not uncommon, especially in older patients (> 40 years) *(52)*.

Patients with APAs have more severe hypertension; have more profound hypokalemia (< 3.0 mEq/L) and higher plasma (> 25 ng/dL) and urinary (> 30 μg/24 h) levels of aldosterone; and are younger (< 50 years) than those with IHA *(8,53)*. Patients fitting at least one of these descriptors are considered to have a high probability of APA (Fig. 7). However, these factors are not absolute predictors of unilateral vs bilateral adrenal disease. With the addition of adrenal venous sampling, unilateral APAs have been found in 36% of those with clinically "high-probability" APA who had normal findings or unilateral adrenal limb thickening on CT *(54)*. Gordon et al. *(44)* reported that CT contributed to lateralization in only 59 of 111 patients with surgically proven APA; CT detected fewer than 25% of the APAs that were less than 1 cm in diameter. Magill et al. *(55)* reported that in 38 patients who had both CT and adrenal venous sampling, CT findings were either inaccurate or provided no additional information for 68% of patients with primary aldosteronism. Therefore, adrenal venous sampling is essential to direct appropriate therapy in patients with primary aldosteronism who have a high probability of APA and CT findings of unilateral adrenal limb thickening.

### Adrenal Venous Sampling

Adrenal venous sampling is the reference standard test to differentiate unilateral from bilateral disease in patients with primary aldosteronism *(56)*. Adrenal venous sampling is a difficult procedure because the right adrenal vein is small; the success rate depends on the proficiency of the angiographer *(44)*. According to a review of 47 reports, the success rate for canulating the right adrenal vein in 384 patients was 74% *(8)*. With experience, the success rate increased to between 90 and 93% *(44,54)*. Some centers perform adrenal venous sampling in all patients diagnosed with primary aldosteronism *(44)*. A more practical approach is the selective use of adrenal venous sampling as outlined in Fig. 7. To minimize stress-induced fluctuations in aldosterone secretion, an infusion of 50 μg of cosyntropin per hour is initiated 30 minutes before adrenal vein catheterization and continued throughout the procedure *(54)*. The adrenal veins are catheterized via the percutaneous femoral vein approach, and the position of the catheter tip is verified by gentle injection of a small amount of nonionic contrast medium and radiographic documentation. Blood is obtained from both adrenal veins and the inferior vena cava (IVC) below the renal veins and assayed for aldosterone and cortisol concentrations. The venous sample from the left side typically is obtained from the inferior phrenic vein immediately adjacent to the entrance of the adrenal vein. The right adrenal vein may be especially difficult to catheterize because it is short and enters the IVC at an acute angle *(57)*. The cumulative failure rate for catheterization of the right adrenal vein reported in the literature is 26% (review of 47 separate reports [384 patients]) *(8)*. More recently, one center reported a 36% failure rate in catheterizing both adrenal veins *(53)*. The cortisol concentrations from the adrenal veins and IVC are used to confirm sucessful catherterization. The adrenal vein/IVC cortisol ratio is typically greater than 10:1 (mean values at the Mayo Clinic are 32:1 on the right and 22:1 on the left). Dividing the right and left adrenal vein PACs by their respective cortisol concentrations corrects for the dilutional effect of the inferior phenic vein flow into the left adrenal vein; these are termed cortisol-corrected ratios (Fig. 9). In patients with APA, the mean cortisol-corrected aldosterone ratio (APA-side PAC/cortisol:normal adrenal PAC/cortisol) is 18:1 (range, 3.7:1 to 79:1). A cutoff of the cortisol-corrected aldosterone ratio from high side to low side of greater than 4:1 is used to indicate unilateral aldosterone excess (Fig. 10). Usually in patients with unilateral aldosterone excess, the contralateral aldosterone/cortisol ratio is less than the IVC aldosterone-cortisol ratios, which reflects a lower proportional contribution of aldosterone from the contralateral adrenal gland. In patients with IHA, the mean cortisol-corrected aldosterone ratio is 2:1 (high side:low side; range, 1:0 to 3:5); a ratio less than 3.0 to 1.0 is suggestive of bilateral aldosterone hypersecretion (Fig. 10). In patients with IHA, the low-side aldosterone-cortisol ratio is usually greater than in the IVC. With the selective use of adrenal venous sampling, unilateral APA has been found in 36% of those with clinically high-probability APA who had normal findings or unilateral adrenal limb thickening on CT. Adrenal venous sampling is essential to direct appropriate therapy for patients with primary aldosteronism who have a high probability of APA and CT findings of unilateral adrenal limb thickening.

#### Subtype Evaluation Tests of Historical Interest

Multiple tests and procedures were used to distinguish between APA and IHA before the development of the combined adrenal CT and adrenal venous sampling approach summarized above. At the Mayo Clinic, [$^{131}$I]-19-iodocholesterol scintigraphy *(58)* was first used in 1973, and

## Results of Bilateral Adrenal Vein Sampling

| Vein | Aldosterone (A) ng/dL | Cortisol (C) mcg/dL | A/C Ratio | Aldosterone Ratio* |
|---|---|---|---|---|
| RT Adrenal Vein | 582 | 1,745 | 0.3 | |
| LT Adrenal Vein | 7,762 | 1,235 | 6.3 | 21.0* |
| IVC | 62 | 45 | 1.4 | |

***Left adrenal vein A/C ratio divided by right adrenal vein A/C ratio.**
**IVC, inferior vena cava**

**Fig. 9.** Adrenal venous sampling data from a 40-year-old man with primary aldosteronism and normal adrenal glands seen with computed tomography. The patient had been hypertensive for 1 year, with poor control; his antihypertensive medication program included a calcium channel blocker and an α-adrenergic blocker. His screening test for primary aldosteronism was positive, with a mildly increased PAC of 25 ng/dL and low PRA at less than 0.6 ng/mL/h (PAC/PRA ratio >41). The 24-hour urinary excretion of aldosterone was increased at 26 μg (urinary sodium = 221 mEq/24 h). Because of his age and severity of hypertension, the possibility of a unilateral aldosterone-producing adenoma was pursued with adrenal venous sampling (AVS). AVS localized the tumor to the left adrenal gland. He had laparoscopic left adrenalectomy and a 0.5 × 1.0 cortical adenoma was found. The postoperative PAC was less than 1.0 ng/dL.

an improved agent, [6β-$^{131}$I]iodomethyl-19-norcholesterol (NP-59), was introduced in 1977 *(59)*. The NP-59 scan, performed with dexamethasone suppression, has the advantage of correlating function with anatomical abnormalities. However, its sensitivity depends heavily on the size of the adenoma *(60,61)*. Because tracer uptake is poor in adenomas less than 1.5 cm in diameter, NP-59 scintigraphy often is not helpful in interpreting micronodular findings obtained with high-resolution CT.

The posture stimulation test, also developed in the 1970s, is based on the finding that blood aldosterone levels in patients with APA have a diurnal variation and are relatively unaffected by changes in angiotensin II (Ang II) levels. In contrast, IHA is characterized by enhanced sensitivity to a small change in Ang II that occurs with standing. In a review of 16 reports in the literature, the accuracy of the posture stimulation test was 85% for 246 patients with surgically verified APA *(8)*. However, it became clear that some APAs are sensitive to Ang II, and some patients with IHA have diurnal variation in aldosterone secretion *(62)*. Also,

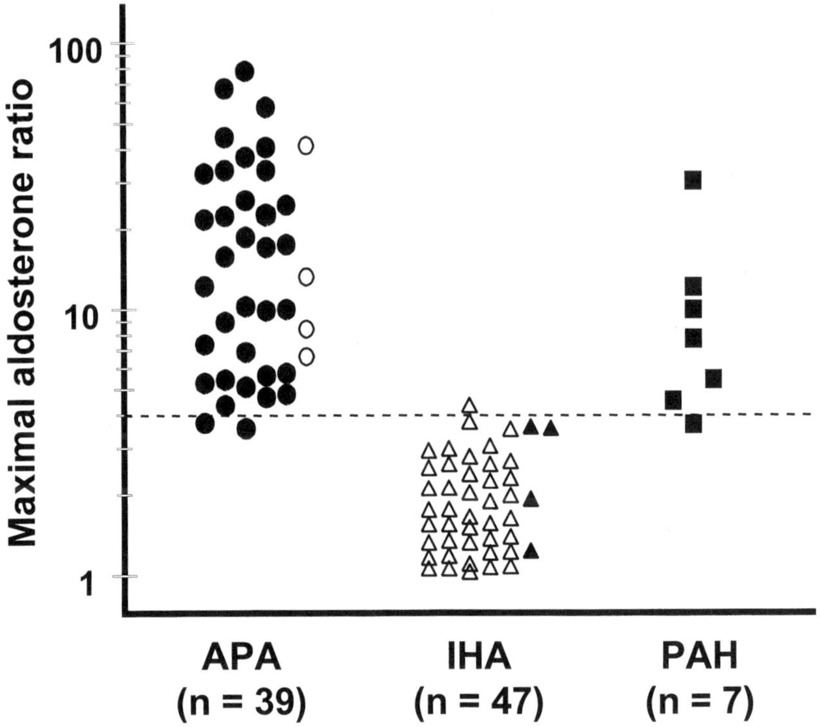


**Fig. 10.** Adrenal vein aldosterone ratios for 93 patients with unilateral APA, bilateral IHA, and unilateral PAH. Aldosterone levels were corrected for dilutional effects by dividing aldosterone concentrations by simultaneously obtained adrenal vein cortisol concentrations. The right adrenal vein was catherterized successfully in 93 of 100 patients. Solid symbols indicate patients with surgically confirmed disease. The dashed line indicates the cutoff of cortisol-corrected aldosterone ratio from high to low side (> 4:1). (Adapted from ref. *54*.).

although the posture stimulation test may predict which patient has APA, it does not assist in localization. Serum 18-hydroxycorticosterone (18-OHB) is considered to be either the immediate precursor of aldosterone or a separate end product formed after 18-hydroxylation of corticosterone *(63)*. Patients with APA generally have recumbent serum 18-OHB levels greater than 100 ng/dL at 0800 hours, whereas patients with IHA usually have less than 50 ng/dL *(64–66)*. The diagnostic accuracy of 18-OHB for APA is approximately 82% *(8)*. Serum 18-OHB levels serve as a surrogate for plasma aldosterone, which is also higher in patients with APA than in those with IHA.

It has become clear that, beyond historical interest, there is no role for many tests (e.g., NP-59 scintigraphy, posture stimulation test, and serum 18-OHB concentration) that have been standards in the subtype evaluation of primary aldosteronism.

### Familial Aldosteronism

Familial hyperaldosteronism type I is GRA and should be suspected in the following clinical situations: (a) primary aldosteronism is diagnosed in the first to third decades of life, (b) there is a family history of primary aldosteronism, or (c) there is a family history of cerebrovascular events at a young age (18% of 167 patients with proven GRA had cerebrovascular complications at an average age of 32 years) *(67)*. The majority of patients with familial hyperaldosteronism type 1 are normokalemic, a finding most likely explained by the diurnal nature of this disorder—"ACTH-dependent aldosterone excess by day and eualdosteronism by night" *(68)*. A 24-hour urine 18-hydroxycortisol excretion greater than 3,000 nmol *(25)* or direct genetic blood testing with Southern blotting or a long polymerase chain reaction technique to detect the chimeric gene *(69,70)* confirms the diagnosis.

Familial hyperaldosteronism type II is an autosomal dominant disorder of both IHA and APA. Thus far, 17 families (44 affected members with familial hyperaldosteronism type II) have been reported. In at least seven families, dominant inheritance is suggested *(71)*. In a recent study, seven patients from one kindred were screened for CYP11B1/CYP11B2 and CYP11B2 (aldo synthase gene on chromosome 8q), and all were negative for the defect *(72,73)*. A genomewide search was completed recently in a large family with familial hyperaldosteronism type II, and genetic linkage was identified with the polymorphic markers D7S511, D7S517, and GATA24F02 on chromosome 7 (7p22) *(72)*. The gene responsible for familial hyperaldosteronism type II has not been identified.

## REFERENCES

1. Conn JW. Presidential address: part I; painting background, Part II. Primary aldosteronism: a new clinical syndrome. J Lab Clin Med 1955;45:3–17.
2. Gordon RD, Stowasser M, Tunny TJ, et al. High incidence of primary aldosteronism in 199 patients referred with hypertension. Clin Exp Pharmacol Physiol 1994; 21:315–318.
3. Loh K-C, Koay ES, Khaw M-C, et al. Prevalence of primary aldosteronism among Asian hypertensive patients in Singapore. J Clin Endocrinol Metab 2000; 85:2854–2859.
4. Young WF Jr. Primary aldosteronism: a common and curable form of hypertension. Cardiology-in-Review 1999;7:207–214.

5. Stowasser M. Primary aldosteronism: rare bird or common cause of secondary hypertension? Curr Hypertens Rep 2001;3:230–239.
6. Schwartz, GL, Turner ST. Prevalence of unrecognized primary aldosteronism in essential hypertension. Am J Hypertension 2002;15:18A (abstract).
7. Calhoun DA, Nishizaka MK, Weissman P, et al. High prevalence of primary aldosteronism among black and white subjects with resistant hypertension. Am J Hypertension 2002;15:20A (abstract).
8. Young WF Jr, Klee GG. Primary aldosteronism: diagnostic evaluation. Endocrinol Metab Clin North Am 1988;17:367–395.
9. Young WF Jr, Hogan, MJ. Renin-independent hypermineralocorticoidism. Trends in Endocrinology and Metabolism 1994;5:97–106.
10. Ganguly A. Primary aldosteronism. N Engl J Med 1998;339:1828–1834.
11. Irony I, Kater CE, Biglieri EG, Shackleton CH. Correctable subsets of primary aldosteronism: primary adrenal hyperplasia and renin responsive adenoma. Am J Hypertens 1990;3:576–582.
12. Lifton RP, Dluhy RG, Powers M, et al. A chimaeric 11β-hydroxylase/aldosterone synthase gene causes glucocorticoid-remediable aldosteronism and human hypertension. Nature 1992;355:262–265.
13. Dluhy RG. Glucocorticoid-remediable aldosteronism. Endocrinologist 2001;11: 263–268.
14. Tanabe A, Naruse M, Naruse K, et al. Left ventricular hypertrophy is more prominent in patients with primary aldosteronism than in patients with other types of secondary hypertension. Hypertens Res 1997;20:85–90.
15. Rossi GP, Sacchetto A, Pava E, et al. Remodeling of the left ventricle in primary aldosteronism due to Conn's adenoma. Circulation 1997;95:1471–1478.
16. Shigematsu Y, Hamada M, Okayama H, et al. Left ventricular hypertrophy precedes other target-organ damage in primary aldosteronism. Hypertension 1997;29: 723–727.
17. Yoshihara F, Nishikimi T, Yoshitomi Y, et al. Left ventricular structural and functional characteristics in patients with renovascular hypertension, primary aldosteronism and essential hypertension. Am J Hypertens 1996;9:523–528.
18. Rizzoni D, Porteri E, Castellano M, et al. Vascular hypertrophy and remodeling in secondary hypertension. Hypertension 1996;28:785–790.
19. Rizzoni D, Muiesan ML, Porteri E, et al. Relations between cardiac and vascular structure in patients with primary and secondary hypertension. J Am Coll Cardiol 1998;32:985–992.
20. Abe M, Hamada M, Matsuoka H, et al. Myocardial scintigraphic characteristics in patients with primary aldosteronism. Hypertension 1994;23:I164–167.
21. Halimi JM, Mimran A. Albuminuria in untreated patients with primary aldosteronism or essential hypertension. J Hypertens 1995;13:1801–1802.
22. Torres VE, Young WF Jr, Offord KP, et al. Association of hypokalemia, aldosteronism, and renal cysts. N Engl J Med 1990;322:345–351.
23. Ogasawara M, Nomura K, Toraya S, et al. Clinical implications of renal cyst in primary aldosteronism. Endocr J 1996;43:261–268.
24. Duprez D, De Buyzere M, Reitzchel ER et al. Aldosterone and vascular damage. Curr Hypertens Rep 2000;2:327–334.
25. Nishimura M, Uzu T, Fujii T, et al. Cardiovascular complications in patients with primary aldosteronism. Am J Kidney Dis 1999;33:261–266.
26. Streeten DHP, Tomycz N, Anderson GH Jr. Reliability of screening methods for the diagnosis of primary aldosteronism. Am J Med 1979;67:403–413.

27. Rich GM, Ulick S, Cook S, et al. Glucocorticoid-remediable aldosteronism in a large kindred: clinical spectrum and diagnosis using a characteristic biochemical phenotype. Ann Intern Med 1992;116:813–820.
28. Gallay BJ, Ahmad S, Xu L, et al. Screening for primary aldosteronism without discontinuing hypertensive medications: plasma aldosterone-renin ratio. Am J Kidney Dis 2001;37:699–705.
29. Hiramatsu K, Yamada T, Yukimura Y, et al. A screening test to identify aldosterone-producing adenoma by measuring plasma renin activity.: results in hypertensive patients. Arch Intern Med 1981;141:1589–1593.
30. McKenna TJ, Sequeira SJ, Hefferanan A, et al. Diagnosis under random conditions of all disorders of the renin-angiotensin-aldosterone axis, including primary hyperaldosteronism. J Clin Endocrinol Metab 1991;73:952–957.
31. Brown MA, Cramp HA, Zammit VC, et al. Primary hyperaldosteronism: a missed diagnosis in "essential hypertensives"? Aust N Z J Med 1996;26:533–538.
32. Fardella C, Mosso L, Gomez-Sanchez C, et al. Primary hyperaldosteronism in essential hypertensives: prevalence, biochemical profile, and molecular biology. J Clin Endocrinol Metab 2000;85:1863–1867.
33. Gordon RD, Ziesak MD, Tunny TJ, et al. Evidence that primary aldosteronism may not be uncommon: 12% incidence among antihypertensive drug trial volunteers. Clin Exp Pharmacol Physiol 1993;20:296–298.
34. Hamlet SM, Tunny TJ, Woodland E, et al. Is aldosterone/renin ratio useful to screen a hypertensive population for primary aldosteronism? Clin Exp Pharmacol Physiol 1985;12:249–252.
35. Kreze A, Okalova D, Vanuga P, et al. Occurrence of primary aldosteronism in a group of ambulatory hypertensive patients. Vnitr Lek 1999;45:17–21.
36. Kumar A, Lall SB, Ammini A, et al. Screening of a population of young hypertensives for primary hyperaldosteronism. J Hum Hypertens 1994;8:731–732.
37. Lazurova I, Schwartz P, Trejbal D, et al. Incidence of primary hyperaldosteronism in hospitalized hypertensive patients. Bratisl Lek Listy 1999;100:200–203.
38. Lim P, Dow E, Jung R, et al. Prevalence of primary aldosteronism in the Tayside Hypertension Clinic population. J Hum Hypertens 2000;14:311–315.
39. Lim PO, Rodgers P, Cardale K, et al. Potentially high prevalence of primary aldosteronism in a primary-care population. Lancet 1999;353:40.
40. Mosso L, Fardella C, Montero J, et al. High prevalence of undiagnosed primary hyperaldosteronism among patients with essential hypertension [Alta prevalencia de hiperaldosteronismo primario no diagnosticado en hipertension catalogados como esenciales]. Rev Med Chile 1999;127:800–806.
41. Rossi GP, Rossi E, Pavan E, et al. Screening for primary aldosteronism with a logistic multivariate discriminant analysis. Clin Endocrinol 1998;49:713–723.
42. Montori VM, Young WF Jr. Use of plasma aldosterone concentration-to-plasma renin activity ratio as a screening test for primary aldosteronism: a systematic review of the literature. Endocrinol Metab Clin North America 2002;31:619–632.
43. Moneva MH, Gomez-Sanchez CE. Establishing a diagnosis of primary aldosteronism. Curr Op Endocrinol Diabetes 2001;8:124–129.
44. Gordon RD, Stowasser M, Rutherford JC. Primary aldosteronism: are we diagnosing and operating too few patients? World J Surg 2001;25:941–947.
45. Montori VM, Schwartz GL, Chapman AB, et al. Validity of the aldosterone-renin ratio used to screen for primary aldosteronism. Mayo Clin Proc 2001;76:877–882.
46. Trenkel S, Seifarth C, Schobel H, et al. Ratio of serum aldosterone to plasma renin concentration in essential hypertension and primary aldosteronism. Exp Clin Endocrinol Diabetes 2002;110:80–85.

47. Hirohara D. Nomura K, Okamoto T, et al. Performance of the basal aldosterone to renin ratio and of the renin stimulation test by furosemide and upright posture in screening for aldosterone-producing adenoma in low renin hypertensives. J Clin Endocrinol Metab 2001;86:4292–4298.
48. Weinberger MH, Fineberg NS. The diagnosis of primary aldosteronism and separation of two major subtypes. Arch Int Med 1993;153:2125–2129.
49. Holland O, Brown H, Kuhnert L, et al. Further evaluation of saline infusion for the diagnosis of primary aldosteronism. Hypertension 1984;6:717–723.
50. Bravo EL, Tarazi RC, Dustan et al. The changing clinical spectrum of primary aldosteronism. Am J Med 1983;74:641–651.
51. Sawka AM, Young WF Jr, Thompson GB, et al. Primary aldosteronism: factors associated with normalization of blood pressure after surgery. Ann Intern Med 2001;135:258–261.
52. Kloos RT, Gross MD, Francis IR, et al. Incidentally discovered adrenal masses. Endocrine Reviews 1995;16:460–484.
53. Blumenfeld JD, Sealey JE, Schlussel Y, et al. Diagnosis and treatment of primary aldosteronism. Ann Intern Med 1994;121:877–885.
54. Young WF Jr, Stanson AW, Grant CS, et al. Primary aldosteronism: adrenal venous sampling. Surgery 1996;120:913–920.
55. Magill SB, Raff H, Shaker JL, et al. Comparison of adrenal vein sampling and computed tomography in the differentiation of primary aldosteronism. J Clin Endocrinol Metab 2001;86:1066–1071.
56. Magill SB. Adrenal vein sampling: an overview. Endocrinologist 2001;11: 357–363.
57. Doppman JL, Gill JR Jr. Hyperaldosteronism: sampling the adrenal veins. Radiology 1996;198:309–312.
58. Conn JW, Beierwaltes WH, Lieberman LM, et al. Primary aldosteronism: preoperative tumor visualization by scintillation scanning. J Clin Endocrinol Metab 1971;33:713–716.
59. Miles JM, Wahner HW, Carpenter PC, et al. Adrenal scintiscanning with NP-59, a new radioiodinated cholesterol agent. Mayo Clin Proc 1979;54:321–327.
60. Hogan MJ, McRae J, Schambelan M, et al. Location of aldosterone-producing adenomas with I-19-iodocholesterol. N Engl J Med 1976;294:410–414.
61. Nomura K, Kusakabe K, Maki M, et al. Iodomethylnorcholesterol uptake in an aldosteronoma shown by dexamethasone-suppression scintigraphy: relationship to adenoma size and functional activity. J Clin Endcrinol Metab 1990;71:825–830.
62. Irony I, Kater CE, Biglieri EG, et al. Correctable subsets of primary aldosteronism: primary adrenal hyperplasia and renin responsive adenoma. Am J Hypertension 1990;3:576–582.
63. Fraser R, Lantos CP. 18-Hydroxycorticosterone: a review. J Steroid Biochem 1978;9:273–286.
64. Kem DC, Tang K, Hanson CS, et al. The prediction of anatomical morphology of primary aldosteronism using serum 18-hydroxycorticosterone levels. J Clin Endocrinol Metab 1985;60:67–73.
65. Phillips JL, Walther MM, Pezzullo JC, et al. Predictive value of preoperative tests in discriminating bilateral adrenal hyperplasia from an aldosterone producing adenoma. J Clin Endocrinol Metab 2000;85:4526–4533.
66. Biglieri EG, Schambelan M. The significance of elevated levels of plasma 18-hydroxy-corticosterone in patients with primary aldosteronism. J Clin Endocrinol Metab 1979;49:87–91.

67. Litchfield WR, Anderson BF, Weiss RJ, et al. Intracranial aneurysm and hemorrhagic stroke in glucocorticoid remediable aldosteronism. Hypertension 1998;31: 445–450.
68. Litchfield WR, Coolidge C, Silva P, et al. Impaired potassium-stimulated aldosterone production: a possible explanation for normokalemic glucocorticoid-remediable aldosteronism. J Clin Endocrinol Metab 1997;82:1507–1510.
69. Mulatero P, Veglio F, Pilon C, et al. Diagnosis of glucocorticoid-remediable aldosteronism in primary aldosteronism: aldosterone response to dexamethasone and long polymerase chain reaction for chimeric gene. J Clin Endocrinol 1998;83:2573–2575.
70. Stowasser M, Gartside MG, Gordon RD. A PCR-based method of screening individuals of all ages, from neonates to the elderly, for familial hyperaldosteronism type I. Aust N Z J Med 1997;27:685–690.
71. Gordon RD, Torpy DJ, Lafferty AR, et al. Familial hyperaldosteronism type II (FH-II) [abstract #S55-2]. In Program and Abstracts of 81st Annual Meeting of the Endocrine Society, San Diego, 1999.
72. Lafferty AR, Torpy DJ, Stowasser M, et al. A novel genetic locus for low renin hypertension: familial hyperaldosteronism type II maps to chromosome 7 (7p22). J Med Genetics 2000;37:831–835.
73. Torpy DJ, Gordon RD, Lin JP, et al. Familial hyperaldosteronism type II: description of a large kindred and exclusion of the aldosterone synthase (CYP11B2) gene. J Clin Endocrinol Metab 1998;83:3214–3218.

# 9 Medical Management of Primary Aldosteronism

*Emmanuel L. Bravo,* MD

*CONTENTS*



## INTRODUCTION

Traditionally, the treatment of choice for primary aldosteronism is the surgical excision of a unilaterally diseased adrenal gland (i.e., either tumor or hyperplasia). Medical therapy is used to reverse the metabolic and hemodynamic sequelae of aldosterone excess before surgery and in the long-term management of patients who are not surgical candidates. The latter include patients with bilateral disease who require bilateral adrenalectomy or who have associated comorbid conditions that preclude surgery. Some patients who are surgical candidates may choose medical management instead.

## PATHOPHYSIOLOGICAL AND THERAPEUTIC OPTIONS

Mineralocorticoids lead to fluid retention and might be expected to increase intravascular volume. Early studies have reported hypervolemia in primary aldosteronism, but this abnormality is not a universal finding. Many subjects have either low or normal intravascular volume (Fig. 1), and there is no correlation between arterial pressure and plasma or total blood volume in either men or women with untreated primary aldoster-

From: *Secondary Hypertension: Clinical Presentation, Diagnosis, and Treatment*
Edited by: G. A. Mansoor © Humana Press Inc., Totowa, NJ

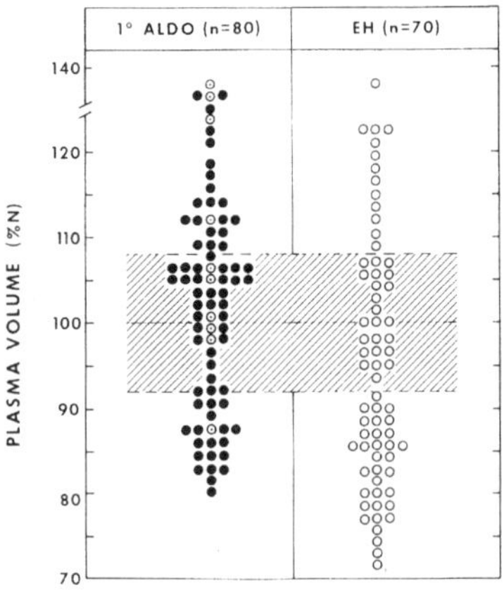


**Fig. 1.** Plasma volume values in patients with primary aldosteronism and age- and gender-matched essential hypertensive patients. Values are expressed as percent of normal because of naturally occurring gender differences. For patients with primary aldosteronism, black dots represent adenomas ($n$ = 70) and open triangles represent hyperplasia ($n$ = 10). The crosshatched area represents the variability of the method (i.e., ± 8%). In primary aldosteronism, there were as many patients who were hypovolemic (25%) as there were those who were hypervolemic (30%). (From ref. *1*.)

onism *(1)*. In contrast, there is an inverse correlation between volume and total peripheral resistance, similar to that reported in essential hypertension, renal arterial disease, and normal subjects. However, for any level of peripheral resistance, plasma volume (PV) is always greater in primary aldosteronism (Fig. 2) *(2)*. Additionally, with diuretic therapy, the arterial pressure response is directly and significantly related to the magnitude of intravascular volume alterations (Fig. 3) *(3)*.

Abnormalities in intravascular volume are associated with drug resistance in some patients with primary aldosteronism. In 12 out of 28 patients with primary aldosteronism (25 with a solitary adenoma) and resistant hypertension who were receiving three to seven drugs but were on small amounts of diuretic agents, hemodynamic studies revealed that PV was either normal or elevated despite marked elevations of total peripheral resistance (Fig. 4) *(4)*. The addition of spironolactone (200 mg/day) and hydrochlorothiazide (50–100 mg/day) to previous multiple-drug therapy reduced blood pressure (BP) significantly in all 28 patients. The reduction in BP was associated with a concomitant decrease in intravascular volume (Fig. 5) *(4)*.

Drugs that suppress sympathetic vasomotor activity have the potential of increasing PV, which diminishes their therapeutic effectiveness *(5)*. The studies that show this emphasize how potent this influence can

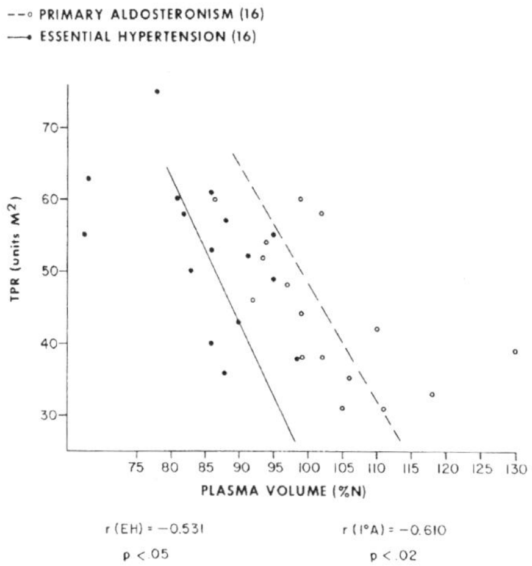


**Fig. 2.** Correlation between plasma volume (PV) and total peripheral resistance (TPR) in patients with primary aldosteronism and those with hypovolemic essential hypertension. The slopes of the regression equations defining the two lines are not significantly different from each other, but the intercepts are. For any level of TPR, PV is always greater in primary aldosteronism. Primary aldosteronism ($n = 16$; $r = -0.531$; $p < 0.05$); essential hypertension ($n = 16$; $r = -0.610$; $p < 0.02$). (From ref. *2*.)

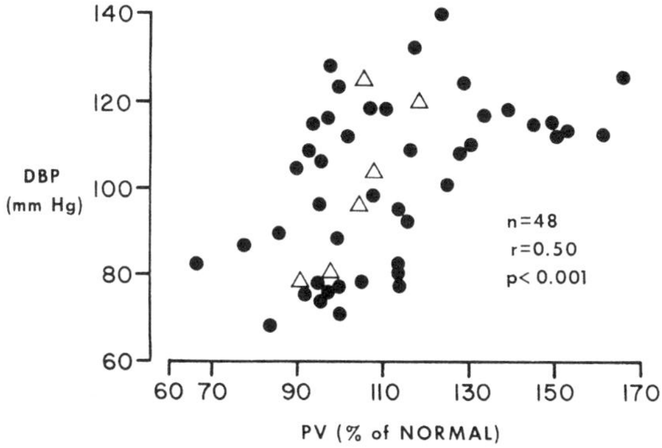


**Fig. 3.** Relationship between diastolic blood pressure (DBP) and plasma volume (PV) in 10 patients (48 determinations) with primary aldosteronism during long-term treatment periods with spironolactone alone (triangles) or in combination with either hydrochlorothiazide or low dietary sodium. Data were obtained over a period of 6 weeks to 6 years. PV is expressed in percent of normal because of naturally occurring gender differences. (From ref. *3*.)

become, given that the amounts of diuretic agents that usually are adequate to prevent fluid retention in essential hypertensives fail to do so in patients with primary aldosteronism. Additionally, they reiterate an

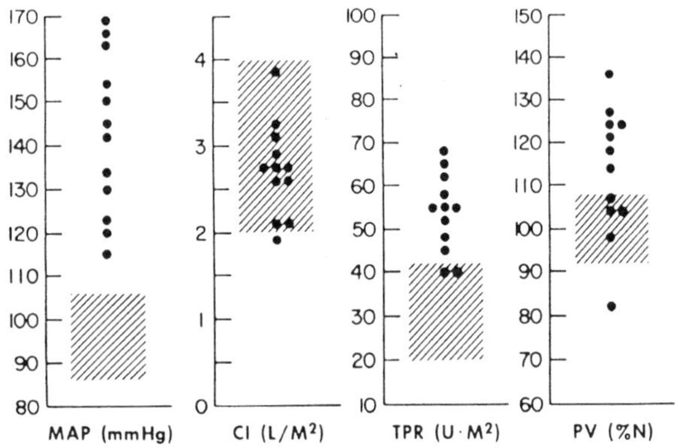


**Fig. 4.** Hemodynamic characteristics of primary aldosteronism ($n$ = 12) with refractory hypertension. At the time of the study, patients were on three to seven different drugs in combination. Despite marked increases in mean arterial pressure, patients were either normovolemic or hypervolemic. MAP, mean arterial pressure; CI, cardiac index; TPR, total peripheral resistance; PV, plasma volume; % *N*, percent of normal. (From ref. *4*.)

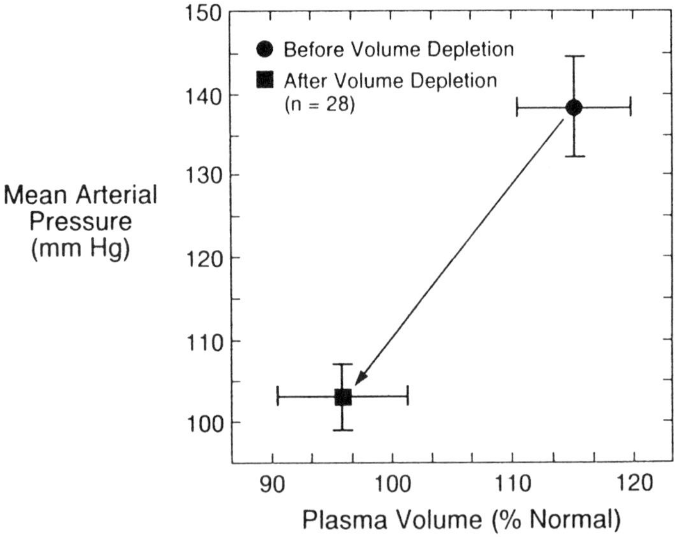


**Fig. 5.** The effect of volume depletion in patients with primary aldosteronism and resistant hypertension. Spironolactone (100 mg BID) and hydrochlorothiazide (25–50 mg BID) were added to current therapy. Blood pressure (mean arterial pressure [MAP]) and plasma volume (PV) were then obtained before and after 8 to 12 weeks of continued therapy. MAP was significantly reduced in all; as a group it fell from 138 ± 2 to 102 ± 9 (SE) mmHg. Associated with reductions in MAP were decreases in PV (from 114 ± 3 to 97 ± 2 [SE] % of normal, $p < 0.01$). (From ref. *4*.)

important therapeutic principle that salt- and water-dependent hypertension responds poorly to antihypertensive agents that cause fluid retention or fail to reduce the existing hypervolemia *(6,7)*. These drugs include those that decrease sympathetic motor activity, angiotension-converting enzyme inhibitors, direct arteriolar vasodilators, and calcium channel blockers.

The aforementioned studies strongly indicate that hypertension associated with primary aldosteronism is salt and water dependent and is best treated by aggressive and sustained salt and water depletion.

### *Short-Term Medical Therapy*

Patients undergoing surgery should receive drug treatment for at least 8 to 10 weeks, both to decrease BP and to correct metabolic abnormalities. These patients have significant potassium deficiency that must be corrected preoperatively because hypokalemia increases the risk of cardiac arrhythmia during anesthesia. Prolonged reduction of arterial BP permits the use of intravenous fluids during surgery without producing hypertension and decreases morbidity. Administration of medications is continued until surgery, and glucocorticoid administration is not needed before surgery.

Spironolactone, 100–200 mg/day, or amiloride, 10–20 mg/day, is administered the first 2 weeks, then either hydrochlorothiazide, 25–50 mg/day, or furosemide, 80–160 mg/day is added. This combination results in prompt correction of hypokalemia and normalization of arterial BP within 1 to 2 weeks (Fig. 6) *(3)*. These agents may be added to current β-blocker or vasodilator therapy.

After removal of an aldosterone-producing tumor, selective hypoaldosteronism usually occurs, even in patients whose plasma renin activity had been stimulated with chronic diuretic therapy *(8)*. Therefore, serum potassium values should be monitored closely and potassium supplementation should be given cautiously, if at all. Sufficient residual mineralocorticoid activity often is left to prevent excessive renal retention of potassium provided that adequate sodium intake is maintained. If serum potassium values rise above 5.5 mEq/L, administration of furosemide, 80–160 mg/day, should be started. Treatment with fludrocortisone is often not necessary. If it is needed, 0.1 mg/day may be used as the initial dose. Abnormalities in aldosterone production can persist for as long as 3 to 6 months after tumor removal.

### *Long-Term Medical Therapy*

The use of potassium-sparing agents along with diuretics and other antihypertensive agents as needed can control BP and maintain normal serum potassium concentration over long periods. The efficacy of long-

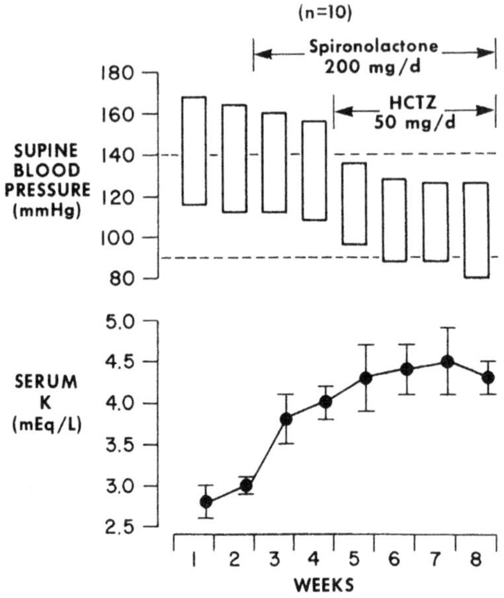


**Fig. 6.** The effect of spironolactone combined with hydrochlorothiazide on blood pressure (BP) and serum potassium concentration in patients with aldosterone-producing tumors ($n = 6$). The mean systolic and diastolic BP were not different from control during administration of spironolactone alone, although a significant rise in serum potassium concentration occurred as early as the first week of therapy. The addition of hydrochlorothiazide significantly decreased BP but did not alter serum potassium concentration. (From ref. *8*.)

term medical management of aldosterone-producing adenomas was recently demonstrated in a retrospective cohort study *(9)* of 24 patients who were treated medically for at least 5 years. The clinical and biochemical data of these patients is shown in Table 1. Patients were followed at 3- to 6-month intervals as outpatients. The final measurement of BP and potassium corresponded with the interim measurements of followup. Therefore, the last measurement taken was used in this study.

At the time of initial diagnosis, the mean systolic BP was 175 ± 2.3 (SE) mmHg (range 150–200 mmHg) and the mean diastolic BP was 106 ± 2.6 (SE) mmHg (range 92–132 mmHg). The mean serum potassium concentration was 3.0 ± 0.07 (SE) nmol/L (range 2.4 to 3.9 nmol/L). The sizes of adrenal tumors on presentation ranged from 0.5 cm to 2.4 cm. The median duration of followup was 8 years (range 5 to 17 years).

At the time of the most recent followup, the mean systolic BP was 129 ± 3.4 (SE) mmHg (range 101–118 mmHg) (95% confidence interval (CI) for difference, 37.1–53 mmHg) and the mean diastolic BP was 79

Table 1
Clinical and Biochemical Data

| Patient | Age (yrs) | Gender | FU (yrs) | BP at presentation* (mmHg) | Most recent BP* (mmHg) | Electrolyte levels at time of diagnosis (mmol/L) | | | | Electrolyte levels at last follow-up (mmol/L) | | | |
|---|---|---|---|---|---|---|---|---|---|---|---|---|---|
| | | | | | | Na | K | Cl– | $CO_2$ | Na | K | Cl– | $CO_2$ |
| 1 | 65 | male | 5 | 170/04 | 120/80 | 145 | 3.1 | 105 | 30 | 140 | 5.2 | 110 | 28 |
| 2 | 69 | male | 12 | 164/65 | 157/86 | 141 | 3.2 | 98 | 35 | 141 | 3.9 | 104 | 30 |
| 3 | 63 | male | 11 | 178/96 | 130/95 | 141 | 2.9 | 100 | 28 | 14 | 4.0 | 107 | 26 |
| 4 | 42 | female | 8 | 180/104 | 124/82 | 140 | 3.0 | 98 | 31 | 137 | 4.1 | 105 | 25 |
| 5 | 39 | female | 5 | 184/132 | 128/80 | 141 | 3.9 | 102 | 29 | 140 | 3.7 | 106 | 28 |
| 6 | 76 | male | 9 | 174/100 | 116/74 | 143 | 2.9 | 104 | 29 | 139 | 4.7 | 103 | 23 |
| 7 | 68 | male | 6 | 180/105 | 155/76 | 140 | 3.1 | 98 | 32 | 142 | 4.2 | 109 | 28 |
| 8 | 69 | male | 5 | 190/95 | 130/70 | 144 | 2.9 | 103 | 29 | 140 | 4.1 | 104 | 21 |
| 9 | 59 | male | 7 | 180/116 | 145/99 | 144 | 2.4 | 102 | 35 | 139 | 4.3 | 104 | 30 |
| 10 | 55 | male | 8 | 180/110 | 140/74 | 145 | 3.0 | 102 | 30 | 142 | 4.6 | 104 | 30 |
| 11 | 59 | male | 6 | 165/102 | 112/68 | 142 | 3.0 | 106 | 30 | 142 | 4.8 | 108 | 30 |
| 12 | 50 | male | 6 | 117/117 | 115/80 | 144 | 3.1 | 102 | 3.1 | 143 | 4.5 | 104 | 27 |
| 13 | 44 | male | 6 | 160/110 | 130/82 | 141 | 3.0 | 106 | 29 | 140 | 4.3 | 103 | 29 |
| 14 | 64 | female | 8 | 160/98 | 142/60 | 144 | 3.4 | 106 | 29 | 142 | 4.7 | 108 | 25 |
| 15 | 52 | female | 13 | 150/104 | 104/76 | 142 | 3.3 | 105 | 24 | 137 | 4.4 | 106 | 25 |
| 16 | 52 | female | 5 | 168/102 | 128/91 | 143 | 2.7 | 102 | 32 | 141 | 3.6 | 106 | 32 |
| 17 | 54 | female | 17 | 180/110 | 101/71 | 143 | 3.0 | 105 | 33 | 139 | 4.4 | 101 | 30 |
| 18 | 59 | male | 8 | 176/116 | 158/78 | 142 | 2.6 | 106 | 29 | 138 | 4.6 | 101 | 27 |
| 19 | 44 | female | 9 | 190/122 | 122/78 | 142 | 2.6 | 98 | 32 | 137 | 3.6 | 98 | 26 |

(continued)

**Table 1 (*Continued*)**
**Clinical and Biochemical Data**

| | *Age* | | *FU* | *BP at presentation** | *Most recent BP** | *Electrolyte levels at time of diagnosis (mmol/L)* | | | | *Electrolyte levels at last follow-up (mmol/L)* | | | |
|---|---|---|---|---|---|---|---|---|---|---|---|---|---|
| *Patient* | *(yrs)* | *Gender* | *(yrs)* | *(mmHg)* | *(mmHg)* | *Na* | *K* | *Cl–* | *$CO_2$* | *Na* | *K* | *Cl–* | *$CO_2$* |
| 20 | 61 | female | 14 | 160/110 | 144/72 | 145 | 2.9 | 103 | 35 | 140 | 3.7 | 113 | 29 |
| 21 | 68 | female | 5 | 166/108 | 111/78 | 143 | 2.6 | 103 | 30 | 146 | 4.6 | 108 | 26 |
| 22 | 66 | male | 11 | 178/108 | 150/92 | 141 | 3.0 | 101 | 31 | 142 | 3.8 | 102 | 26 |
| 23 | 73 | male | 10 | 178/100 | 107/66 | 143 | 3.8 | 99 | 31 | 143 | 4.8 | 105 | 24 |
| 24 | 56 | male | 15 | 200/125 | 128/85 | 141 | 3.2 | 102 | 32 | 139 | 4.6 | 102 | 26 |

* Blood pressure values are the average of at least three measurements. From ref. *9*.
BP, blood pressure; Cl–, chloride; $CO_2$, carbon dioxide; FU, follow-up; K, potassium; Na, sodium.

± 1.9 (range 60–99 mmHg) (95% CI for difference, 20.8–33.9 mmHg). After treatment, the mean serum potassium concentration was 4.3 ± 0.09 (SE) nmol/L (range 3.6–5.2 nmol/L) (95% CI for difference, 1.1–1.5 nmol/L). Four patients were receiving a single potassium-sparing diuretic, 13 were receiving a potassium-sparing diuretic and one other antihypertensive agent, six were receiving a total of three antihypertensive agents, and one was receiving four antihypertensive medications.

During followup, there were no incidences of strokes, myocardial infarctions, or cardiac failures. None of the patients experienced any malignant transformation of their tumors. Only 5 of the 24 patients had a noticeable (≥ 0.5 cm) increase in size of the adrenal tumor as measured by computed tomography.

The morbidity seen with medical management of aldosterone-producing adenomas relates to the side-effect profiles of potassium-sparing diuretics. The most common side effects noted for spironolactone therapy were breast tenderness, breast engorgement, and muscle cramps. Less frequent adverse effects include decreased libido, inability to sustain an erection, menstrual irregularity, axillary hair loss, and irritability. These adverse events were unrelated to dose. The only side effect noted with amiloride was muscle cramping.

These observations show that medical management of aldosterone-producing adenomas in reliable patients is an acceptable alternative to surgery if such therapy is warranted by overriding comorbid conditions or strong preferences. However, if surgery can eliminate the need for medication altogether, it should be considered foremost, before medical treatment is chosen *(10)*.

## REFERENCES


1. Bravo EL, Tarazi RC, Dustan HP, et al. The changing clinical spectrum of primary aldosteronism. Am J Med 1983;74:641–651.
2. Tarazi RC, Ibrahim MM, Bravo EL, Dustan HP. Hemodynamic characteristics of primary aldosteronism. N Engl J Med 1973;289:1330–1335.
3. Bravo EL, Dustan HP, Tarazi RC. Spironolactone as a nonspecific treatment for primary aldosteronism. Circulation 1973;48:491–498.
4. Bravo EL, Fouad-Tarazi FM, Tarazi RC, Pohl M, Gifford RW Jr, Vidt DG. Clinical implications of primary aldosteronism with resistant hypertension. Hypertension 1988;11:I207–I211.
5. Dustan HP, Tarazi RC, Bravo EL. Dependence of arterial pressure on intravascular volume in treated hypertensive patients. N Engl J Med 1972;286:861–866.
6. Bravo EL, Tarazi RC, Dustan HP, Fouad FM. The sympathetic nervous system and hypertension in primary aldosteronism. Hypertension 1985;7:90–96.
7. Bravo EL, Fouad FM, Tarazi RC. Calcium channel blockade with nifedipine in primary aldosteronism. Hypertension 1986;8(Suppl I):I191.

8. Bravo EL. Primary aldosteronism: issues in diagnosis and management. Endocrinol Metab Clin N Am 1994:23(2):271–283.
9. Ghose RP, Hall PM, Bravo EL. Medical management of aldosterone-producing adenomas. Ann Intern Med 1999;131:105–108.
10. Brown JJ, Davies DL, Ferriss JB, et al. Comparison of surgery and prolonged spironolactone therapy in patients with hypertension, aldosterone excess, and low plasma renin. Br Med J 1972;2:729–734.

# 10 Primary Aldosteronism

## *Surgical Approaches*

*Mihir M. Desai,* MD
*and Inderbir S. Gill,* MD

**CONTENTS**



## INTRODUCTION

Primary hyperaldosteronism, the hypersecretion of aldosterone by the adrenal gland, most commonly results from a unilateral adrenocortical adenoma (aldosteronoma). Less frequently, primary hyperaldosteronism may result from bilateral adrenal hyperplasia or an adrenocortical carcinoma. Although relatively uncommon, aldosteronoma represents a surgically correctable cause of secondary hypertension. The advent of laparoscopy has resulted in a significant change in the surgical management of aldosteronoma. In this chapter, we describe the indications, various surgical approaches, and worldwide results of the surgical management of primary hyperaldosteronism.

From: *Secondary Hypertension: Clinical Presentation, Diagnosis, and Treatment*
Edited by: G. A. Mansoor © Humana Press Inc., Totowa, NJ

## INDICATIONS FOR SURGERY

### *Unilateral Adrenal Adenoma*

Surgical excision is indicated in all cases of primary hyperaldosteronism caused by a unilateral adrenal adenoma, which may account for approximately 60% of cases of primary hyperaldosteronism. Currently, sensitive imaging techniques such as thin slice spiral computed tomography and magnetic resonance imaging are sensitive methods for diagnosing an adrenal adenoma in a patient with biochemical evidence of aldosterone hypersecretion. The majority of aldosteronomas are small, with more than 80% being less than 3 cm in size. As a result, these tumors are particularly amenable to surgical excision.

### *Adrenal Hyperplasia*

Adrenal hyperplasia, usually accounting for 40% of cases of primary hyperaldosteronism, is generally treated medically with spironolactone or another potassium-sparing diuretic. A certain variant of adrenal hyperplasia, which is unresponsive to angiotensin II (Ang II), may be cured by surgical excision if there is lateralization to one adrenal gland. Postural biochemical testing, estimation of C-18 methyl oxidation metabolites of cortisol (18-oxocortisol and 18-hydroxycortisol) in the urine, and selective adrenal vein aldosterone sampling may be beneficial in identifying this subset of patients with angiotensin-unresponsive adrenal hyperplasia that may be cured after a unilateral adrenalectomy *(1)*. Rarely, bilateral adrenalectomy may be indicated in patients with bilateral adrenal hyperplasia and severe hypertension and/or hypokalemia that are refractory to medical treatment.

### *Adrenocortical Carcinoma*

Occasionally, adrenocortical carcinoma may present with features of mineralocorticoid excess. These tumors are generally large (>5 cm), and are best treated with wide surgical excision, whenever technically feasible.

## SURGICAL ANATOMY

The adrenal glands are paired retroperitoneal organs that lie within Gerota's fascia, separated from the upper pole of the kidney by a fibrous layer. Both adrenal glands differ in their location, size and shape, anatomical relations, and vascular supply.

The right adrenal gland is triangular in shape and lies above the upper pole of the kidney. Despite the right kidney being lower than the left, the right adrenal gland is located higher in the retroperitoneum compared to the left side. The right adrenal gland is related to the liver superiorly, kidney inferolaterally, inferior vena cava medially, duodenum and liver anteriorly, and diaphragm and pleura posteriorly. The right adrenal gland derives its arterial supply from the inferior phrenic artery (superior supply), aorta (middle supply), and right renal artery (inferior supply). The arterial branches arborize near the adrenal gland, forming a vascular network, which enters the gland at the superior and medial aspect *(2)*. The right adrenal gland is drained by a single short and wide adrenal vein, which exits the superior pole of the adrenal gland and enters the posterolateral aspect of the inferior vena cava.

The left adrenal gland is crescentic in shape and is situated lower than the right adrenal gland along the medial border of the upper pole of the left kidney. It is related to the spleen superiorly, tail of the pancreas anteriorly, diaphragm and pleura posteriorly, and aorta medially. The left adrenal gland lies at a slight distance from the aorta in contrast to the right adrenal gland, which is much more closely approximated to the wall of the inferior vena cava. The arterial supply to the left adrenal gland is similar to the right side, being derived from the left inferior phrenic artery, aorta, and left renal artery. The left adrenal vein, in contrast to the right side, is longer and narrower, and drains via the inferior phrenic vein into the superior border of the main left renal vein.

## SURGICAL APPROACHES

Recently, laparoscopic techniques have largely supplanted open adrenalectomy for the surgical management of hyperaldosteronism.

### *Laparascopic Adrenalectomy*

Since Gagner's initial report in 1992 *(3)*, laparoscopic adrenalectomy has evolved as the current standard of care for most adrenal tumors with the possible exception of large, infiltrating cancers. Aldosteronomas, owing to their small size, are particularly amenable to laparoscopic excision. Laparoscopic adrenalectomy has been successfully performed both transperitoneally and retroperitoneally.

#### Transperitoneal Laparoscopic Adrenalectomy *(4,5)*

The transperitoneal technique is performed with the patient secured in the 45° oblique position. Pneumoperitoneum is initially created by either the veress needle or open technique. Typically the procedure is performed using three to five ports, which are illustrated in Fig. 1.

**Transperitoneal Right Adrenalectomy (Fig. 2).** The liver is retracted cephalad, and a transverse incision is made in the posterior parietal peritoneum parallel to and 1 to 2 cm below the inferior edge of

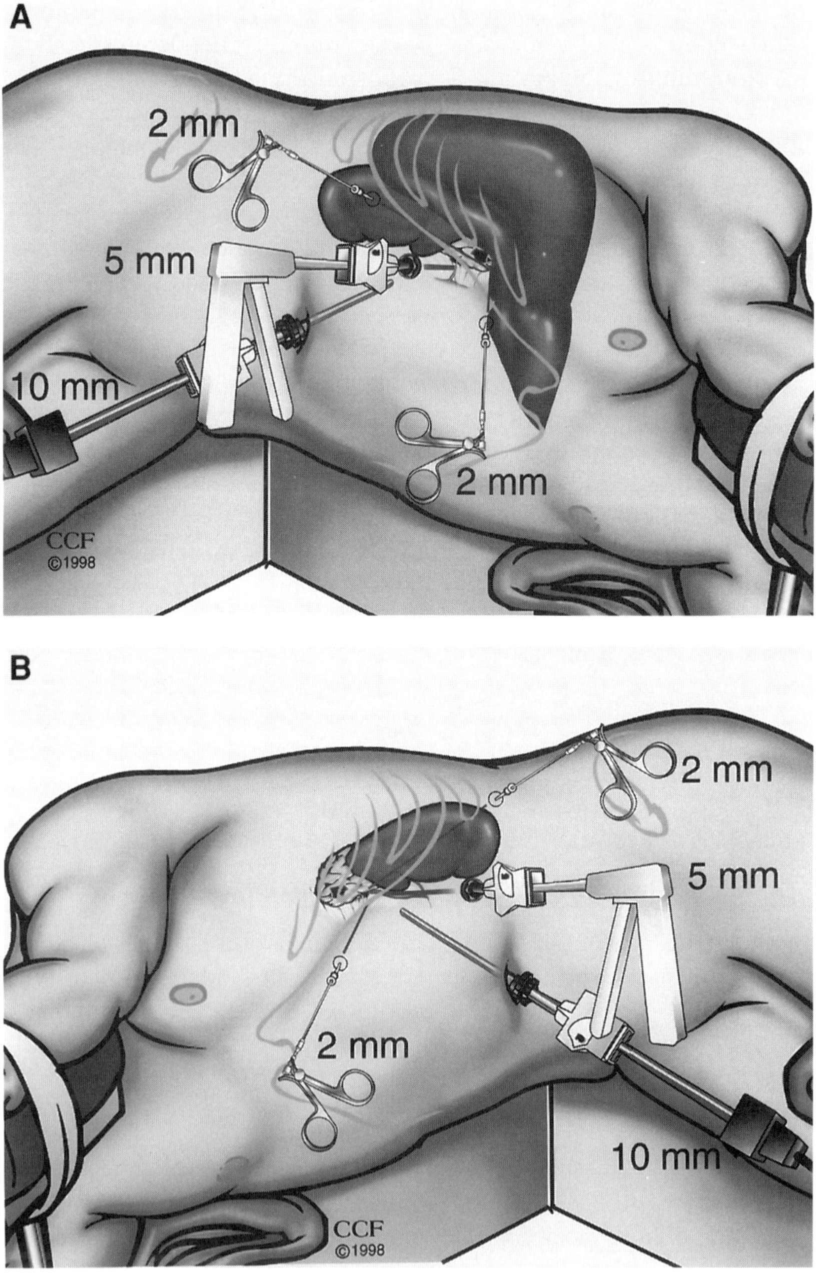


**Fig. 1.** Patient positioning and port placement for transperitoneal laparoscopic adrenalectomy. **(A)** Right-sided transperitoneal adrenalectomy is performed with the patient in a 45° flank position using four ports. A 12 mm primary camera port, a 5 mm left-hand port, a 12 mm right-hand port, and a 5 mm liver

the liver. Extending from the line of Toldt laterally to the inferior vena cava medially, this incision allows access into the retroperitoneum directly onto the anterior surface of the adrenal gland. Virtually no mobilization of the hepatic flexure of the colon is required to expose the right adrenal gland. Typically, dissection is initiated between the medial border of the adrenal gland and the right lateral edge of the inferior vena cava, where the main adrenal vein is identified, clipped, and divided. Superiorly, the gland is freed from the undersurface of the diaphragm by clipping the branches from the inferior phrenic vessels. Inferiorly, adrenal branches of the renal artery are controlled and the gland is completely freed. The adrenal gland is entrapped within an impermeable sac and extracted intact.

**Transperitoneal Left Adrenalectomy (Fig. 3).** In contrast to the right side, the transperitoneal approach to the left adrenal gland requires formal mobilization of the spleen, splenic flexure, descending colon, and tail of the pancreas. The procedure begins with identification and clipping of the adrenal vein draining into the superior border of the left renal vein. Multiple aortic, renal hilar, and inferior phrenic branches supplying the adrenal gland are meticulously controlled, completely freeing the adrenal gland.

Basso et al recently reported on a technique of supragastric left adrenalectomy *(6)*. This technique involves division of the gastro-phrenic ligament and one or two short gastric vessels in order to mobilize the gastric fundus. The gastric fundus is then pulled down, thereby exposing the left

---

**Fig. 1.** (*continued*) retraction port. An additional 2 mm port may be placed in the flank laterally to aid retraction. **(B)** Patient position for a left-sided transperitoneal adrenalectomy is identical to that on the right side. The 5 mm port for liver retraction, however, is not required.

**Fig. 2.** (*Figures on next page*) Right transperitoneal laparoscopic adrenalectomy. **(A)** Initially, a peritoneal incision is made inferior to the liver to expose the suprarenal vena cava and main adrenal vein. The liver is retracted cephalad during the entire procedure to provide optimal exposure of the adrenal gland. Very minimal mobilization of the right colon and hepatic flexure is required on the right side. **(B)** The adrenal gland is gradually dissected from the vena cava to which it is closely approximated. During this part of the mobilization, small aortic branches, entering the adrenal gland from behind the vena cava, are controlled and divided. This exposes the main adrenal vein. **(C)** The main adrenal vein is clipped and the adrenal gland completely mobilized after dividing the superior (inferior phrenic) and inferior (renal) adrenal vascular supply. **(D)** The completely mobilized adrenal gland is entrapped in an impermeable 10 mm Endocatch bag and extracted intact.

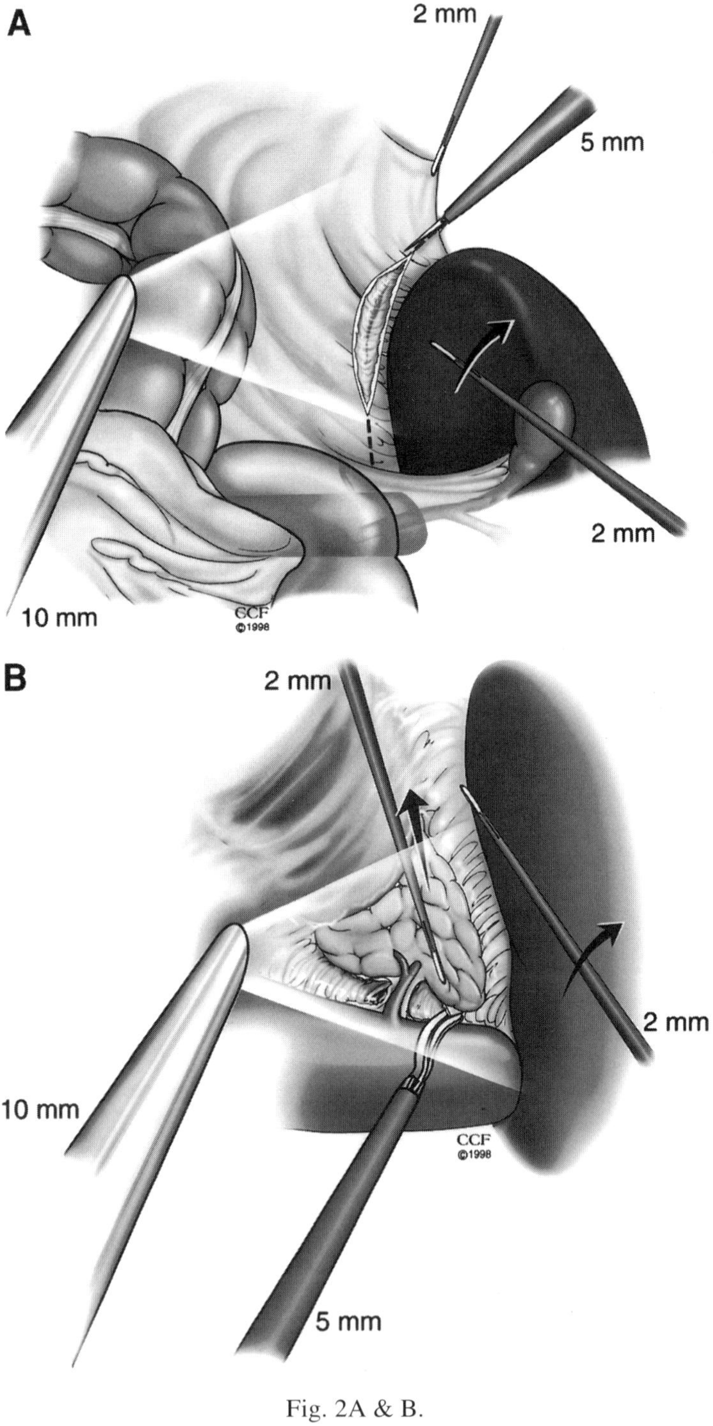


Fig. 2A & B.

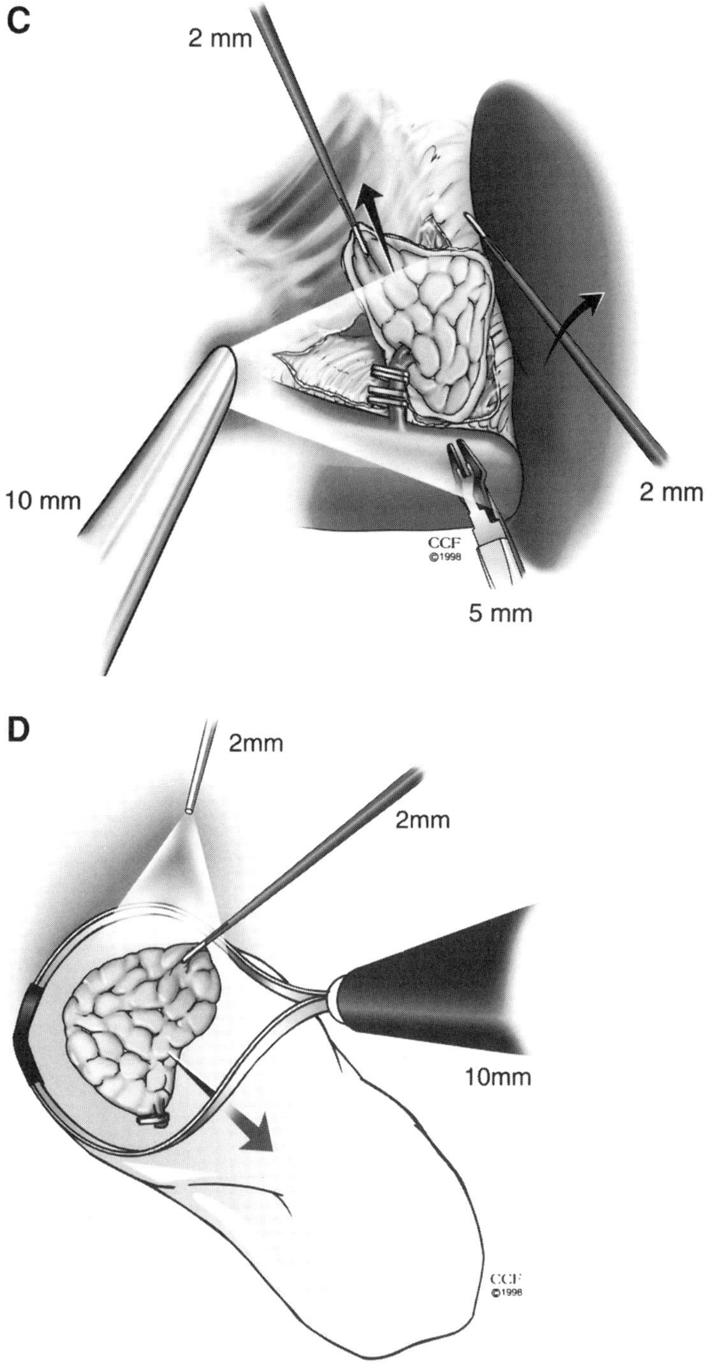


Fig. 2C & D.

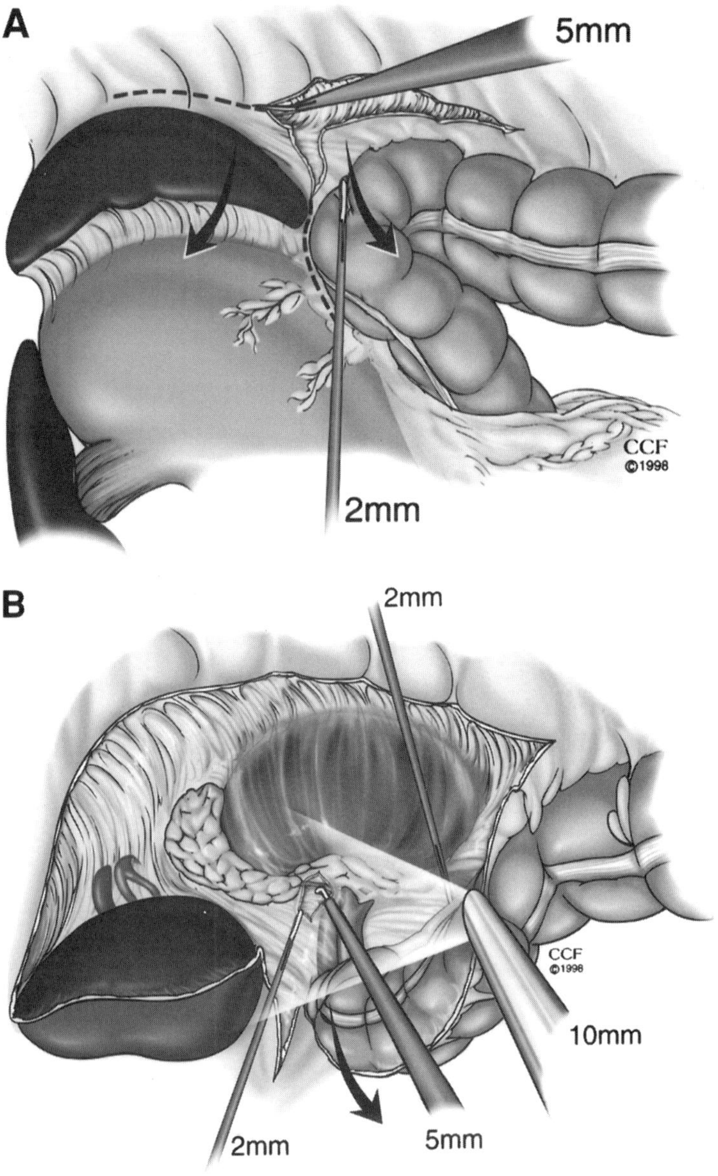


**Fig. 3.** Laparoscopic transperitoneal left adrenalectomy. **(A)** A T-shaped peritoneal incision is made as shown in the figure. The left colon and spleen require significant mobilization for adequate exposure of the left adrenal gland. **(B)** The main adrenal vein is identified at the superior border of the main left renal vein. **(C)** The main adrenal vein is clipped and divided. The adrenal gland is dissected from the upper pole of the kidney by dividing the arterial supply from the renal artery. Subsequently, the posterior surface of the adrenal is mobilized in an avascular plane. **(D)** The medial border of the adrenal gland is

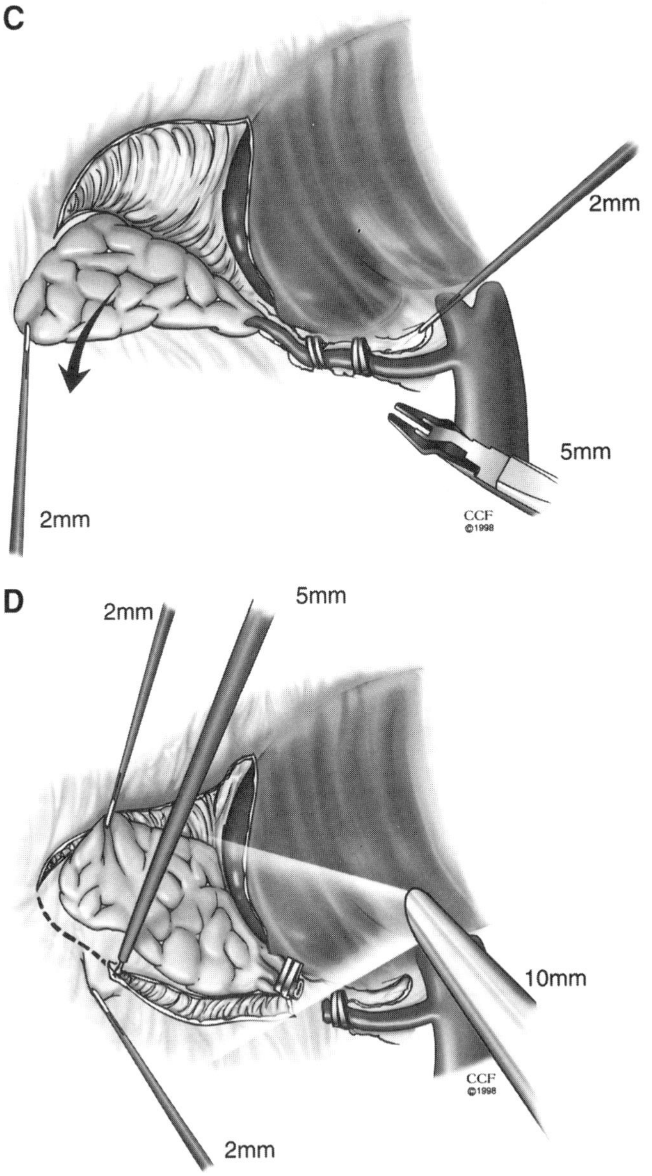


**Fig. 3.** (*continued*) mobilized by dividing aortic branches, and the superior pole is mobilized by dividing the inferior phrenic branches, thereby completing the adrenalectomy. (**Note:** The 2 mm instruments shown in Figs. 3 and 4 are used during needlescopic adrenalectomy, which is the author's preference for most transperitoneal adrenalectomies. However, 5 mm instruments may be employed in place of the 2 mm instruments for performing a transperitoneal adrenalectomy. The operative steps, as outlined above, remain the same regardless of whether 2 mm instruments are used.)

adrenal gland. The authors suggested that the supragastric approach avoided mobilization of the spleen, splenic flexure, and descending colon, which may be a potential advantage over conventional transperitoneal left adrenalectomy. They reported the use of this approach in six patients. The mean operative time was 126 minutes and the mean hospital stay was 4.1 days, and there were no conversions or complications. However, this is the only report of this approach in the literature, and a comparative analysis with conventional laparoscopic adrenalectomy is necessary to objectively assess the proposed merits of the supragastric approach.

**Technical Results of Transperitoneal Laparoscopic Adrenalectomy.** At the time of this writing, more than 500 laparoscopic transperitoneal adrenalectomies have been reported in the literature. A recent review analyzing 147 transperitoneal laparoscopic adrenalectomies reported a mean operative time of 3.4 hours, mean blood loss of 191 mL, and intraoperative transfusion rate of 2%. Mean hospital stay and mean convalescence were 2.9 days and 16 days, respectively *(7)*. Major and minor complications occurred in 3 and 20%, respectively. A multi-institutional study by Yoshida et al analyzed complications occurring in 369 laparoscopic adrenalectomies performed at nine centers from January 1992 to September 1996 *(8)*. No mortality was reported. Thirty-two intraoperative complications occurred in 31 patients (9%). Vascular injuries occurred in 20 cases (5%) and included injury to the inferior vena cava (2), renal vein (2), main adrenal vein (4), and other adrenal vessels (12). Organ injuries occurred in 11 patients (3%) and included liver (4), spleen (3), pancreas (2), gall bladder (1), and ipsilateral adrenal gland (1). Postoperative complications occurred in 24 patients (6.5%): hemorrhage (6), wound infection (4), atelectasis (3), ileus (2), chylocele (1), asthma (1), pulmonary effusion (1), angina (1), hyperventilation (1), delirium (1), compartment syndrome (1), urinary retention (1), and peritonitis (1). The authors concluded that the majority of the complications were minor in nature and could be managed either conservatively or laparoscopically. Conversion to open surgery was necessary in 14 patients (3.8%).

### Retroperitoneal Laparoscopic Adrenalectomy

Retroperitoneal adrenalectomy can be performed through either the lateral *(9)* or posterior approach *(10–12)*, the former being more commonly used.

**Lateral Approach.** In the lateral approach, the patient is secured in the standard (90°) flank position. Initial retroperitoneal access is obtained, by finger dissection, through an incision placed below the tip of the 12th rib. A working space is created in the retroperitoneum, between the Gerota's fascia and transversalis fascia, with the balloon dilation technique using a PDB Balloon Dilator (Origin Medical, Menlo Park, CA). A 10 mm blunt-tip balloon port is placed through the initial access site, and the balloon is inflated and cinched down to create a tight seal around the abdominal wall and prevent leakage of gas. Two additional working ports are placed under direct laparoscopic vision for the right- and left-hand instruments.

**Posterior Approach.** In the posterior approach, the patient is placed prone in a semi jackknife position, and three ports are placed directly posterior along the undersurface of the 12th rib.

**Retroperitoneoscopic Right Adrenalectomy (Fig. 4).** After obtaining retroperitoneal access, the dissection initially commences at the level of the psoas muscle to identify pulsations of the renal artery. The inferior vena cava is identified just cephalad to the renal artery, and dissection proceeds along the superior margin of the inferior vena cava. Small aortic arterial branches to the right adrenal gland are clipped and divided, and the main adrenal vein is identified entering the adrenal gland at its superior pole. The main right adrenal vein is clipped and divided. The adrenal gland is then freed from the undersurface of the diaphragm, peritoneum, and upper pole of the kidney, dividing the inferior phrenic, aortic, and renal arterial branches. The freed specimen is entrapped in an impermeable Endocatch bag (USSC, Norwalk, CT), and extracted intact.

**Retroperitoneoscopic Left Adrenalectomy (Fig. 5).** Similar to the technique on the right side, the initial step of a left retroperitoneoscopic adrenalectomy consists of identification of the left main renal artery. Dissection along the cephalad aspect of the renal artery usually identifies the main left adrenal vein, which is then clipped and divided. Occasionally, the main adrenal vein may not be identified early on in the operation, and in such instances is identified and clipped after mobilizing the upper pole of the kidney and adrenal gland. On the left side, mobilization of the adrenal gland requires exposure and caudolateral mobilization of the upper pole of the kidney. The adrenal gland usually lies along the medial aspect of the upper pole of the kidney. The adrenal gland, once exposed, is mobilized by clipping the adrenal branches of the aorta, renal artery, and inferior phrenic vessels. The completely freed adrenal gland is then entrapped and extracted intact.

**Results.** Retroperitoneal adrenalectomy is a more recent technique than its transperitoneal counterpart. A recently conducted survey of 166 retroperitoneal laparoscopic adrenalectomies (107 lateral, 59 posterior) revealed a mean operative time of 2.8 hours, blood loss of 105 mL, and

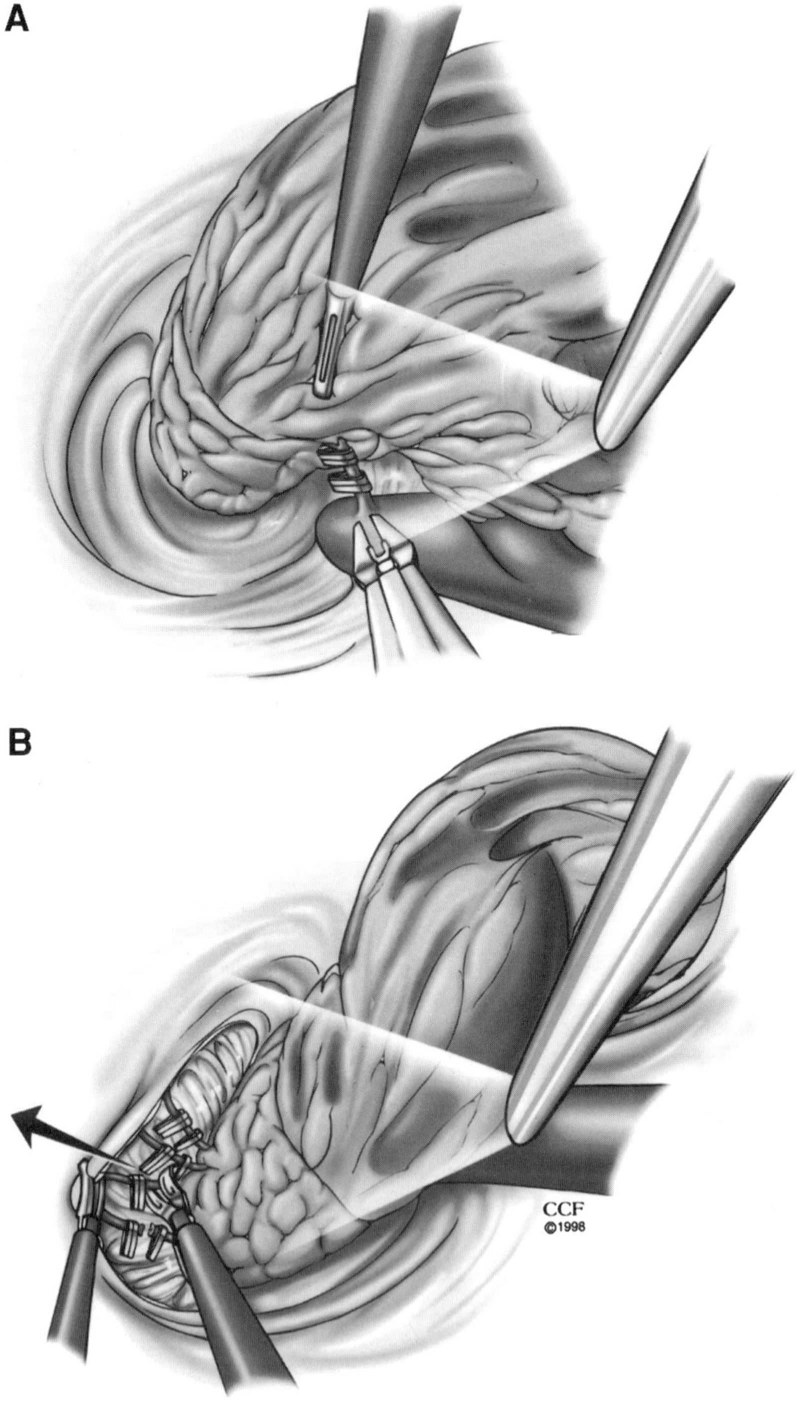
A
B
CCF
©1998

C

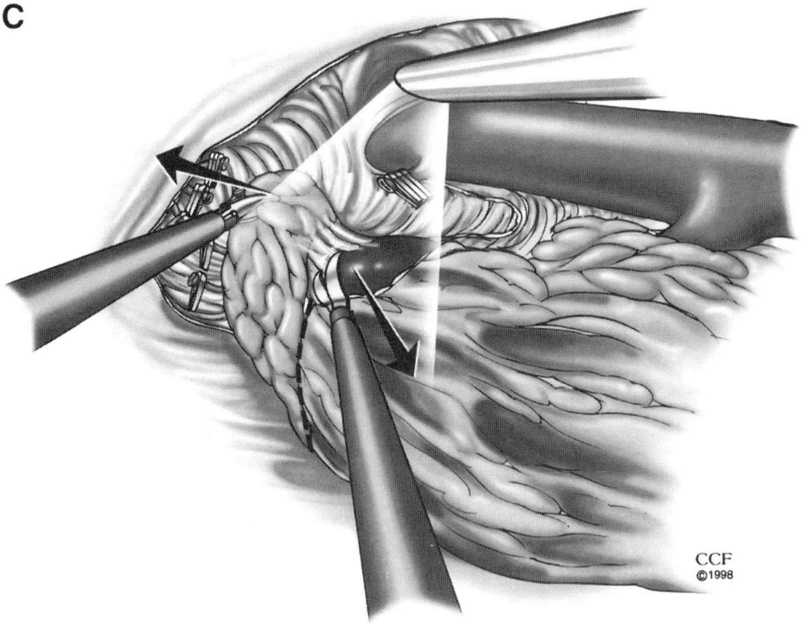


**Fig. 4.** Retroperitoneoscopic right adrenalectomy. **(A)** The initial step in a right retroperitoneoscopic adrenalectomy consists of identifying the suprarenal inferior vena cava. The dissection proceeds along the upper border of the vena cava, carefully dividing the aortic branches to the adrenal gland, until the main right adrenal vein is identified in the region of the upper pole of the adrenal gland. The adrenal vein is clipped and divided. **(B)** The superior attachments of the adrenal gland are divided after clipping the inferior phrenic vascular supply. **(C)** The kidney is mobilized inferolaterally and the adrenal gland is carefully separated from the upper pole of the kidney, thereby completing the adrenalectomy.

**Fig. 5.** (*Next page*) Retroperitoneoscopic left adrenalectomy. **(A)** The Gerota's fascia along the upper pole is incised as shown in the figure. **(B)** The adrenal gland is carefully mobilized from the medial border of the upper pole, ligating the vascular supply from the renal artery. **(C)** The upper pole of the kidney is mobilized laterally and inferiorly. This exposes the main adrenal vein. The superior attachments of the adrenal are also divided (dotted line). **(D)** The main adrenal vein is clipped and the adrenal gland mobilization is completed.

mean hospital stay of 4 days. Mean tumor size was 3.3 cm, convalescence averaged 15.8 days, conversion to open surgery occurred in 7% of cases and complications occurred in 15%of cases *(7)*.

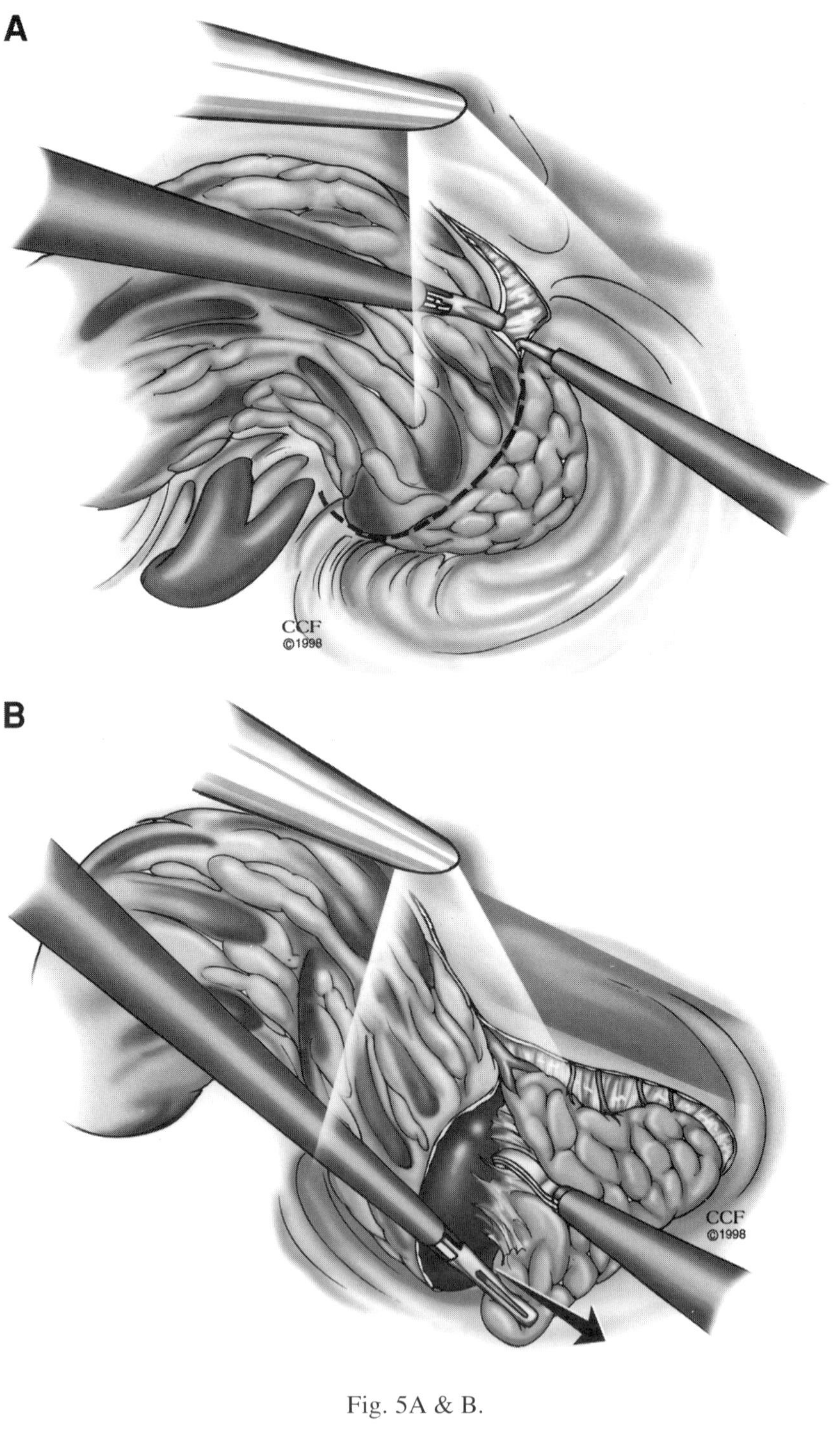


Fig. 5A & B.

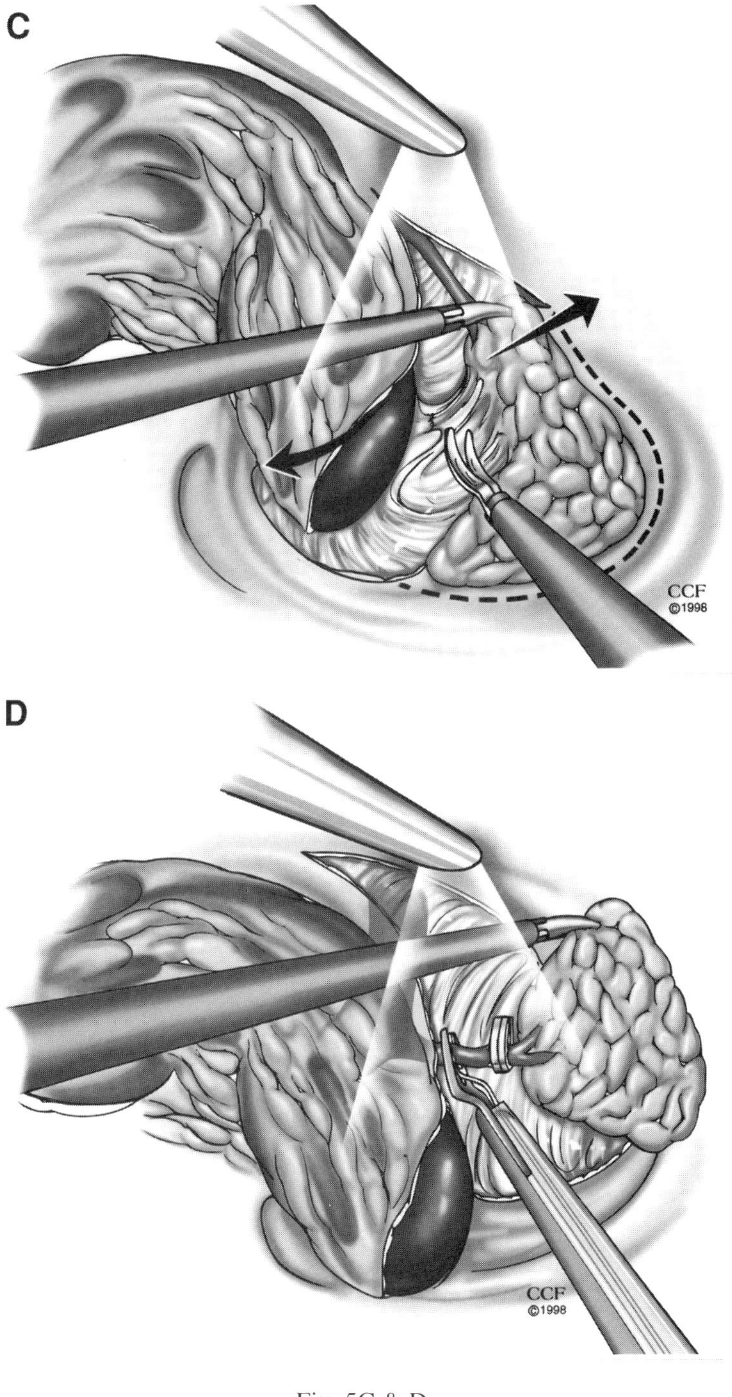


Fig. 5C & D.

### Needlescopic Adrenalectomy

Two-millimeter "needlescopic" instruments and optics are currently available *(13)*. The port needed for 2 mm instruments is similar in caliber to a 14-gage angiocatheter needle and requires a minute skin puncture for insertion, is associated with better cosmesis, and requires only a single adhesive Steri-Strip (3M, St. Paul, MN) for closure. Earlier reserved for diagnostic purposes only, needlescopic techniques are now being employed for definitive therapeutic procedures as well *(14)*.

**Technique of Needlescopic Adrenalectomy.** The current technique of needlescopic adrenalectomy employs four ports: one 10/12 mm umbilical port (camera/specimen extraction), one 5 mm port (dominant hand of the surgeon), and two 2 mm ports (nondominant hand of the surgeon or assistant). The latter three ports lie along the costal margin. The solitary 5 mm port is currently required for the use of certain essential 5 mm instruments (clip applicator, hook, scissors, suction irrigator). The 2 mm versions of these instruments are at present either unavailable or technically inadequate. The mandatory 1.5 to 2 cm skin incision for ultimate extraction of the specimen is well concealed within the umbilical crease and is used to advantage by placing a 10 mm, 45° laparoscope at that site. The subsequent steps of the needlescopic procedure are similar to those of the conventional transperitoneal technique.

**Results of Needlescopic Adrenalectomy.** We retrospectively compared needlescopic ($n = 15$) with conventional laparoscopic adrenalectomy ($n = 21$) *(14)*. The needlescopic group had a shorter operative time (169 vs 220 minutes) and a decreased blood loss (61 vs 183 cc). These benefits of the needlescopic group were thought to reflect the improved learning curve rather than a true benefit of the needlescopic technique. However, the needlescopic technique was associated with a shorter hospital stay (1.1 vs 2.7 days, $p < 0.001$), quicker convalescence (2.1 vs 3.1 weeks, $p < 0.001$), and a superior cosmetic result when compared with the conventional laparoscopic group, which does seem to represent a true benefit of the needlescopic technique. At the current time, needlescopic adrenalectomy only partially incorporates 2 mm technology, in that one 5 mm port is still used. Anticipated advances in instrumentation are likely to render the 5 mm ports unnecessary. The 10/12 mm umbilical port, however, will continue to be used, given our preference for intact removal of the specimen. Needlescopic adrenalectomy is currently our technique of choice in suitable patients who are considered candidates for transperitoneal laparoscopic adrenalectomy.

### Robotic-Assisted Laparoscopic Adrenalectomy

Recently, remote robotic telemanipulators have been used to perform a variety of laparoscopic procedures including adrenalectomy. We recently reported on robotic-assisted laparoscopic adrenalectomy (one on the right, one on the left) using the da Vinci Remote Surgical System (Intuitive Surgical, Sunnyvale, CA) in two patients with an adrenal tumor *(15)*. The ability to perform delicate maneuvers using such remote robotic telemanipulators adjacent to vital organs and major vascular structures opens the possibility of performing remote surgery by an experienced surgeon located at a geographically distant place.

### Thoracoscopic Transdiaphragmatic Adrenalectomy

This radical approach can be employed for the occasional patient with multiple prior transperitoneal and retroperitoneal operations in whom adrenalectomy is indicated. We reported thoracoscopic transdiaphragmatic adrenalectomy in three patients (two with metastatic adrenal mass, one with adrenal myelolipoma) *(16)*. All patients had had multiple abdominal operations on the kidney, thereby rendering transperitoneoscopic or retroperitoneoscopic adrenalectomy extremely hazardous. Thoracoscopic adrenalectomy is performed through four ports, with the patient positioned prone and under single-lung anesthesia. After gaining thoracoscopic access, the diaphragm is incised directly over the adrenal mass using real-time thoracoscopic ultrasound control. The adrenal mass is then mobilized and removed and the diaphragm is suture repaired with continuous sutures using laparoscopic freehand intracorporeal suturing. All three procedures were performed successfully without any major complications. Although this approach has not been utilized specifically for excising aldosteronomas, it does provide an additional tool in the armamentarium of the laparoscopic surgeon in the occasional patient where prior multiple open surgery on the kidney renders conventional laparoscopic adrenalectomy, both trans- and retroperitoneal, prohibitive.

### Choice of Laparoscopic Approach: Transperitoneal vs Retroperitoneal

As mentioned earlier, both the transperitoneal and retroperitoneal approaches are efficacious for performing laparoscopic adrenalectomy. The transperitoneal approach has the advantage of having definite anatomic landmarks and a greater working space. The retroperitoneoscopic approach, though limited by less defined anatomical landmarks and a smaller working space, potentially offers a quicker recovery, less paralytic ileus, shorter hospital stay, and reduced analgesia requirements. Factors that govern the choice of approach include prior open surgery in the quadrant of interest and body habitus. The transperitoneal approach is preferred in patients with prior retroperitoneal surgery and vice versa. Morbid obesity, especially when associated with a large abdominal pannus, may render transperitoneal laparoscopy difficult or even impossible. During retroperitoneoscopy, the abdominal pannus falls forward and hence does not significantly increase the technical difficulty of the procedure. The retroperitoneal approach, in our opinion, may therefore be preferred in patients with morbid obesity *(17)*. In practice, the choice between transperitoneal and retroperitoneal approach for laparoscopic adrenalectomy is chiefly determined by individual surgeon preference and comfort. Both approaches, obesity and prior surgery notwithstanding, are equally efficacious in performing laparoscopic adrenalectomy. However, facility and experience with both approaches enables the laparoscopic surgeon to optimally tailor the operation to the individual patient.

## *Open Adrenalectomy* (18)

Currently, open adrenalectomy has been largely supplanted by laparoscopic approaches for surgical treatment of benign adrenal lesions. Aldosteronomas are generally small and therefore ideally suited for laparoscopic excision. Open adrenalectomy can be performed through retroperitoneal, transperitoneal, and thoracoabdominal approaches. In the past, the retroperitoneal flank or dorsal approaches were the most commonly used approaches for surgical excision of aldosteronomas. Transperitoneal and thoracoabdominal approaches are rarely used for aldosteronomas and are typically employed for pheochromocytomas and large infiltrating adrenal cancers.

### Technique of Open Adrenalectomy

Because aldosteronomas are typically small in size and are accurately localized preoperatively, most open surgical excisions are via the retroperitoneal approach, posterior or flank.

**Posterior Approach.** The posterior approach provides direct access to either adrenal gland with minimal disturbance of the surrounding viscera and without cutting muscle, thereby minimizing operative morbidity. The patient is positioned prone on a laminectomy frame, thereby providing flexion at the hips and allowing gentle dorsal curvature of the lower thoracic and lumbar spine. The left adrenal gland can be approached through the 12th rib bed. The right adrenal, located superiorly, is approached through the 11th rib bed. The rib is exposed in its entirety and resected subperiosteally. Medial retraction of the sacrospinalis muscle helps in resecting the medial portion of the rib. The diaphragm and pleura can be safely mobilized cephalad on the right side. However, this dissection may be tedious through the 11th rib bed on the left side, whereas opening the pleural and diaphragmatic layers of the thorax expeditiously provides access to the adrenal gland without creating significant pleurotomies. At this point, opening the Gerota's fascia exposes the posterior surface of the upper pole of the kidney and adrenal gland.

On the left side, the adrenal gland is left attached to the upper pole of the kidney, so that gentle caudad traction on the upper pole can be used to expose the adrenal gland. Initially, the superior and lateral attachments are divided, taking care to ligate the branch from the inferior phrenic vein. The adrenal gland is then retracted medially to expose the main adrenal vein as it courses anteromedial to the upper pole of the kidney to enter the superior border of the left renal vein. The adrenal vein is ligated and the adrenal gland is further mobilized by ligating the renal arterial branches to the adrenal gland. Finally, the medial border of the adrenal gland is dissected by ligating the aortic branches to the adrenal gland, thereby completely freeing the adrenal gland.

On the right side, the liver is retracted cephalad and the upper pole of the kidney is retracted caudad to expose the adrenal gland. The lateral and inferior aspects of the adrenal gland are easily mobilized. The anterior surface of the gland is mobilized up to the inferior vena caval margin. Lateral retraction of the gland identifies the short main adrenal vein, which enters the gland at its superior pole. After ligating the main adrenal vein, the arterial branches from the aorta are divided, thus completing the adrenalectomy.

Once the adrenalectomy is complete, the diaphragm and pleura are sutured if required. A chest film is routinely obtained in the recovery room to rule out a pneumothorax.

**Flank Approach.** Although the posterior approach provides direct exposure to the adrenal gland with minimal morbidity in most patients with aldosteronoma, the flank approach may be indicated in the obese patient for obtaining adequate surgical exposure. The patient is positioned in the conventional flank position. A generous flank incision through the bed of the 11th or 12th rib provides optimal exposure to the adrenal gland.

On the left side, the colon is mobilized medially, and the tail of the pancreas and the spleen are retracted superiomedially to expose the anterior surface of the kidney and the adrenal gland. The upper pole of the kidney is then retracted caudad to better expose the adrenal gland.

The adrenal gland is then dissected along its avascular anterior and posterior surfaces. The main adrenal vein is then identified as it exits the superior border of the renal vein just lateral to the aorta. The main adrenal vein is divided such that it leaves a generous stump toward the adrenal gland, which is subsequently used as a handle to facilitate manipulation of the adrenal gland. Downward traction on the adrenal gland identifies the inferior phrenic vascular supply, which is clipped and divided. The adrenal gland is now attached only at its medial margin. The direct aortic branches to the adrenal gland are divided to complete the adrenalectomy.

On the right side, the colon and duodenum are mobilized medially to expose the kidney and adrenal gland. Downward traction on the kidney pulls the adrenal gland into view. The adrenal gland is mobilized bluntly on its anterior and posterior surface. The apical vessels from the inferior phrenic veinare clipped and divided. The inferior surface is mobilized from the kidney, dividing the arterial branches from the renal artery. The adrenal gland is subsequently mobilized along its medial border, ligating aortic arterial branches. The main adrenal vein is identified entering the gland at its superior pole and then divided. The few remaining superior attachments to the adrenal gland are divided, thus completing the adrenalectomy.

### *Postoperative Considerations*

Most patients undergoing adrenalectomy for aldosteronomas experience uneventful recovery. Especially with the laparoscopic approach, morbidity is minimal and convalescence short. Suppression of aldosterone production from the contralateral normal adrenal gland by the aldosteronoma may result in temporary postoperative hypoaldosteronism characterized by a moderate diuresis, natriuresis, and potassium retention. Proper attention to fluid and electrolyte balance is essential. Rarely, severe postoperative hypoaldosteronism may warrant temporary mineralocorticoid replacement.

## RESULTS OF ADRENALECTOMY FOR ALDOSTERONOMA

Currently, laparoscopic adrenalectomy may be considered the gold standard for surgical treatment of aldosteronoma. Reports from various centers worldwide have attested to the lower morbidity, shorter hospital stay, better cosmesis, and a quicker recovery of the laparoscopic approach as compared to the open approach for treatment of benign hyperfunctioning adrenal tumors (Table 1) *(19–24)*. Laparoscopic excision is particularly suited for surgical treatment of aldosteronomas owing

Table 1
Laparoscopic vs Open Adrenalectomy

| *Author/ year* | *Tech* | *No. of Pts.* | *Age (years)* | *Diagnosis* | *App* | *O.R. time (hrs)* | *EBL (mL)* | *Hosp. stay (days)* | *Specimen size (cm)* | *Conval (days)* | *Complications Minor* | *Major* |
|---|---|---|---|---|---|---|---|---|---|---|---|---|
| Guzzoni 1995 *(19)* | Open | 20 | 39 | Pheo 10<br>Conn's 7<br>Cushing's 3 | Various incisions | 2.4 | 450 | 9 | 3.1 | 16 | 4 (20%) | 1 (5%) |
| | Laparo | 20 | 41 | Conn's 10<br>Pheo 7<br>Cushing's 3 | Trans | 2.8 | 100 | 3.4 | 3.0 | 9.7 | 0 | 1 (5%) |
| Suzuki | Open | 11 | – | – | – | 2.6 | 297 | – | – | 23.1 | – | – |
| 1993 *(20)* | Laparo | 12 | – | – | – | 4.6 | 397 | – | – | 10.4 | 7 (58%) | – |
| Staren 1996 *(21)* | Open | 19 | 42 | Pheo 12<br>Cancer 7<br>Other 4 | Anterior 15<br>Posterior<br>Thoracoabd 3 | 3.0 | – | 6.1 | 9.2 | – | – | – |
| | Laparo | 20 | 50 | Pheo 7<br>Conn's 5<br>Cushing's 6<br>Other 2 | Trans 17<br>Retro 4 | 2.8 | 100 | 3.4 | 3.0 | 9.7 | 0 | 1 (5%) |
| Brunt 1996 *(22)* | Open | 42 | 49 | Pheo 19<br>Conn's 8<br>Other 15 | Anterior 25<br>Posterior 17 | Ant 2.4<br>Post 2.3 | | 3.2 | 9.2 | – | Anterior<br>11 (44%)<br>Posterior<br>7 (47%) | Anterior<br>8 (32%)<br>Posterior<br>2 (12%) |
| | Laparo | 24 | 50 | Pheo 11<br>Conn's 6<br>Other 7 | Trans | 3.1 | 104 | 6.2 | 2.7 | 10.6 | 2 (8%) | 2 (8%) |

*(continued)*

Table 1 (*Continued*)
Laparoscopic vs Open Adrenalectomy

| *Author/ year* | *Tech* | *No. of Pts.* | *Age (years)* | *Diagnosis* | *App* | *O.R. time (hrs)* | *EBL (mL)* | *Hosp. stay (days)* | *Specimen size (cm)* | *Conval (days)* | *Complications Minor* | *Complications Major* |
|---|---|---|---|---|---|---|---|---|---|---|---|---|
| Winfield 1998 *(23)* | Open | 17 | 53 | Pheo 7<br>Conn's 6<br>Other 4 | Various incisions | 2.3 | 266 | 2.7 | 2.5 | 45 | 9 (53%) | 9 (53%) |
| | Laparo | 21 | 52 | Conn's 16<br>Adenoma 3 | Trans | 3.7 | 183 | 5.7 | 1.8 | 22 | 6 (29%) | 0 |
| Thompson 1997 *(23)* | Open | 50 | 51 | Conn's 25<br>Conn's 6<br>Other 4 | Dorsal | 2.1 | – | 3.7 | 2.9 | 42 | 9 (18%) | 0 |
| | Laparo | 50 | 50 | Conn's 24<br>Cushing's 10<br>Pheo 10<br>Adenoma 6 | Trans | 2.8 | – | 4.4 | 2.9 | 26 | 3 (6%) | 0 |

App, approach; Conval, convalescence; EBL, estimated blood loss; Retro, retroperitoneal; Tech, technique; Trans, transperitoneal .

to their relatively small size. The results of laparoscopic adrenalectomy for primary hyperaldosteronism are summarized in Table 2 *(25–31)*. Our review included 92 patients with primary hyperaldosteronism who underwent laparoscopic adrenalectomy (transperitoneal 60, retroperitoneal 32). Mean operative time was 196.7 minutes, estimated blood loss was 221 cc, hospital stay was 3.2 days, and convalescence was 11.9 days. There were three complications (3.7%), and blood pressure (BP) cure was reported in 64 of 70 patients (91.4%).

## *Factors Predicting Response to Surgery*

The single most important factor associated with a favorable response after adrenalectomy in a patient with primary hyperaldosteronism is the presence of an adrenal adenoma on postoperative pathology. Although some cases with adrenal hyperplasia may be cured or improved with surgery, possibly because of a reduction in the number of glomerulosa cells, the results are generally inferior to those with an adrenal adenoma. In addition to the presence of adenoma or adrenal hyperplasia on pathology, several other factors have been correlated to the presence of a favorable response to adrenalectomy. Celen et al studied the various factors influencing the outcome of surgery in 42 patients with primary hyperaldosteronism *(32)*. Over a mean followup of 106 months, surgery cured hypertension in 62% of cases with adenoma and 16% of cases with hyperplasia. Using univariate analysis, factors associated with complete response to surgery included adenoma classification (odds ratio [OR] = 9.6, $p = 0.002$), preoperative response to spironolactone (OR = 8.3, $p = 0.007$), age less than 44 years (OR = 6.2, $p = 0.009$), and duration of hypertension (OR = 5.1, $p = 0.03$). Using multivariate logistic regression, presence of adenoma on pathologic classification, response to spironolactone, and duration of hypertension less than 5 years correlated independently to a complete response to surgery. Sawka et al also studied factors associated with normalization of BP after adrenalectomy for hyperaldosteronism *(33)*. The authors reported on 97 patients undergoing adrenalectomy for primary hyperaldosteronism. Overall cure of hypertension, defined as a postoperative BP of less than 140/90 mmHg occurred in 31 of 93 cases (35%). Of the 62 patients with unresolved hypertension, 61 patients (98%) had improved BP control. The factors that were independently associated with BP cure included absence of a strong family history of hypertension (OR = 10.9, $p < 0.001$), and preoperative use of two or fewer antihypertensive drugs (OR = 4.7, $p = 0.005$). Factors associated with resolution of hypertension on univariate analysis included younger age, shorter duration of hypertension, higher preoperative ratio of plasma aldosterone to plasma renin

**Table 2**
**Laparoscopic Adrenalectomy for Aldosteronomas**

| *Author/year* | *No. of pts.* | *Mean age (years)* | *Approach* | *Mean O.R. time (minutes)* | *EBL[3] (cc)* | *Hosp. stay (days)* | *Conv[5] (days)* | *Complic[1] (%)* | *Cure of BP (%)* | *Pathology* | *Weight /size* |
|---|---|---|---|---|---|---|---|---|---|---|---|
| Takeda 1994 *(25)* | 10 | 48.2 | TP | 295 | 270.5 | – | – | 1 (bleeding) | 10 (100) | Adenoma 10 | 6.6 |
| Shen 1999 *(26)* | 42 | 50 | TP 28<br>RP 14 | – | – | – | – | 0 | 37 (88) | Adenoma 41<br>Hyperplasia 1 | – |
| Siren 1999 *(27)* | 12 | 51 | – | 126 | – | 3.4 | 13 | 0 | 12 (100) | – | – |
| Go 1994 *(28)* | 11 | 47.6 | TP | 269 | 256.8 | – | – | 1 (bleeding) | – | – | 6.6 gm |
| Uchida 1994 *(29)* | 6 | – | RP | 196 | 94 | – | – | 1 (pneumothorax) | 6 (100) | – | – |
| Fernandez Cruz 1996 *(30)* | 11 | 53 | TP | 121.4 | 210 | 3 | 11.7 | – | – | – | 2.3 |
| Total | 92 | 51.2 | TP 60<br>RP 20 | 196.7 | 221.1 | 3.2 | 11.9 | 3 (3.7) | 64/70<br>(91.4) | – | 6.6 gm |

[1]Complic, complications; [2]Conv, convalescence; [3]EBL, estimated blood loss; [4]RP, retroperitoneal; [5]TP, transperitoneal.

activity, and a higher 24-hour urinary aldosterone level ($p < 0.05$). In summary, pathological evidence of an adrenal adenoma correlates best with the likelihood of cure of hypertension after surgery in patients with primary hyperaldosteronism. Complete cure of hypertension occurs in 30 to 60% of cases of aldosteronomas, based on the criteria defining cure (Table 3) *(1,27,32)*. Nevertheless, the majority of patients experience improvement of BP control, as defined as a reduction in BP and/or number and dosage of antihypertensive medications.

## PARTIAL ADRENALECTOMY

Adrenal-sparing surgery has been advocated for select patients with benign adrenal disease whom a total adrenalectomy could potentially render without any functional adrenal tissue, thereby necessitating lifelong steroid replacement. In an excellent study by Nakada et al., 48 patients with aldosteronoma were randomized to undergo either open adrenalectomy or enucleation of the adenoma *(34)*. Over a followup of five years, both groups had similar responses in BP and serum potassium. The plasma renin and serum aldosterone response to ambulation and furosemide in the enucleation group was markedly enhanced ($p < 0.001$), and similar to that of normal healthy individuals, whereas that in the adrenalectomy group was slight ($p < 0.05$ and $< 0.01$). Additionally, the authors reported that the serum aldosterone secretion in response to Ang II infusion and cortisol secretion in response to adrenocorticotropic hormone stimulation was more pronounced in the enucleation group compared to the adrenalectomy group. Moreover, there was no recurrence of hyperaldosteronism in any patient in either group. The authors concluded that, physiologically, adenoma enucleation may be preferred to total adrenalectomy for surgical treatment of aldosteronoma.

Recently, adrenal-sparing surgery has also been reported laparoscopically *(35)*. Walz et al. reported retroperitoneoscopic partial adrenalectomy in 22 patients (11 Conn adenomas, 4 pheochromocytomas, 4 Cushing's adenomas, and 3 hormonally inactive tumors) *(36)*. The authors found no difference in operative times or blood loss in the partial adrenalectomy group when compared with total adrenalectomy. None of the patients with Conn's syndrome or pheochromocytomas required steroid replacement. The four patients with Cushing's syndrome required decreasing amounts of steroid replacement, while of the two patients with multiple endocrine neoplasia II, one is on low-dose replacement and the other does not require replacement. Thus, it seems that partial adrenalectomy may be a viable and effective option in patients at risk of developing adrenocortical insufficiency with total adrenalectomy.

Table 3

**Long-Term Results of Surgical Treatment of Primary Hyperaldosteronism**

| *Author & Year* | *No of Patients* | *Surgical Approach* | *Systolic BP (mmHg)* | | *Diastolic BP (mmHg)* | | *Serum K (μeq/L)* | | *Pathology* | *Followup (months)* | *Blood Pressure* | | |
|---|---|---|---|---|---|---|---|---|---|---|---|---|---|
| | | | *Pre* | *Post* | *Pre* | *Post* | *Pre* | *Post* | | | *Cured* | *Improved* | *Same* |
| Shen et al., 1999 *(26)* | 80 | Open 38<br>Lap 42 | NA | NA | NA | NA | 2.6<br>3.3 | 3.6–5.0<br>3.5–4.9 | Adenoma 32<br>Adenoma 41 | 6–36%<br>4–36 | 30 (81%)<br>37 (88%) | NA | NA |
| Celen et al., 1996 *(31)* | 42 | Open 42 | 181 | 131 | 114 | 85 | 2.8 | 4.2 | Adenoma 27<br>Hyperplasia 15 | 106 | 25 (60%) | 17 (40%) | – |
| Blumenfeld et al., 1994 *(1)* | 51 | Open 51 | 184<br>161 | 131<br>144 | 112<br>105 | 86<br>93 | 3.0<br>3.5 | 4.5<br>4.3 | Adenoma 43<br>Hyperplasia 8 | 2 weeks–<br>15 years | 15 (35%)<br>3 (38% | 24 (56%)<br>1 (12%) | 4(9%)<br>4 (50%) |

NA, not available.

## CONCLUSIONS

Currently, laparoscopic adrenalectomy can be considered the standard of care for treatment of aldosteronomas. Aldosteronomas, owing to their relatively small size, are particularly amenable to laparoscopic excision by either the transperitoneal or retroperitoneal approach. Worldwide data attest to the safety and efficacy of laparoscopic adrenalectomy for aldosteronomas. Adrenalectomy results in either cure or better control of hypertension and resolution of hypokalemia in most patients with aldosteronomas.

## REFERENCES

1. Blumenfeld JD. Diagnosis and treatment of primary hyperaldosteronism [see comments]. Ann Intern Med 1994;121:877–885.
2. Bravo EL, Steward, BH. The adrenal: anatomy and physiology. Urology Update Series 1978;1:1.
3. Gagner M, Lacroix A, Bolte E. Laparoscopic adrenalectomy in Cushing's syndrome and pheochromocytoma. N Engl J M 1992;327:1033.
4. Winfield HN, Hamilton BD, Bravo EL. Technique of laparoscopic adrenalectomy. Urol Clin N Am 1997;24:459–465.
5. Terachi T, Matsuda T, Terai A, et al. Transperitoneal laparoscopic adrenalectomy: experience in 100 patients. J Endourol 1997;11:361–365.
6. Basso N, De Leo A, Fantini A, Genco A, Rosato P, Spaziani E. Laparoscopic direct supragastric left adrenalectomy. Am J Surg 1999;178:308–310.
7. Gill IS, Novick, AC. Laparoscopic versus open adrenal surgery. AUA Update Series 1999;18:258–263.
8. Yoshida O, Terachi,T, Matsuda,T, et al. Complications in 369 laparoscopic adrenalectomies: a multiinstitutional study in Japan. J Urol 1997;157:282.
9. Gasman D, Droupy S, Koutani A, et al. Laparoscopic adrenalectomy: the retroperitoneal approach. J Urol 1998;159:1816–1820.
10. Baba S. Laparoscopic adrenalectomy: posterior approach. Biomed Pharmacother 2000;54 Suppl 1:161s–163s.
11. Duh QY, Siperstein AE, Clark OH, et al. Laparoscopic adrenalectomy: comparison of the lateral and posterior approaches. Arch Surg 1996;131:870–875; discussion 875–876.
12. Walz MK, Peitgen K, Hoermann R, Giebler RM, Mann K, Eigler FW. Posterior retroperitoneoscopy as a new minimally invasive approach for adrenalectomy: results of 30 adrenalectomies in 27 patients. World J Surg 1996;20:769–774.
13. Soble JJ, Gill IS. Needlescopic urology: incorporating 2-mm instruments in laparoscopic surgery [see comments]. Urol 1998;52:187–194.
14. Gill IS, Soble JJ, Sung GT, Winfield HN, Bravo EL, Novick AC. Needlescopic adrenalectomy—the initial series: comparison with conventional laparoscopic adrenalectomy [see comments]. Urol 1998;52:180–186.
15. Desai MM, Gill IS, Kaouk JH, Matin SF, Sung GT, Bravo EL. Robotic-assisted laparoscopic adrenalectomy. Urol 2002;60:1104–1107.
16. Gill IS, Meraney AM, Thomas JC, Sung GT, Novick AC, Lieberman I. Thoracoscopic transdiaphragmatic adrenalectomy: the initial experience [see comments]. J Urol 2001;165:1875–1881.

17. Fazeli-Matin SF, Gill IS, Hsu TH, et al. Laparoscopic renal and adrenal surgery in obese patients: comparison to open surgery. J Urol 1999;162:665.
18. Novick AC. Surgery for primary hyperaldosteronism. Urol Clin N Am 1989;16: 535–545.
19. Guzzoni G, Montorsi F, Bocciardi A, et al. Transperitoneal laparoscopic versus open adrenalectomy for benign hyperfunctioning adrenal tumors: a comparative study. J Urol 1995;153:1597–1600.
20. Suzuki K, Kageyama S, Ueda D, et al. Laparoscopic adrenalectomy: clinical experience with 12 cases. J Urol 1993;150:1099.
21. Staren ED, Prinz RA. Adrenalectomy in the era of laparoscopy. Surg 1996;120: 706–711.
22. Brunt LM, Doherty GM, Norton JA, Soper NJ, Quasebarth MA, Moley JF. Laparoscopic adrenalectomy compared to open adrenalectomy for benign adrenal neoplasms. J Am College Surg 1996;183:1–10.
23. Winfield HN, Hamilton BD, Bravo EL, Novick AC. Laparoscopic adrenalectomy: the preferred choice? A comparison to open adrenalectomy. J Urol 1998;160: 325–329.
24. Thompson GB, Grant CS, Van Heerden JA, et al. Laparoscopic versus open posterior adrenalectomy: a case control study of 100 patients. Surg 1997;122:1132–1136.
25. Takeda M, Go H, Imai T, Nishiyama T, Morishita H. Laparoscopic adrenalectomy for primary aldosteronism: report of initial 10 cases. Surg 1994;115(5):621–625.
27. Shen WT, Lim RC, Siperstein AE, et al. Laparoscopic versus open adrenalectomy for the treatment of primary hyperaldosteronism. Arch Surg 1999;134:628–632.
28. Siren J, Haglund C, Huikuri K, Sivula A, Haapiainen R. Laparoscopic adrenalectomy for primary aldosteronism: clinical experience in 12 patients. Surg Laparosc Endosc Percutan Tech 1999;9(1):9–13.
29. Go H, Takeda M, Imai T, Komeyama T, Nishiyama T, Morishita H. Laparoscopic adrenalectomy for Cushing's syndrome: comparison with primary aldosteronism. Surg 1995;117:11–17.
30. Uchida M, Imaide Y, Yoneda K, et al. Endoscopic adrenalectomy by retroperitoneal approach for primary aldosteronism. Honiyokika Kiyo-Acta Urol Jap 1994; 40(1):43–46.
31. Fernandez-Cruz L, Taura P, Saenz A, Benarroch G, Sabater L. Laparoscopic approach to pheochromocytoma: hemodynamic changes and catecholamine secretion. World J Surg 1996;20(7):762–768; discussion 768.
32. Celen O. Factors influencing outcome of surgery for primary aldosteronism. Arch Surg 1996;131:646–650.
33. Sawka AM. Primary aldosteronism: factors associated with normalization of blood pressure after surgery. Ann Intern Med 2001;135:258–261.
34. Nakada T. Therapeutic outcome of primary aldosteronism: adrenalectomy versus enucleation of aldosterone-producing adenoma [see comments]. J Urol 1995;153: 1775–1780.
35. Janetschek G, Lhotta K, Gasser R, Finkenstedt G, Jaschke W, Bartsch G. Adrenal-sparing laparoscopic surgery for aldosterone-producing adenoma. J Endourol 1997;11:145–148.
36. Walz MK, Peitgen K. Laparoscopic partial adrenalectomy. Surg Endosc 2000; 14:1089–1090.

# 11 Nonprimary Aldosteronism

## *Mineralocorticoid Disorders*

*William T. Kendrick,* MD,
*Jean-Michel Achard,* MD, PhD
*and David G. Warnock,* MD

*CONTENTS*



## INTRODUCTION

Our understanding of sodium ($Na^+$) transport defects has greatly expanded in the last few years, providing unique insights into epithelial

From: *Secondary Hypertension: Clinical Presentation, Diagnosis, and Treatment*
Edited by: G. A. Mansoor © Humana Press Inc., Totowa, NJ

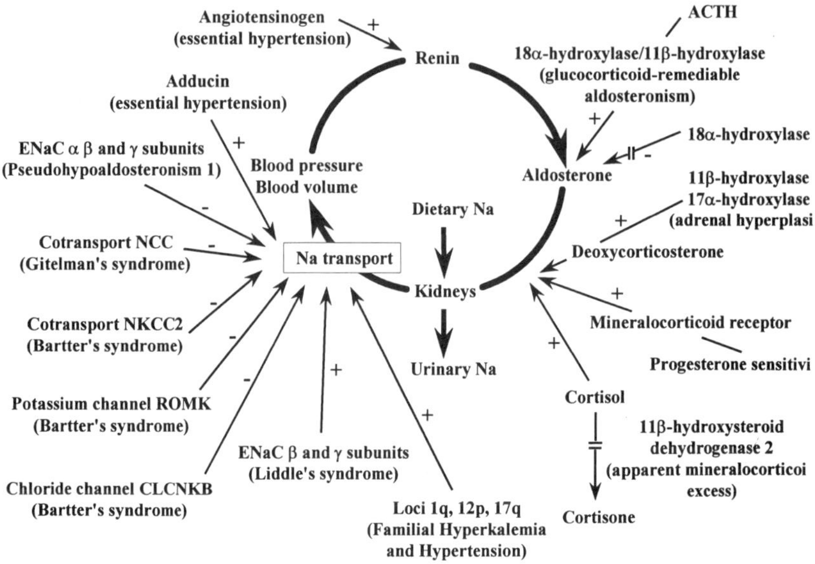


**Fig. 1.** Mutations and polymorphisms altering BP in humans. All the genes are involved directly or indirectly in the control of renal $Na^+$ reabsorption. The mutations have been found in monogenic human diseases associated with disorders of BP regulation. (Reprinted from ref. *2* with permission.)

transport processes and unusual clinical syndromes resulting from mutations of specific ion transporters. These genetic disorders affect $Na^+$ balance, with $Na^+$ retaining and wasting conditions as the consequence *(1)*. The epithelial sodium channel (ENaC) can be directly affected by mutations or by changes in the response to or production of mineralocorticoid hormones. As a result, there are clearly defined syndromes in which ENaC activity is "dysregulated" with subsequent disorders of systemic blood pressure (BP) that can be attributed to a primary renal mechanism. In fact, every presently defined genetic syndrome that affects BP regulation affects some specific aspect of renal sodium chloride (NaCl) handling (Fig. 1). These findings reinforce Guyton's view of the renal regulation of fluid volume and BP (for review see refs. *1–3*, and are supported by observations in a large number of human clinical disorders and parallel studies of "knock-out" models in mice *(2,3)*. With these previous efforts in mind, a more clearly focused view of the regulation of $Na^+$ transport in the aldosterone-responsive distal nephron has emerged and is depicted in Fig. 2.

This chapter surveys the human monogenic forms of hypertension, nearly all of which represent a form of hereditary low-renin hyperten-

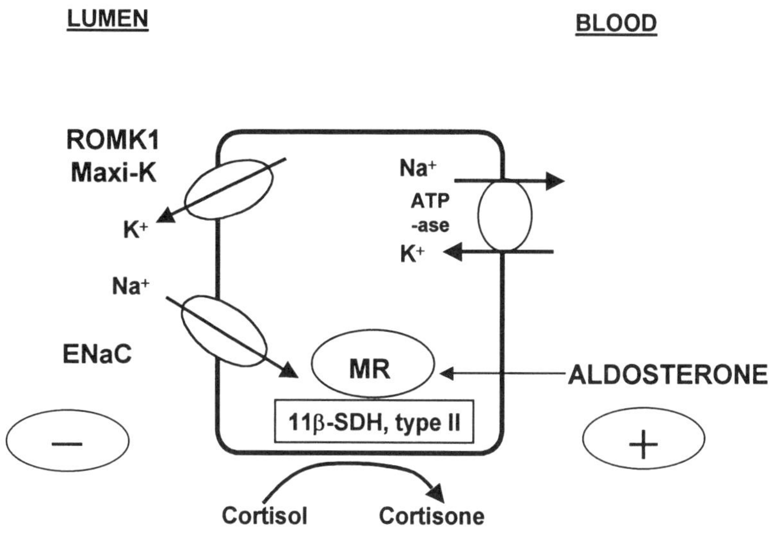


**Fig. 2.** Mineralocorticoid action in renal cells of the distal tubule and cortical collecting duct. When aldosterone enters the cell, it binds to the mineralocorticoid receptor (MR); thereafter, the ligand-receptor complex is translocated into the nucleus. Binding to nuclear response elements increases the transcription of genes encoding specific aldosterone-inducible proteins, such as the subunits of the apical epithelial sodium channel (ENaC). In turn, this stimulates sodium ($Na^+$) reabsorption; the resulting lumen-negative electrical gradient is an important driving force for $K^+$ secretion through apical $K^+$ channels (ROMK1 and maxi-K). The MR is protected from occupation by glucocorticoids because the 11β OH SDH type II oxidizes cortisol into its receptor-inactive form cortisone.

sion. In the classical presentation of Liddle's syndrome, low-renin hypertension and low aldosterone secretion rates have been described. The clinical phenotype strongly resembles primary aldosteronism, yet the measured levels of aldosterone are dramatically reduced, accounting for the descriptor "pseudoaldosteronism" (PA1) *(1)*. In other forms, these inherited syndromes present with many of the features of primary aldosteronism, yet the actual aldosterone levels may be somewhat suppressed because of the presence of a novel mineralocorticoid, such as 18-oxocortisol in the syndrome of glucocorticoid-remediable aldosteronism (GRA), or an inappropriate mineralocorticoid response to endogenous steroids such as cortisol in the apparent mineralocorticoid excess syndrome, or progesterone in the syndrome associated with a mutation in the steroid binding domain of the mineralocorticoid receptor. Finally, recent information concerning the familial hyperkalemia and hypertension syndrome implicates mutations in a specific family of serine/threonine kinases that regulate specific aspects of NaCl reabsorption in the aldosterone-sensitive portion of the distal tubule. Although the clinical aspects of these disorders resemble many aspects of primary aldosteronism, the familial inheritance and distinct pathophysiologic features distinguish these syndromes and proscribe somewhat unique therapeutic approaches to the individual patient.

## MUTATIONS AND POLYMORPHISMS OF ENaC

Mutations of the ENaC subunits can result in a gain of function (Liddle's syndrome) with the predictable clinical phenotype of low-renin hypertension and suppressed aldosterone secretion *(1)*. These mutations were originally described as truncations or frame-shifts in the β or γ subunits of ENaC *(2)*. These mutations delete a critical proline-rich region of the cytosolic tail that interacts with a cytoskeletal protein called Nedd4 *(4–7)*. Several pedigrees with mutations of critical amino acids in this proline-rich region have been described, which are also associated with a gain of ENaC function, resulting in the familiar clinical phenotype of hypertension with metabolic alkalosis and renal potassium wasting *(8,9)*. Despite the promise of defining an important cause of human low-renin hypertension, numerous screening efforts of various ethnic populations have not changed the original view that Liddle's syndrome is a rare cause of human hypertension.

Although activating mutations of ENaC subunits are uncommon in patients with "essential" hypertension, there may be polymorphisms in these genes that could have important effects on the regulation of ENaC activity. It is important to characterize such polymorphisms, especially in defined patients with hypertension and relatively low levels of aldosterone secretion. An extensive survey was undertaken with hypertensive families in the HYPERGENE data set *(10)*. Sequence analysis of the β ENaC subunit was carried out in 532 hypertensive probands, including 101 probands with low-renin hypertension. Mis-sense mutations were identified in seven unrelated individuals; three probands of African ancestry had mutations that changed threonine to methionine at position 594 (T594M), with an overall incidence of 6% of the hypertensive probands of African ancestry. A glycine to valine (G442V) β subunit variant was identified in 19 probands; all but 1 was of African ancestry and 8 of the probands were from the subset of low-renin hypertension. Although of low incidence in whites, G442V was found in 34.8% of the low-renin hypertensive probands of African ancestry. A larger case-control study confirmed these findings *(11)*, however, there could have been a selection bias in defining the hypertensive subjects *(12,13)*.

Although of potential importance at the epidemiological level, none of these mis-sense mutations or polymorphisms have had any demonstrable effects in the in vitro expression systems used to examine ENaC activity.

Ambrosius et al. *(14)* evaluated human ENaC polymorphisms, BP and the renin-angiotensin-aldosterone system in a group of young (mean age 13.4 years) white and African American subjects. Because direct measurements of ENaC activity in the collecting tubule are not obtainable in humans, a surrogate marker is needed for the effects of activated ENaC activity. An increase in urinary calcium excretion is one possibility and has been associated with the M594T polymorphism in a small group of patients *(12)*. In the characterization of the extended original pedigree with Liddle's syndrome, it was reported that overnight urinary potassium excretion was high and the urinary aldosterone excretion was low in affected individuals, giving very low urinary aldosterone/potassium ratios, consistent with the physiologic effect of activated ENaC activity at the potassium secretory site in the collecting tubule *(15)*. Ambrosius et al. *(14)* also used this approach to estimate the intrinsic level of ENaC activity in their studies. In overnight urine samples collected from 249 white and 181 black subjects, the urinary aldosterone/potassium ratio was lower in black than in white subjects: 0.42 ( 0.02 (mean ( SE) vs 0.58 ( 0.02 nmol/mmol ($p < 0.0001$). In addition, four out of five ENaC polymorphisms were found to be much more common in black than in white individuals. G442V in the β subunit was present in 16% of the blacks and in only one white individual, and was associated with indices of greater $Na^+$ retention and potentially greater ENaC activity: lower plasma aldosterone concentration, lower urinary aldosterone excretion rate, higher potassium excretion, and a lower urinary aldosterone/potassium ratio ($p = 0.027$). On the basis of these findings, it was suggested that ENaC activity is higher in blacks than in whites and that this activity could contribute to racial differences in $Na^+$ retention and the subsequent risk of developing low-renin hypertension *(14)*. These findings were supported by the findings of BP-lowering effects of ENaC inhibitors (amiloride), in combination with mineralocorticoid receptor antagonism with spironolactone *(16)*.

## ALDOSTERONE SYNTHASE AND LOW-RENIN HYPERTENSION

It has long been recognized that low-renin hypertension in African Americans is associated with relatively normal plasma aldosterone levels *(17,18)*. If suppressed plasma renin activity is regarded as an index of effective circulating arterial volume, then these "normal" aldosterone levels could be regarded as inappropriately high. Although a number of factors directly affect aldosterone secretion, polymorphisms in the 18-hydroxylase gene ("aldosterone synthase," or CPY11B2) have also been described that appear to be associated with variations in plasma aldosterone levels *(19)*; C344T polymorphism of the CYP11B2 gene has been described, with the T allele significantly associated with higher plasma aldosterone levels. Polymorphisms of the 18-hydroxylase gene need to be defined in African Americans with low-renin hypertension to determine whether a similar association could explain the nonsuppressed (albeit low normal) level of plasma aldosterone despite the suppression of plasma renin activity *(17)*. Aldosterone secretion remains under control of angiotensin II (Ang II) in African American individuals although the plasma aldosterone response to Ang II infusion is blunted compared to that of white controls *(20)*. Recent insights into these issues have been obtained from studies of the original Liddle's pedigree *(17)*. Gas chromatograpic-mass spectrometry *(21)* was used to examine the urinary steroid metabolite profile in these patients. A marked suppression of aldosterone metabolite excretion, as well as all of the adrenal 18-hydroxylase urinary steroid metabolites, was observed, denoting a chronic, global suppression of aldosterone synthase activity in the adrenal zona glomerulosa in Liddle's syndrome *(17)*. Of note was the fact that, in the original proband studied two years after successful renal transplantation, the plasma renin activity and aldosterone excretion were restored to normal *(15)*, confirming that suppression of aldosterone synthase activity in Liddle's syndrome and the suppressed plasma renin activity are simply indices of chronic sustained volume expansion *(17)*. The lack of down-regulation of ENaC activity in the face of persistent volume expansion underlies the pathophysiology of Liddle's syndrome. A similar lack of down-regulation of ENaC activity, especially in the face of dietary salt excess, could underlie more common forms of low-renin hypertension. Liddle's syndrome can be regarded as the phenotypic extreme of low-renin hypertension *(17)*. In the original studies of the index case, aldosterone secretion was markedly suppressed, accounting for the descriptor "pseudoaldosteronism" *(22)*. The studies following renal transplantation of the proband *(15)* suggested that the suppression of the plasma renin activity was the result of ENaC gain of function in Liddle's syndrome. Continued suppression of aldosterone excretion despite rigorous dietary salt restriction is best explained by chronic suppression of 18-hydroxylase (adrenal aldosterone synthase) as a consequence of chronic volume expansion *(17)*.

## S810L MUTATION IN THE MINERALOCORTICOID RECEPTOR

A second form of PA1 has recently been described that results from a mutation in the hormone-binding domain of the mineralocorticoid receptor *(23)*. Although the phenotype of this autosomal dominant disorder strongly resembles Liddle's syndrome with hypertension and suppressed peripheral renin activity and aldosterone secretion, there is also an especially severe presentation during pregnancy *(23)*. In recognition of the classical description of Liddle's syndrome as PA1 *(1,22)*, it would be reasonable to refer to the activating mutations in the mineralocortidoid receptor as pseudoaldosteronism, type II (PA2) *(24)*. Geller et al. *(23)* reported that a serine to leucine mutation at position 810 (S810L) in the hormone-binding domain of the mineralocorticoid receptor changes the affinity of the mineralocorticoid receptor for a number of steroids: progesterone in particular has an exceptionally high affinity for the mutated receptor, thus accounting for the especially severe presentation during pregnancy. Geller et al. *(23)* screened for this mineralocorticoid receptor mutation in 75 patients with early onset of severe hypertension. Twenty-three relatives of a 15-year-old boy proband, who had severe hypertension and was heterozygous for a mis-sense mutation giving a S810L substitution in the mineralocorticoid receptor were evaluated. Upon evaluation, 11 of these 23 were diagnosed with severe hypertension before age 20, with three relatives dying of early heart failure before the age of 50 *(23)*.

Spironolactone is an agonist for the mutated receptor; therefore, spironolactone is ineffective in PA1 *(22)* and contraindicated in PA2 *(23)*. It appears that the mutated receptor has constitutively activated basal activity or may be responding to other endogenous steroids (e.g., 19-norprogesterone or 17-OH progesterone) to account for the clinical phenotype in males and nonpregnant females with PA2.

## NOVEL MINERALOCORTICOIDS AND LOW-RENIN HYPERTENSION

PA1 and PA2 are examples of constitutive alterations of ENaC activity occurring independently of mineralocorticoid hormones, in which mineralocorticoid receptor antagonist has no beneficial effect whatsoever. Are there novel or unusual mineralocorticoid hormones involved in low-renin hypertension? If so, then these syndromes would be responsive to mineralocorticoid receptor antagonists, in contrast to PA1 and PA2.

Pratt et al. *(25)* examined mineralocorticoid and $Na^+$ excretion in young black and white subjects. Black individuals appear, on average, to retain more $Na^+$ than white individuals; a higher production rate of mineralocorticoids could explain the greater $Na^+$ retention in blacks compared with whites. Although production of aldosterone has been shown to be lower in blacks, the level of another mineralocorticoid could potentially be increased, as has been described in a population of hypertensive Japanese subjects *(26)*. Blacks had lower plasma renin activity and aldosterone levels, and lower urinary aldosterone excretion rates. In a larger cohort of 407 young whites and 247 young blacks, 18-hydroxycortisol excretion rates were also lower in blacks compared to whites ($p = 0.021$). Such studies indicated that the increased $Na^+$ retention in black individuals does not appear to be secondary to increased production of aldosterone, deoxycorticosterone, cortisol, or 18-hydroxycortisol *(25)*. A primary renal mechanism may mediate the increase in $Na^+$ reabsorption in blacks, which could include constitutive activation of ENaC, or enhanced sensitivity to what would otherwise be relatively low levels of circulating mineralocorticoid hormones, or even activation of $Na^+$ reabsorption sites proximal to the distal site of ENaC expression. The finding of elevated urinary aldosterone/potassium excretory ratios *(14)* in these black subjects lends credence to this interpretation. Further detailed studies or urinary steroid metabolite profiles, including free cortisol *(27)* and free cortisone (*vida infra*) would be of great interest.

## GLUCOCORTICOID REMEDIABLE ALDOSTERONISM (GRA)

GRA results from a chimeric gene product that places 18-hydroxylase ("aldosterone synthase") under the control of an adrenocorticotrophic hormone (ACTH) promoter, which regulates its level and cellular site of expression. As a consequence, ACTH-regulated 18-hydroxylase activity is aberrantly expressed in the zona fasciculata and acts on cortisol, which is normally produced in this zone to form 18-hydroxycortisol (18-OH F) and 18-oxocortisol *(28)*. These 18-oxygenated steroids are greatly overproduced (between 20 and 30 times normal levels) and can be measured in the urine to help in the diagnosis of this syndrome *(29)*.

GRA is an important cause of human genetic hypertension that is relatively common, and represents the first example of successful application of the "new" genetics to define an inherited human hypertensive syndrome. The continuing stimulation of adrenal steroidogenesis by

ACTH and the suppressive effects of modest doses of dexamethasone are usual features of the syndrome. The normal renin-angiotensin-aldosterone system is restored by dexamethasone therapy, giving rise to increased plasma renin activity and Ang II generation, with normal stimulation of aldosterone production in the zona glomerulosa.

Recent studies have used genetic testing to prospectively identify affected family members and further define the clinical phenotype. Complete linkage analysis of GRA indicates that the physiological abnormalities of GRA arise from a gene duplication, an unequal crossing over on chromosome 8q, that fuses 5' regulatory region of 11-β hydroxylase to the coding sequences of aldosterone synthase *(28,30)*. Hypertension in affected individuals is diagnosed earlier in life (often in teenage years or prior to age 25 to 30), is difficult to control with conventional therapy, and is often accompanied by a family history of early death or morbidity from cerebral hemorrhages from underlying intracranial aneurysms *(31)*. Known GRA individuals should be screened in early adulthood and before pregnancy with magnetic resonance angiography for intracranial aneurysms. Furthermore, infants born to mothers affected with GRA should be screened for the disorder, because many develop clinically significant hypertension in childhood *(31)*.

Although pregnant women with GRA do not appear to be more prone to pre-eclampsia, they do have chronic hypertension, are at increased risk for exacerbation of their hypertension during pregnancy, and have a Cesarean section rate twice that of other general or even hypertensive obstetrical populations *(32)*.

## APPARENT MINERALOCORTICOID EXCESS (AME) SYNDROME

Renal 11β-hydroxysteroid dehydrogenase, type II (11β-OH SDH type II) is an enzyme in the kidney that is responsible for inactivating 11-hydroxy steroids, thus protecting type I mineralocorticoid receptors from being occupied by glucocorticoids *(33)*. The adrenal cortex produces cortisol in large amounts (10 to 20 mg/day) and aldosterone in lesser amounts (0.10 to 0.15 mg/day) to serve their physiological roles in cell growth, adaptation, and homeostasis. Cortisol and aldosterone have the same affinity for the type I mineralocorticoid receptors, and it has been proposed that the 11β OH SDH type II enzyme serves to maintain the aldosterone selectivity of the mineralocorticoid receptors by inactivating cortisol to cortisone, thus preventing cortisol-mediated mineralocorticoid hypertension (Fig. 2) *(33–35)*.

We now have much more precise knowledge of the underlying pathophysiology of the AME syndrome *(1)*. AME results from inactivation of 11β OH SDH type II enzyme, causing reduced metabolism of cortisol to cortisone, and local cortisol excess and mineralocorticoid response in aldosterone-target cells that express 11β OH SDH type II enzyme and type I mineralocorticoid receptors. The balance between cortisol and cortisone metabolism determines whether cortisol will exert any mineralocorticoid effect at the target tissue level. Although plasma cortisol levels are not necessarily elevated, the metabolic clearance of cortisol is prolonged in AME, and there is an excess urinary excretion of the reduced metabolites of cortisol compared to cortisone.

Features of the syndrome of AME include early onset of hypertension, with low-renin and aldosterone levels, hypokalemia, and severe salt-sensitive hypertension often accompanied by low birth weight, polyuria, failure to thrive, and nephrocalcinosis *(33,34)*. The syndrome of AME is of autosomal recessive inheritance; the mineralocorticoid receptor antagonist spironolactone is effective in treating this genetic cause of low-renin, low-aldosterone hypertension *(36)*.

Dietary salt excess does not appear to affect 11β OH SDH type II enzyme activity *(37)*, but there may be hypertensive patients who have mild 11β OH SDH type II enzyme deficiency and are therefore especially susceptible to the effects of exogenous inhibitors *(38)*. Salt-sensitive hypertension has recently been associated with reduced 11β OH SDH type II enzyme activity and with a specific polymorphism in the 11β OH SDH type II gene *(39)*. The allelic frequency of 11β OH SDH type II polymorphisms needs to be more fully described in human populations because there could be genetically determined differences in the levels of 11β OH SDH type II enzyme activity or in its response to exogenous inhibitors. More information is needed concerning the intrinsic activity and the regulation of 11β OH SDH type II enzyme in human hypertensive populations *(33,38)*.

An addition insight into the role of 11β OH SDH type II enzyme activity in regulating renal salt handling was obtained from studies of a patient with the AME syndrome who developed renal failure and then underwent renal transplantation *(40)*. Renal failure is distinctly uncommon in Liddle's syndrome and AME; nevertheless, renal transplantation corrects the underlying disorder in both syndromes. Palermo et al. *(40)* reported resolution of the AME syndrome in a 38-year-old female following renal transplantation. Although the abnormal ratio of the reduced metabolites of cortisol to cortisone in the urine was not corrected by renal transplantation, the ratio of urinary-free cortisol to cortisone was corrected and correlated with the resolution of the syndrome. This report suggests that the AME syndrome is a disorder of the metabolism of cortisol in the renal tubule that is best reflected by the measurement of urinary free cortisol and cortisone rather than the urinary excretion of hepatic tetrahydro-reduced metabolites that were not affected by renal transplantation. More extensive evaluations of these measurements are needed in a larger population of patients.

## FAMILIAL HYPERKALEMIA AND HYPERTENSION (FHH)

This is an autosomal-dominant disorder(s) with persistent hyperkalemia with normal glomerular filtration rate (GFR), reduced renal $K^+$ secretion, hyperchloremic metabolic acidosis, and, especially in adults, low-renin hypertension. Although formerly referred to as Gordon's syndrome or pseudohypoaldosteronism, type 2, the current descriptor (FHH) is now preferred *(41)*.

The first two descriptions of this syndrome mentioned hypertension as a prominent feature *(42,43)*, but subsequent reports of pediatric cases laid greater emphasis on the hyperkalemia with normal GFR *(44,45)*. Hyperchloremic metabolic acidosis is also a feature of the syndrome, but this can be relatively mild and is clearly affected in its severity by the hyperkalemia *(46)*.

Farfel et al. *(47)* and Nahum et al. *(48)* suggested that a proximal acidification defect could be superimposed on the basic distal renal tubular acidosis; hyperkalemia can suppress renal ammoniagenesis and proximal bicarbonate reabsorption and appears to play a major role in the acidification defect that causes the hyperchloremic metabolic acidosis in this syndrome.

Subsequent descriptions detailed the development of low-renin hypertension in this syndrome with low or normal levels of plasma aldosterone or aldosterone secretion *(46,49–57)*. Nahum et al. *(48)* reported that the serum aldosterone was high and plasma renin completely suppressed during severe hyperkalemia, but the serum aldosterone level was normalized when the hyperkalemia was corrected. Throckmorton and Bia *(57)* reported a 41-year-old male with hyperkalemia, mild hypertension, normal aldosterone levels, and no metabolic acidosis. Careful studies of the largest pedigree yet reported demonstrate that hypertension appears to become more severe as the subjects age, and initially the BP may, in fact, be normal *(58,59)*.

The low-renin state, as an index of volume expansion, is a manifestation of altered chloride reabsorption in the distal nephron *(55,56)*. There is an important relation between chloride ($Cl^-$) delivery to the aldosterone-responsive distal nephron and potassium ($K^+$) secretion. With this apparent increase in $Cl^-$ avidity, net NaCl reabsorption is favored and $K^+$ secretion (and to some extent, $H^+$ secretion) is reduced. If other anions are substituted, as during $Na_2SO_4$ or $NaHCO_3$ infusions, $K^+$ secretion will be enhanced and the hyperkalemia will improve *(55,56)*. A similar effect is seen with thiazide diuretics in this syndrome *(41)*; hyperkalemia is improved, presumably by inhibition of NaCl reabsorption in the distal convoluted tubule. Gordon et al. reported that dietary $Na^+$ restriction can also completely reverse the suppressed renin and aldosterone and hyperkalemia *(50)*. Schambelan et al. proposed that the underlying pathophysiologic mechanism, an inward $Cl^-$ absorptive rate in the distal nephron, might shunt the electrogenic current generated by $Na^+$ transport and thereby reduce $K^+$ secretion *(55)*. Although this shunt pathway was explicitly viewed as a paracellular route for $Cl^-$ permeation, and recent studies of the determinants of paracellular ion permeability in the thick ascending limb support this interpretation *(60,61)*, it is also worth noting that other recent studies have demonstrated apical expression of a cystic fibrosis transmembrane regulator-related protein *(62)* that could provide a transcellular route for transepithelial $Cl^-$ transport in the distal nephron. This transporter may provide another candidate gene for linkage efforts and studies of its regulation.

A third explanation for the syndrome focuses on a primary derangement of $K^+$ secretion in the distal nephron. This hypothesis accounts for the initial hyperkalemic presentation in childhood *(44,45,58,59)*, with subsequent development of systemic hypertension. It is not obvious how a primary derangement in the $K^+$ secretory process could eventuate in systemic hypertension through a primary increase in renal NaCl reabsorption and volume expansion. Further studies are clearly needed in this area.

The longitudinal studies *(58,59)* support this view that there is a primary derangement in the $K^+$ secretory pathway(s) in FHH. Nahum et al. *(48)* have reported that dDAVP appears to stimulate renal $K^+$ secretion and can correct the hyperkalemia, thus supporting the view of a primary impairment of $K^+$ secretion. Gordon et al *(51)* reported that stopping therapy in a patient treated with thiazide for 23 years was promptly followed by recurrence of all of the biochemical derangements, but the BP remained normal. Although the deranged $K^+$ secretion probably reflects a functional limitation on the apical K conductances in the distal tubule, the K conductive pathway still appears to be responsive to hyperpolarization of the transmembrane electrical potential when $SO4^{=}$ or $HCO3^{-}$ are substituted by $Cl^{-}$ *(49,50)* and can be stimulated by dDAVP *(42)*. Increasing distal NaCl delivery with furosemide after stimulation with desmopressin acetate *(64)* improves hyperkalemia. High-dose exogenous steroids can improve the hyperkalemia and metabolic acidosis *(65,66)*. In these settings, increases in luminal flow play an important role in $K^{+}$ secretion (Fig. 2). Recent studies have suggested that a $Ca^{++}$-regulated "maxi"-K channel may play a critical role in the flow-dependent $K^{+}$ secretory process *(63,64)*.

Recently, linkage studies have allowed significant progress. Although gain-of-function mutations of the NaCl cotransporter in the connecting tubule could explain the entire syndrome, all the linkage studies so far performed in various families have ruled out this gene, which is located on chromosome 16q13 *(41)*. Analysis of affected pedigrees showed autosomal dominant inheritance of the trait, and genetic linkage had been reported for chromosomes 1 *(65)* and 17 *(65,66)*. Further genetic heterogeneity was later established by the analysis of a large French pedigree, demonstrating linkage to chromosome 12 *(58,59)*. International collaborative efforts have allowed identification of two members, WNK1 and WNK4, of a novel family of serine/threonine kinases (*W*ith *N*o Lysine) *(67)*) as the genes causing the disease at two of these loci *(68)*. Both gene products have been shown to localize in the distal nephron, confirming this segment of the nephron as the anatomical and functional origin of FHH syndromes *(68)*. Disease-causing mutations in the WNK1 gene are large deletions in the first intron leading to a 5- to 10-fold increased gene expression. Transcripts of WNK1 are found in many tissues with two predominant isoforms: a 10-kb transcript, lacking the first exon, is expressed at high levels in the kidney, and a 12-kb transcript is predominant in the heart, vessels, and skeletal muscle. The large deletion in the first intron results in increased abnormal ubiquitous expression of the short kidney-specific transcript, and it is expected that the deleted sequence would contain a silencer element possibly interacting with a kidney-specific transcription factor. Mutations in the WNK4 gene are mis-sense mutations (single base substitutions) clustering in a short negatively charged domain highly conserved among this kinases family, which putatively alter the catalytic activity of the enzyme or modify its interactions with partners *(68)*.

It may not be coincidental that three distinct genetic loci have been defined by linkage studies. It is possible that each of these distinct sites on chromosome 1q31-42 *(65)*, chromosome 12p13.3 *(59)*, and chromosome 17p11-q21 *(65,66)* code for a specific transport process corresponding to the three pathophysiologic processes. Indeed, the apparent phenotypic versatility in the various cases reported worldwide since 1964 is consistent with the genetic heterogeneity and supports the possibility that this syndrome actually encompasses a variety of related but distinct tubular dysfunctions. Additional genetic heterogeneity may emerge as the currently defined loci are identified and investigated in pedigree studies. In fact, there are reported FHH pedigrees in which linkage to the three previously identified loci has been ruled out, implying the existence of at least a fourth locus for FHH *(69)*.

The recent identification of two genes responsible for FHH has still not allowed a complete definition of the underlying pathophysiology(ies) of FHH because the regulators, effectors, and targets of WNK kinases are so far unknown. The identification of this novel family of kinases *(67)* and linkage to some forms of FHH *(68)* represents, however, a crucial step toward the characterization of new regulatory pathways of ion transport in the distal part of the nephron and BP control *(58)*. It is even possible that these loci may be related to more common forms of essential hypertension. Soubrier *(70)* has suggested that this locus may account for a linkage of hypertension to chromosome 17 observed in the Framingham study *(66)*.

## CONCLUSIONS

Recent advances in understanding the molecular pathophysiology of Mendelian hypertensive disorders occurred with the convergence of elegant genetic linkage efforts, informative and willing pedigrees, and astute insights about the underlying clinical and physiologic processes. In many cases, the latter insights have provided the obvious candidate gene for directed linkage efforts. Although the described Mendelian forms of human hypertension are quite rare, all converge on renal mechanisms of sodium reabsorption as a final common pathway *(71)*. It is important to determine whether there are contributions of these pathways to the more common forms of hypertension. Of note to our overall understanding of the various causes of human essential hypertension, we now have clear-cut examples whereby disorders of systemic BP regulation can be attributed to primary renal mechanisms. Future studies are needed to define the specific interactions of dietary mineral constituents with the renal NaCl transport pathways.

## ACKNOWLEDGMENT

Grant support from the National Institutes of Health (DK19407, DK53161) is acknowledged.

## REFERENCES

1. Scheinman SJ, Guay-Woodford LM, Thakker RV, Warnock DG. Genetic disorders of renal electrolyte transport. N Engl J Med 1999;340:1177–1187.
2. Meneton P, Oh YS, Warnock DG. Genetic renal tubular disorders of renal ion channels and transporters. Sem Nephrol 2001;21:81–93.
3. Meneton P, Warnock DG. Involvement of renal apical Na transport systems in the control of blood pressure. Am J Kidney Dis 2001;37:S39–S47.
4. Staub O, Dho S, Henry PC, et al. WW domains of Nedd4 bind to the proline-rich PY motifs in the epithelial $Na^+$ channel deleted in Liddle's syndrome. EMBO J. 1996;15:2371–2380.
5. Abriel H, Loffing J, Rebhun JF, et al. Defective regulation of the epithelial Na+ channel by Nedd4 in Liddle's syndrome. J Clin Invest 1999;103:667–673.
6. Kamynina E, Debonneville C, Bens M, Vandewalle A, Staub O. A novel mouse Nedd4 protein suppresses the activity of the epithelial Na+ channel. Faseb J 2001;15:204–214.
7. Debonneville C, Flores SY, Kamynina E, et al. Phosphorylation of Nedd4-2 by Sgk1 regulates epithelial Na(+) channel cell surface expression. Embo J 2001;20: 7052–7059.
8. Warnock DG. Liddle syndrome: genetics and mechanisms of Na+ channel defects. Am J Med Sci 2001;322:302–307.
9. Warnock DG. Liddle syndrome: an autosomal dominant form of human hypertension. Kidney Int 1998;53:18–24.
10. Persu A, Barbry P, Bassilana F, et al. Genetic analysis of the beta subunit of the epithelial $Na^+$ channel in essential hypertension. Hypertension 1998;32:129–137.
11. Baker EH, Dong YB, Sagnella GA, et al. Association of hypertension with T594M mutation in beta subunit of epithelial sodium channels in black people resident in London. Lancet 1998;351:1388–1392.
12. Baker EH, Dong YB, Sagnella GA, MacGregor GA. T594M mutation in the ENaC beta subunit and low-renin hypertension in blacks: author's reply. Am J Kidney Dis 1999; 34:583-587.
13. Warnock DG. T594M mutation in the ENaC beta subunit and low-renin hypertension in blacks. Journal Club. Am J Kidney Dis 1999;34:579–587.
14. Ambrosius WT, Bloem LJ, Zhou L, et al. Genetic variants in the epithelial sodium channel in relation to aldosterone and potassium excretion and risk for hypertension. Hypertension 1999;34:631–637.
15. Botero-Velez M, Curtis JJ, Warnock DG. Brief report: Liddle's syndrome revisited: a disorder of sodium reabsorption in the distal tubule. N Engl J Med 1994;330:178–181.
16. Pratt JH, Eckert GJ, Newman S, Ambrosius WT. Blood pressure responses to small doses of amiloride and spironolactone in normotensive subjects. Hypertension 2001;38:1124–1129.
17. Warnock DG. The epithelial sodium channel in hypertension. Curr Hypertens Rep 1999;1:158–163.
18. Griffing GT, Wilson TE, Melby JC. Alterations in aldosterone secretion and metabolism in low renin hypertension. J Clin Endocrinol Metab 1990;71: 1454–1460.
19. Paillard F, Chansel D, Brand E, et al. Genotype-phenotype relationships for the renin-angiotensin-aldosterone system in a normal population. Hypertension 1999;34:423–429.
20. Fisher ND, Gleason RE, Moore TJ, Williams GH, Hollenberg NK. Regulation of aldosterone secretion in hypertensive blacks. Hypertension 1994;23:179–184.

21. Shackleton CH. Mass spectrometry in the diagnosis of steroid-related disorders and in hypertension research. J Steroid Biochem Mol Biol 1993;45:127–140.
22. Liddle GW, Bledsoe T, Coppage WSJ. A familial renal disorder simulating primary aldosteronism but with negligible aldosterone secretion. Trans Assoc Am Physicians 1963;76:199–213.
23. Geller DS, Farhi A, Pinkerton N, et al. Activating mineralocorticoid receptor mutation in hypertension exacerbated by pregnancy. Science 2000;289:119–123.
24. Warnock DG. Genetic forms of human hypertension. Curr Opin Neph Hyperten 2001;10:493–499.
25. Pratt JH, Rebhun JF, Zhou L, et al. Levels of mineralocorticoids in whites and blacks. Hypertension 1999;34:315–319.
26. Komiya I, Yamada T, Aizawa T, et al. Inappropriate elevation of the aldosterone/plasma renin activity ratio in hypertensive patients and 18-hydroxy-11-deoxycorticosterone: a subtype of essential hypertension? Cardiology 1991;78:99–110.
27. Litchfield WR, Hunt SC, Jeunemaitre X, et al. Increased urinary free cortisol: a potential intermediate phenotype of essential hypertension. Hypertension 1998; 31:569–574.
28. Lifton RP, Dluhy RG, Powers M, et al. A chimaeric 11 β-hydroxylase/aldosterone synthase gene causes glucocorticoid-remediable aldosteronism and human hypertension. Nature 1992;355:262–265.
29. Rich GM, Ulick S, Cook S, Wang JZ, Lifton RP, Dluhy RG. Glucocorticoid-remediable aldosteronism in a large kindred: clinical spectrum and diagnosis using a characteristic biochemical phenotype. Ann Intern Med 1992;116:813–820.
30. Lifton RP, Dluhy RG, Powers M, et al. Hereditary hypertension caused by chimaeric gene duplications and ectopic expression of aldosterone synthase. Nat Genet 1992;2:66–74.
31. Litchfield WR, Anderson BF, Weiss RJ, Lifton RP, Dluhy RG. Intracranial aneurysm and hemorrhagic stroke in glucocorticoid-remediable aldosteronism. Hypertension 1998;31:445–450.
32. Wycoff JA, Seely EW, Hurwitz S, Anderson BF, Lifton RP, Dluhy RG. Glucocorticoid-remediable aldosteronism and pregnancy. Hypertension 2000;35:668–672.
33. Ferrari P, Krozowski ZS. Role of 11 beta-hydroxysteroid dehydrogenase type 2 in blood pressure regulation. Kidney Int 2000;57:1374–1381.
34. Ferrari P. Genetics of the mineralocorticoid system in primary hypertension. Curr Hypertens Rep 2002;4:18–24.
35. Stewart PM, Corrie JE, Shackleton CH, Edwards CR. Syndrome of apparent mineralocorticoid excess. A defect in the cortisol-cortisone shuttle. J Clin Invest 1988;82:340–349.
36. Nunez BS, Rogerson FM, Mune T, et al. Mutants of 11beta-hydroxysteroid dehydrogenase (11-HSD2) with partial activity: improved correlations between genotype and biochemical phenotype in apparent mineralocorticoid excess. Hypertension 1999;34:638–642.
37. Ingram MC, Wallace AM, Collier A, Fraser R, Connell JMC. Sodium status, corticosteroid metabolism and blood pressure in normal human subjects and in a patient with abnormal salt appetite. Clin Exp Pharmacol Physiol 1996;23:375–378.
38. Warnock DG. Low renin hypertension in the next millennium. Sem Nephrol 2000;20:40–46.
39. Lovati E, Ferrari P, Dick B, et al. Molecular basis of human salt sensitivity: the role of the 11beta-hydroxysteroid dehydrogenase type 2. J Clin Endo Metab 1999; 84:3745–3749.

40. Palermo M, Cossu M, Shackleton CHL. Cure of apparent mineralocorticoid excess by kidney transplantation. N Engl J Med 1998;339:1787–1788.
41. Warnock DG. Genetic forms of renal potassium and magnesium wasting. Am J Med 2002;112:235–236.
42. Paver WKA, Pauline GJ. Hypertension and hyperpotassemia without renal disease in a young male. Med J Aust 1964;2:305–306.
43. Arnold JE, Healy JK. Hyperkalemia, hypertension and systemic acidosis without renal failure associated with a tubular defect in potassium excretion. Am J Med 1969;47:461–472.
44. Spitzer A, Edelmann CM, Jr., Goldberg LD, Henneman PH. Short stature, hyperkalemia and acidosis: a defect in renal transport of potassium. Kidney Int 1973;3:251–257.
45. Weinstein SF, Allan DM, Mendoza SA. Hyperkalemia, acidosis, and short stature associated with a defect in renal potassium excretion. J Pediatr 1974;85:355–358.
46. Brautbar N, Levi J, Rosler A, et al. Familial hyperkalemia, hypertension, and hyporeninemia with normal aldosterone levels: a tubular defect in potassium handling. Arch Intern Med 1978;138:607–610.
47. Farfel Z, Iaina A, Levi J, Gafni J. Proximal renal tubular acidosis: association with familial normaldosteronemic hyperpotassemia and hypertension. Arch Intern Med 1978;138:1837–1840.
48. Nahum H, Paillard M, Prigent A, et al. Pseudohypoaldosteronism type II: proximal renal tubular acidosis and dDAVP-sensitive renal hyperkalemia. Am J Nephrol 1986;6:253–262.
49. Farfel Z, Iaina A, Rosenthal T, Waks U, Shibolet S, Gafni J. Familial hyperpotassemia and hypertension accompanied by normal plasma aldosterone levels: possible hereditary cell membrane defect. Arch Intern Med 1978;138:1828–1832.
50. Gordon RD, Geddes RA, Pawsey CG, O'Halloran MW. Hypertension and severe hyperkalaemia associated with suppression of renin and aldosterone and completely reversed by dietary sodium restriction. Austr Ann Med 1970;19:287–924.
51. Gordon RD. The syndrome of hypertension and hyperkalaemia with normal GFR: a unique pathophysiological mechanism for hypertension? Clin Exp Pharmacol Physiol 1986;13:329–333.
52. Gordon RD. The syndrome of hypertension and hyperkalemia with normal glomerular filtration rate: Gordon's syndrome. Aust NZ J Med 1986;16:183–184.
53. Gordon RD, Hodsman GP. The syndrome of hypertension and hyperkalaemia without renal failure: long term correction by thiazide diuretic. Scott Med J 1986;31:43–44.
54. Isenring P, Lebel M, Grose JH. Endocrine sodium and volume regulation in familial hyperkalemia with hypertension. Hypertension 1992;19:371–377.
55. Schambelan M, Sebastian A, Rector FC, Jr. Mineralocorticoid-resistant renal hyperkalemia without salt wasting (type II pseudohypoaldosteronism): role of increased renal chloride reabsorption. Kidney Int 1981;19:716–727.
56. Take C, Ikeda K, Kurasawa T, Kurokawa K. Increased chloride reabsorption as an inherited renal tubular defect in familial type II pseudohypoaldosteronism. N Engl J Med 1991;324:472–476.
57. Throckmorton DC, Bia MJ. Pseudohypoaldosteronism: case report and discussion of the syndrome. Yale J Biol Med 1991;64:247–254.
58. Disse-Nicodème S, Achard J-M, Fiquet-Kempf B, et al. Hypertension familiale hyperkaliemique: analyse de la variabilité phenotypique par l'étude de 7 familles.

In: Grunfield JP, ed. Actualités Néphrologiques de l'Hôpital Necker. Paris: Medicine-Sciences Flammarion, 2001:60–71.
59. Disse-Nicodème S, Achard JM, Desitter I, et al. A new locus on chromosome 12p13.3 for pseudohypoaldosteronism type II, an autosomal dominant form of hypertension. Am J Hum Genet 2000;67:302–310.
60. Simon DB, Lu Y, Choate KA, et al. Paracellin-1, a renal tight junction protein required for paracellular $Mg^{2+}$ resorption. Science 1999;285:103–106.
61. Yu AS. Paracellular solute transport: more than just a leak? Curr Opin Nephrol Hypertens 2000;9:513–515.
62. Van Huyen JP, Bens M, Teulon J, Vandewalle A. Vasopressin-stimulated chloride transport in transimmortalized mouse cell lines derived from the distal convoluted tubule and cortical and inner medullary collecting ducts. Nephrol Dial Transplant 2001;16:238–245.
63. Woda CB, Leite M, Jr., Rohatgi R, Satlin LM. Effects of luminal flow and nucleotides on $[Ca^{(2+)}]_{(i)}$ in rabbit cortical collecting duct. Am J Physiol Renal Physiol 2002;283:F437–F446.
64. Woda CB, Bragin A, Kleyman TR, Satlin LM. Flow-dependent K+ secretion in the cortical collecting duct is mediated by a maxi-K channel. Am J Physiol Renal Physiol 2001;280:F786–F793.
65. Mansfield TA, Simon DB, Farfel Z, et al. Multilocus linkage of familial hyperkalaemia and hypertension, pseudohypoaldosteronism type II, to chromosomes 1q31-42 and 17p11-q21. Nat Genet 1997;16:202–205.
66. O'Shaughnessy KM, Fu B, Johnson A, Gordon RD. Linkage of Gordon's syndrome to the long arm of chromosome 17 in a region recently linked to familial essential hypertension. J Hum Hypertens 1998;12:675–678.
67. Xu B, English JM, Wilsbacher JL, Stippec S, Goldsmith EJ, Cobb MH. WNK1, a novel mammalian serine/threonine protein kinase lacking the catalytic lysine in subdomain II.PG - 16795-801. J Biol Chem 2000;275:16795–16801.
68. Wilson FH, Disse-Nicodeme S, Choate KA, et al. Human hypertension caused by mutations in WNK kinases. Science 2001;293:1107–1112.
69. Achard JM, Disse-Nicodeme S, Fiquet-Kempf B, Jeunemaitre X. Phenotypic and genetic heterogeneity of familial hyperkalaemic hypertension (Gordon syndrome). Clin Exp Pharmacol Physiol 2001;28:1048–1052.
70. Soubrier F. Gordon's syndrome, renal tubule, chromosome 17 and essential hypertension: a credible link? J Hum Hypertens 1998;12:663–664.
71. Lifton RP, Gharavi AG, Geller DS. Molecular mechanisms of human hypertension. Cell 2001;104:545–56.

# 12 Hypertension in Cushing's Syndrome

*Judith A. Whitworth,* MD, PhD,
*George J. Mangos,* MD,
*and John J. Kelly,* MD

*Contents*



## INTRODUCTION

The adrenal glands were discovered by Bartolommeo Eustachio in 1563—the "glandular renibus incumbentes." Adrenal disease was first recognized by Addison in 1855. Hypertension caused by adrenal disease has been recorded only in the last 100 years.

The name of Harvey Cushing (1869–1939), a US neurosurgeon, is given to two clinical syndromes: acoustic neuroma and glucocorticoid (GC) excess *(1)*. He was best known in his day for his pioneering work in reducing neurosurgical mortality and for his Pulitzer Prize winning biography of Osler. He published his classical monograph, "The pituitary body and its disorders," in 1912. Cushing believed the disorder was caused by overactivity of the adrenal cortex secondary to a pituitary basophil disorder. "The basophil adenomas of the pituitary body and their clinical manifestations (pituitary basophilism)," a compilation of

From: *Secondary Hypertension: Clinical Presentation, Diagnosis, and Treatment*
Edited by: G. A. Mansoor © Humana Press Inc., Totowa, NJ

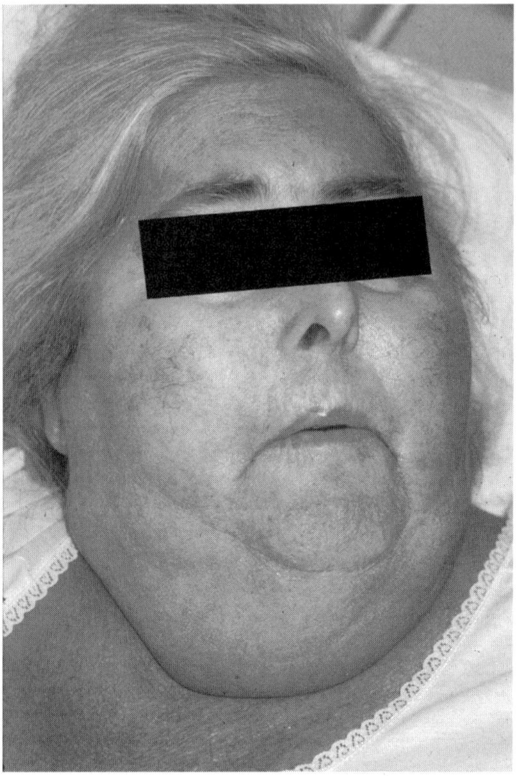

**Fig. 1.** Classical Cushingoid face.

previously reported cases, was published in 1932 *(2)*. Hypertension was a feature in 9 of 12 of the original cases *(3)*. Cushing's name was given to the syndrome by Bishop and Close *(4)*.

Cushing's syndrome of GC excess is characterized by moon face (Fig. 1), truncal obesity, abdominal striae, plethora, hirsutism, glucose intolerance and diabetes, hypogonadism, neuropsychiatric disorders including depression and psychosis, osteoporosis, cataracts, renal calculi, senile purpura, proximal myopathy, susceptibility to infection, particularly fungal and opportunistic infections, and hypertension (Table 1).

Cortisol has also been implicated in other forms of hypertension, including essential hypertension *(5)* but this is beyond the scope of this chapter, which focuses on the hypertension of Cushing's syndrome.

### *Adrenocorticotropic Hormone (ACTH) Excess*

Cushing's disease is responsible for some two-thirds of cases and is thus the commonest cause of Cushing's syndrome *(6)*. Pituitary ACTH

Table 1
Classification of Cushing's Syndrome

| | |
|---|---|
| *Spontaneous* | |
| ACTH excess | |
| Pituitary ACTH excess (Cushing's disease) | ~ 2/3 |
| Ectopic ACTH production | ~ 15% |
| Ectopic CRF production | Very rare |
| Adrenal Cushing's syndrome | ~ 9% |
| Adrenal adenoma | |
| Gardner's syndrome | |
| Adrenal carcinoma | ~ 8% |
| Primary adrenal hyperplasia | Rare |
| Carney's syndrome | |
| McClure-Albright syndrome | |
| Food-dependent Cushing's | |
| *Iatrogenic/factitious* | |
| ACTH administration | Rare |
| Glucocorticoid therapy | Common |
| Pseudo-Cushing's syndrome | |
| Alcohol induced | |
| Depression | |
| AIDS/HIV therapy (protease inhibitor–associated lipodystrophy) | |

Percentages from ref. *3*.

secretion (Fig. 2) is increased *(7)* and plasma ACTH concentrations are often elevated, leading to bilateral adrenal hyperplasia. Pituitary microadenomas are present in most cases and the disease is gradual in onset. Some 10% of patients have discrete pituitary adenomas, either chromophobe or basophil, and enlargement of the pituitary fossa, which can present with visual defects or pituitary hypofunction. Most pituitary adenomas are monoclonal, suggesting a primary pituitary disorder *(3)*.

### Ectopic ACTH Secretion

ACTH secretion from primary tumors leads to bilateral adrenal hyperplasia with suppression of pituitary ACTH secretion. Ectopic ACTH secretion is often associated with carcinoma of the lung but other cancers and carcinoid and endocrine tumors, including pheochromocytoma, also cause ectopic ACTH production *(8)*. Ectopic ACTH accounts for around 15% of cases of Cushing's syndrome *(6)*. Hypertension has been reported to be less common in Cushing's syndrome secondary to ectopic ACTH production than in other forms *(9)* but can also be a

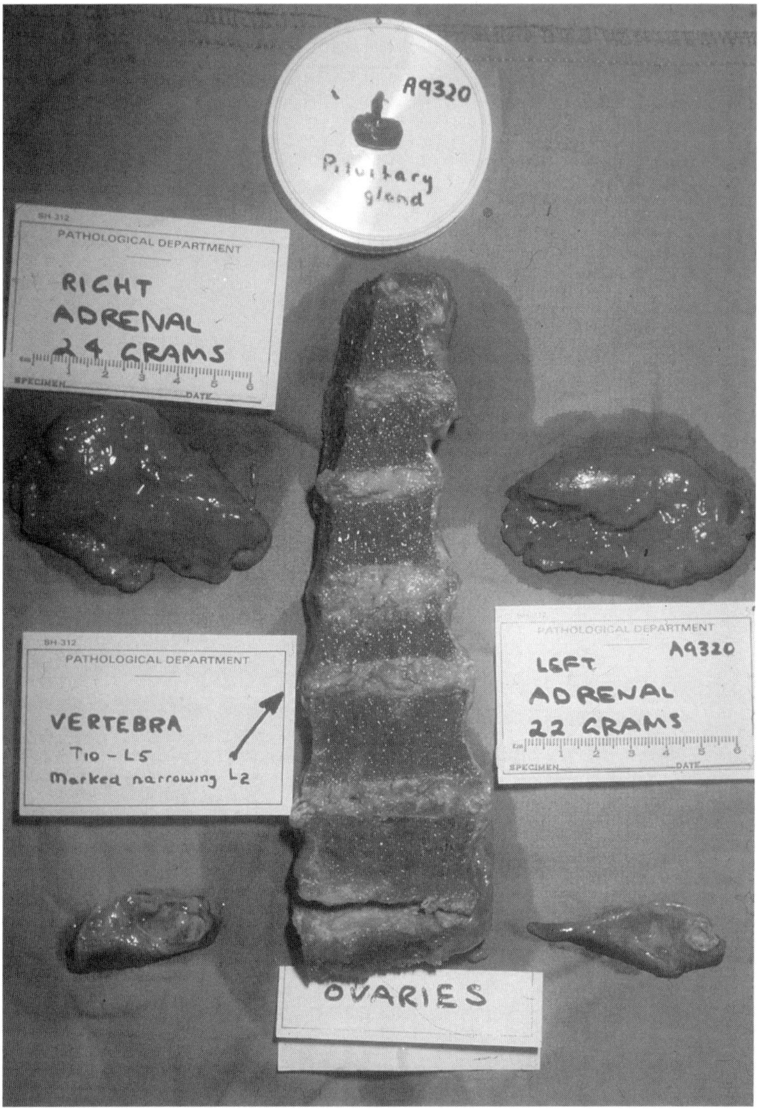


**Fig. 2.** Autopsy findings in a patient with Cushing's disease, with adrenal hyperplasia, pituitary microadenoma, and vertebral collapse.

prominent feature *(3)*. Men are more commonly affected than women and hypokalemic alkalosis, weakness, and pigmentation are prominent. Signs of GC excess may be lacking. In these patients onset may be sudden and progression rapid.

#### Ectopic Corticotrophin-Releasing Factor

Ectopic corticotrophin-releasing factor (CRF) production from nonhypothalamic tumors has been reported as an extremely rare cause of ACTH-dependent Cushing's syndrome.

### *Cushing's Syndrome Secondary to Adrenal Pathology*

#### Adrenal Adenoma

Adrenal adenoma has been reported to account for around 9% of cases of Cushing's syndrome *(6)*. Commonly, there is a single adenoma with atrophy of ipsilateral normal adrenal tissue and the normal contralateral adrenal as a consequence of suppression of pituitary ACTH secretion. Multiple bilateral adrenal adenomas are very rare *(10)*.

Most adrenal adenomas are found by incidental scanning and most are nonfunctioning. A small proportion (up to 12%) do have excess cortisol production with little evidence of clinical features of Cushing's syndrome. This is sometimes called pre-Cushing's syndrome *(11)*.

Cortisol-producing adrenal adenoma has also been reported as a manifestation of Gardner's syndrome (desmoid tumors, osteomas, pigmented retinal lesions, and familial adenomatous polyposis) *(12)*.

A case of adrenocortical–pituitary hybrid tumor, with an adrenal adenoma secreting both cortisol and ACTH precursors, suggests genetic and phenotypic plasticity in the hypothalamic–pituitary–adrenal axis *(13)*. Transition from pituitary-dependent to adrenal-dependent Cushing's syndrome has also been described *(14)*.

#### Adrenal Carcinoma

Carcinoma of the adrenal is reported to cause around 8% of cases of Cushing's syndrome *(6)* and is more common in younger patients. Hypertension and electrolyte abnormalities may be prominent. Adrenal carcinomas usually present with large (> 4 cm) aggressive masses. In a large series, 85% of the adrenal carcinomas produced glucocorticoids either alone or in combination with other steroids *(15)*.

#### Adrenal Hyperplasia (Primary)

Rarely, patients with apparently autonomous cortisol overproduction are found to have bilateral adrenal hyperplasia. It is more common in children and young adults *(16)*. Inappropriate adrenal sensitivity to gastric inhibitory polypeptide—so-called food-dependent Cushing's syndrome—is one such cause *(17)*. Other cases of abnormal adrenal receptors to a variety of hormones, e.g., vasopressin, catecholamines, and serotonin, have been recognized in causing Cushing's syndrome

*(18)*. Development of pigmented micronodular adrenocortical hyperplasia may be caused by circulating adrenal stimulating immunoglobulins *(14)*. Cushing's syndrome with unilateral nodular adrenal hyperplasia has also been reported *(19)* and may represent transition from pituitary-dependent disease with bilateral adrenal hyperplasia developing into nodular hyperplasia after which nodules may become autonomous and suppress ACTH secretion *(14)*.

Carney's syndrome is a rare autosomal dominant condition characterized by skin pigmentation and a range of tumors (peripheral nerve, endocrine, and mesenchymal), which can include adrenal pigmented multinodular adrenocortical dysplasia. It may be caused by ACTH receptor antibody stimulation. McCune-Albright syndrome is characterized by a triad of polyostotic fibrous dysplasia, café-au-lait spots, and precocious puberty. Endocrine hyperfunction may involve the adrenal. The genetic defect is mutation of the gene coding for the signaling units of the G protein linked to adenyl cyclase *(20)*.

## *Iatrogenic Cushing's Syndrome*

### Exogenous ACTH Administration

Recognition that ACTH administration was an important cause of hypertension occurred soon after its introduction into clinical practice *(21,22)*. ACTH is used for some neurological conditions (for example, infantile spasms) where development of hypertension may limit therapy *(23)*, but rarely for inflammatory conditions. ACTH is also used in endocrine diagnosis and may raise blood pressure (BP) even under these short-term conditions *(24)*.

### GC Administration

Synthetic GCs have been used extensively in clinical practice over many years, orally, topically, intranasally, and into joints and are now the most common cause of Cushing's syndrome. GC therapy is known to be associated with severe hypertension *(25,26)*. Hypertension is reported in around 20% of patients who receive exogenous GC *(22,27)*. In experimental studies synthetic GCs invariably increase pressure to at least some extent *(28)*. Factitious cases are characterized by typical symptoms and signs but low serum and urinary cortisol, consequent on abuse of synthetic GCs *(29)*.

### Pseudo-Cushing's Syndrome

A pseudo-Cushing's syndrome occurs in association with depression, stress, and alcohol abuse *(30)*. Hypertension is common. The alcohol-induced syndrome is reversed on withdrawal of alcohol *(31)*.

## Clinical Features of Cushing's Syndrome

The classic patient with Cushing's syndrome is described as a lemon on sticks. This reflects the truncal obesity (the lemon) with steroid-induced myopathy and limb muscle wasting (the sticks) (Fig. 3). The skin may exhibit striae, purpura, ecchymoses, hirsutism, and acne. Around 80% of patients with idiopathic Cushing's syndrome are hypertensive (58–85%) *(32)* but as indicated above it is likely that all patients have at least some elevation of BP. Glucose intolerance and diabetes, menstrual irregularity, sterility, loss of libido, osteoporosis, polycythemia, edema, peptic ulceration, polyuria, nephrocalcinosis, renal stones, tendency to infection and poor wound healing, cataracts, and mood alteration may all be prominent *(33)*. The clinical features of greatest value in making the diagnosis are said to be hypertension, myopathy, and bruising *(34)*. Hyperlipidemia is common, and with the hypertension, hyperglycemia, and obesity, accelerated atherosclerosis accounts for the substantial cardiovascular morbidity and mortality.

Hypokalemia is unusual unless malignancy is present *(8)*, but polycythemia, neutrophilia, lymphopenia, and eosinopenia are common. The naturally occurring disease is relatively rare and affects women in the third and fourth decades, with a male to female ratio around 1:4. In Cushing's disease, the clinical symptoms and signs are usually insidious and duration of illness prior to diagnosis some 3 to 6 years *(32)*. Rapid onset of symptoms suggests malignancy, either adrenal carcinoma or ectopic ACTH production.

## Hypertension in Cushing's Syndrome

Cushing's syndrome is a rare cause of hypertension, said to affect less than 0.1% of the general population and around 1 in 400 hypertensives. In a study from Denmark, the incidence was 1.2–1.7 per million per year (Cushing's disease), 0.6 per million per year (adrenal adenoma), and 0.2 per million per year (adrenal carcinoma). Other types were rare *(35)*. A Spanish study reported 2.4 per million per year for Cushing's disease, with a prevalence of 39.1 per million *(32)*. Given that the prevalence of hypertension in Western countries is around 15%, it seems likely that on a population basis, Cushing's syndrome accounts for less than 1 in 1000 cases—higher figures probably reflect a selected population of hypertensives.

The patient with hypertension caused by Cushing's syndrome is usually not a problem in the investigation of hypertension, as the diagnosis is apparent on clinical grounds. However, the diagnosis may be considered in the obese hypertensive patient.

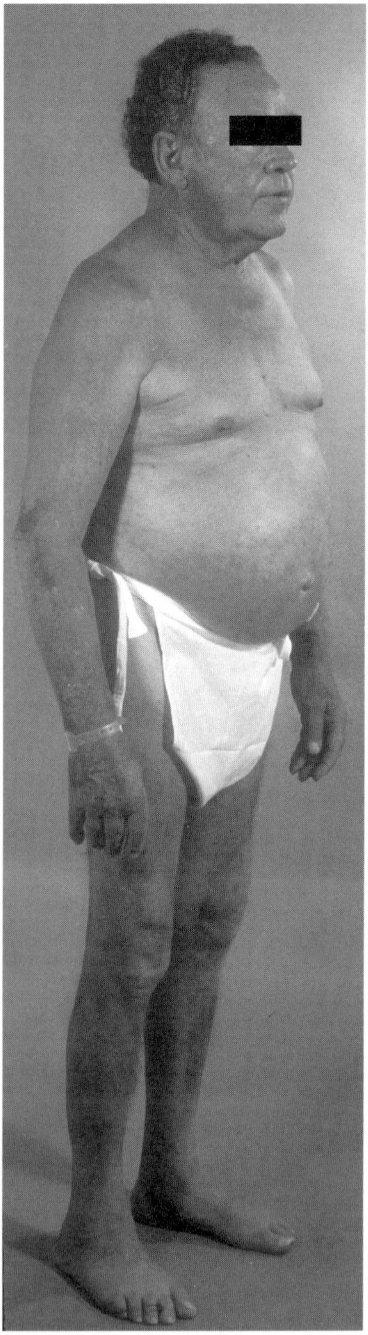

**Fig. 3.** Classical Cushingoid habitus.

Hypertension is very frequent in Cushing's syndrome, and around 80% of patients have clinical hypertension *(36)*. Hypertension is a major contributor to the excess cardiovascular morbidity and mortality of Cushing's syndrome along with age and persistence of diabetes *(32)*. In a study of 148 patients with Cushing's syndrome from Padua, 72% of whom were hypertensive, hypertensive patients were significantly older *(37)*. Cardiovascular damage (abnormal fundoscopy, left ventricular hypertrophy) was observed in a high proportion of hypertensive patients, but also some normotensives *(37)*.

Cardiac output and peripheral resistance are increased in Cushing's syndrome *(38)* as is plasma volume, but total exchangeable sodium was normal *(39)*. Left ventricular hypertrophy is reportedly more severe, and the frequency of asymmetric septal hypertrophy greater in Cushing's syndrome than in other types of hypertension *(40)*. Long exposure to increased cortisol appears to be the major determinant of left ventricular concentric remodeling *(41)*. Dilated cardiomyopathy can also be caused by Cushing's disease *(42)*. Prolonged corticosteroid excess accelerates atherosclerosis, and hypertension, hypercholesterolemia, hypertriglyceridemia, and impairment of glucose tolerance are all implicated *(43)*. Loss of the normal nocturnal fall in BP on ambulatory monitoring is a feature of Cushing's syndrome and GC-induced hypertension, but is of limited diagnostic use *(44,45)* and may relate at least in part to the sleep disturbance that is a common feature of the condition *(46)*. In contrast to the altered BP rhythmicity, heart rate variability is preserved *(45)*.

It is not clear whether the prevalence and severity of the hypertension in Cushing's syndrome depends on etiology *(47)*. Ross et al. *(33)* reported that all 15 patients with adrenal adenoma or carcinoma were hypertensive compared with 87% of patients with adrenal hyperplasia. Greminger et al. reported 100% of patients with adrenal carcinoma were hypertensive compared with 83% with adrenal adenoma and 64% with Cushing's disease *(48)*. Sonino et al. reported 64% of pituitary-dependent patients were hypertensive and 70% of those with adrenal adenoma or hyperplasia *(37)*. Hypertension is claimed to be more severe in the patients with adrenal malignancy *(48)*. In contrast, Welbourn et al. *(49)* reported that 93% of their patients with Cushing's syndrome were hypertensive and that the underlying lesion had no effect on incidence of severity. Forty percent of their patients had cardiovascular complications. It is generally agreed that patients with ectopic ACTH production are less likely to be hypertensive *(9)*. This may reflect the lower BP frequently seen in patients with severe malignant disease, the fact that the disease course is usually quite short, or possibly a different steroid profile.

Cortisol excess is the hallmark of Cushing's syndrome and cortisol excess correlates with the hypertension in some *(50,51)* but not all studies *(37)*. Aldosterone is usually normal or low *(52,53)*, but rarely in patients with adrenal adenoma aldosterone may be increased *(54)*. There is no relationship between mineralocorticoids and BP, and very high levels of mineralocorticoids were found in some normotensive patients with Cushing's syndrome *(37)*. Corticosterone *(55,56)*, deoxycorticosterone (DOC), and 11-deoxycortisol may all be increased *(56)*, as may 18-hydroxy-DOC *(57)* and 19-nor-DOC *(58)*. Dihydroepiandrostenedione sulfate is normal or high in Cushing's disease and low in adenoma *(59)*. Plasma levels of aldosterone, corticosterone, 18-hydroxycorticosterone, and 18-hydroxy-DOC were similar in patients with Cushing's disease and essential hypertension, suggesting they were unlikely to be involved in the pathogenesis of the hypertension *(60)*. Corticotrophin-releasing hormone (CRH) is normal or low in plasma and cerebrospinal fluid in pituitary-dependent Cushing's *(37)*.

Increased pressor responses to noradrenaline and angiotensin II (Ang II) have been reported in patients with Cushing's syndrome *(61,62)*. Cardiac sensitivity to isoprenaline was increased in Cushing's disease in one study and there was no increase in β-adrenoreceptor density *(39)*. $\alpha_2$-Adrenoceptor density and affinity on platelets was normal; $\beta_2$-adrenoceptor density on lymphocytes was normal but affinity was decreased *(39)*. Catecholamines were generally normal *(37)*. Plasma neuropeptide Y concentrations were also normal *(63)*.

Axelrod *(64)* proposed that GC inhibition of phospholipase with inhibition of prostacyclin production would lead to increases in vascular tone, but whether this mechanism does play a role is unclear. Urinary kallikrein and prostaglandin $E_2$ were reduced in patients with Cushing's syndrome because of adrenal adenoma *(62)*, but urinary total kininase, kininase I and II, and neutral endopeptidase were higher in patients with Cushing's syndrome than in normotensives *(65)*. In the one patient tested, urinary excretion of nitrate and nitrite was low, even after L-arginine administration *(66)*.

GCs have important effects on the renin-angiotensin system (RAS). GCs increase renin substrate *(67)* and reduce plasma renin concentration and Ang II *(68)*. Renin substrate may be elevated in Cushing's syndrome *(69)* but the RAS is usually normal *(39,62,70)*. Saralasin was variously reported to lower BP in Cushing's syndrome *(71)* or have no effect *(72)*, depending on sodium status. Similarly, captopril has been found to lower *(62)* or not lower pressure *(48)*.

Catecholamine concentrations in plasma and urine are normal *(39,69)* and atrial natriuretic peptide is increased in Cushing's syndrome *(73,74)*. Cushing's syndrome is associated with an increase in erythrocyte sodium potassium adenosine triphosphatase (ATPase). Ouabain-sensitive uptake of rubidium is increased, intracellular sodium concentration is lower, and potassium is higher in erythrocytes from patients with Cushing's syndrome *(75)*. The endogenous digitalis-like substance is within the normal range *(73)*.

Urinary tetrahydrocortisol/tetrahydrocortisone ratio is elevated in Cushing's disease but similar in normotensives and hypertensives *(76)*. In ectopic ACTH syndrome, these ratios are higher, and hypertension has been attributed in part to cortisol inactivation overload giving rise to mineralocorticoid-type hypertension through cortisol occupancy of mineralocorticoid receptors *(77)*. However, whether mineralocorticoid receptor occupancy contributes to the hypertension is unresolved *(78)*. Administration of spironolactone did not reduce BP significantly in five patients with Cushing's syndrome tested *(66)*.

## *Diagnosis of Cushing's Syndrome (Fig. 4)*

Diagnosis is a two-step process: first, the diagnosis of GC excess, and second, definition of the etiology.

The diagnosis of GC excess can be difficult but in patients with Cushing's syndrome who present with hypertension it is often obvious clinically. In practice the obese hypertensive patient with syndrome X may be difficult to distinguish from the patient with Cushing's syndrome. Obesity can elevate urinary 17- hydroxycorticosteroids but urinary free cortisol is usually normal. Polycystic ovary syndrome presenting with central obesity, glucose intolerance, irregular menses, and hirsutism should also be considered.

Oversecretion of cortisol is the characteristic feature of Cushing's syndrome. Twenty-four-hour urinary-free cortisol (UFF) excretion is increased; this is a useful screening test but it is normal in around 10% of patients with Cushing's *(79)*. With three 24-hour urine collections and simultaneous measurement of urine creatinine, sensitivity of 95–100% and specificity of 94–98% has been reported *(16)*. Plasma cortisol levels may or may not be elevated but circadian rhythm disappears. To be reliable, diurnal plasma cortisol measurements require evening cortisol, which make it unsuitable as a screening test. A cortisol level at midnight below 50 nmol/L is said to be 100% sensitive in excluding active Cushing's syndrome *(80)*. The overnight dexamethasone suppression

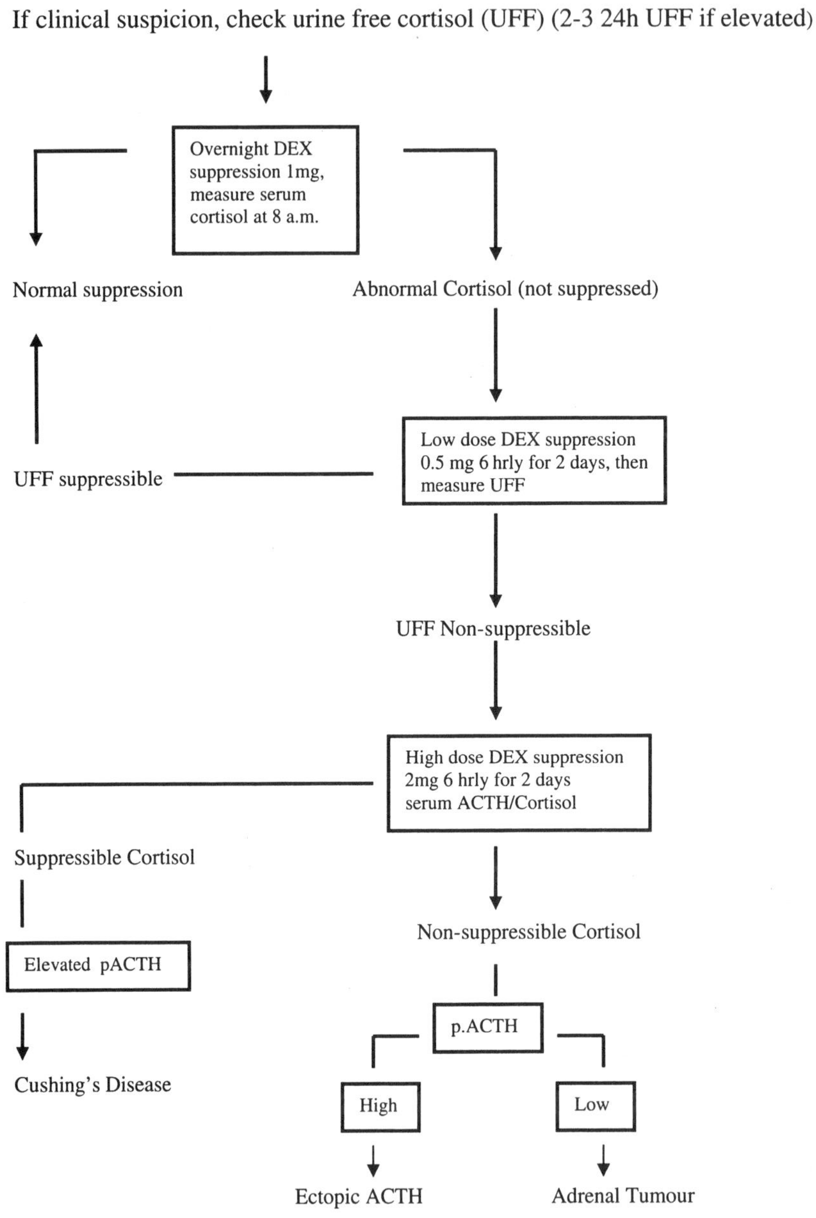


**Fig. 4.** A clinical schema for diagnosis of Cushing's syndrome.

test, which involves 1 mg of dexamethasone at bedtime and a plasma cortisol sample taken at around 8 or 9 AM, is a simple and popular screening test. A cortisol level < 50 nmol/L at 9 AM is said to exclude the diagnosis with 98% sensitivity *(80)*. Salivary cortisol correlates with plasma free cortisol and can be collected easily at home *(16)*.

Cushing's disease is characterized by increased or upper-normal plasma ACTH concentrations, enhanced ACTH stimulation of cortisol, and suppression of plasma cortisol by higher dose dexamethasone (2 mg every 6 hours). In ectopic ACTH, plasma ACTH concentration may be very high, ACTH-stimulated cortisol production is normal, and plasma cortisol does not suppress with high-dose dexamethasone (2 mg every 6 hours). With adrenal adenoma, plasma ACTH concentration is usually normal, and there is little suppression of plasma cortisol following high-dose dexamethasone. Patients with adrenal carcinoma have elevation of plasma cortisol concentrations, no response to ACTH, and low plasma ACTH concentrations.

The low-dose dexamethasone suppression test (0.5 mg every 6 hours for 48 hours) followed by plasma cortisol measurement is used to distinguish patients with Cushing's syndrome from those without the diagnosis *(81,82)*. It is highly sensitive and more specific than the overnight test *(79)*. Suppression may not be seen in patients with depression, alcoholism, pregnancy, and a range of drugs, and false-positives are seen in renal failure and hypothyroidism *(16)*. The high-dose dexamethasone suppression test (2 mg every 6 hours for 48 hours) is used to distinguish Cushing's disease (which is pituitary dependent) from adrenal tumor. Classically, Cushing's disease suppresses with high-dose but not low-dose dexamethasone, whereas patients with adrenal tumor do not suppress following high-dose dexamethasone. An alternative to the high-dose dexamethasone test is dexamethasone infusion (1 mg/hour for 6 hour). Some patients with ectopic ACTH or autonomous adrenal lesions will also suppress with high-dose dexamethasone. The accuracy of dexamethasone suppression tests will depend on appropriate absorption of the drug (impaired in chronic renal failure) and metabolism (accelerated by certain drugs, e.g., anticonvulsants) *(3)*.

Plasma ACTH concentrations are helpful in distinguishing patients with ectopic secretion (elevated ACTH levels) and Cushing's disease (high or normal ACTH concentrations) from those with adrenal tumor (low to undetectable ACTH concentrations) *(83)*, but there may be significant overlap *(16)*.

Selective venous sampling may be useful in experienced hands in identifying an ectopic source of ACTH or in lateralizing pituitary microadenoma (Table 2). Both inferior petrosal sinuses should be sampled. In Cushing's disease, the ratio of sinus to peripheral plasma ACTH is greater than 2, and in ectopic ACTH less than 1.5 *(84)*. Sampling at various levels within the vena cava may be helpful *(85)*. Ovine

Table 2
Selective Venous Sampling for ACTH (pg/ml) (range 0–50) in an Obese Woman With Hypertension, Type 2 Diabetes, and Elevated Urine-Free Cortisol That Suppressed With High-Dose Dexamethasone

| | |
|---|---|
| Inferior vena cava | 44 |
| Superior vena cava | 57 |
| Left internal jugular vein | 46 |
| Right peripheral venous blood | 46 |
| Right internal jugular vein | 61 |
| Right inferior petrosal sinus | 54 |
| Left inferior petrosal sinus | 2379 |
| Diagnosis: Left pituitary microadenoma, confirmed at surgery | |

CRF has been reported to increase diagnostic accuracy *(86,87)*, with gradients greater than 3 being regarded as most useful *(80,86)*. Naloxone, an opioid antagonist, which probably stimulates ACTH secretion through release of CRH has also been used during petrosal sinus sampling *(88)*. The venous sampling procedure is technically difficult, and brain stem stroke has been reported so that it should be reserved for diagnostic uncertainty *(16)*.

CRF administration increased both plasma ACTH and cortisol concentrations in patients with Cushing's syndrome *(89)* but not those with adrenal adenoma *(89)*.

In patients with adrenal tumor, pheochromocytoma must be excluded because these may produce ACTH, and the diagnosis is very important for management *(90)*.

Pituitary and adrenal imaging is key in localization. Differential diagnosis from pituitary and adrenal "incidentalomas" is important, because these are not uncommon. Computed tomography (CT) can detect some microadenomas as well as larger pituitary tumors, but corticotroph adenomas are often only a few millimeters in diameter and may not be seen even with magnetic resonance imaging and enhancement *(79)*. Furthermore, about 10% of subjects have pituitary "incidentalomas." Radionuclide scanning of the adrenals using $^{131}$ I-iodomethyl nor-cholesterol may distinguish bilateral adrenal hyperplasia from adrenal cortical adenoma *(86)*.

A study of the cost effectiveness and accuracy of the tests used in the differential diagnosis concluded that once Cushing's syndrome is diagnosed, low ACTH concentrations and abdominal CT correctly identified an adrenal origin *(83)*. With ACTH-dependent Cushing's syndrome, inferior petrosal sinus sampling was the best predictive test to differentiate Cushing's disease from ectopic ACTH secretion *(92)*. A control to peripheral gradient of >3 following stimulation is said to have 98% sensitivity in confirming a pituitary origin *(80)*.

It is important to recognize that diagnosis may be very difficult; e.g., sometimes ectopic ACTH cases may have features typical of Cushing's disease. Atypical presentation and laboratory shortcomings may further confuse the diagnosis *(16)*.

Cushing's syndrome is rare in pregnancy because ovulatory dysfunction is common and fertility decreased. Striae, obesity, and glucose intolerance are frequent in both pregnancy and Cushing's syndrome. Cortisol production and plasma cortisol concentrations are also increased in pregnancy, but diurnal rhythm and dexamethasone suppressibility are retained. Pregnancy in untreated Cushing's syndrome has been associated with substantial maternal morbidity and perinatal mortality *(93)*.

Both preclinical Cushing's syndrome (cases caused by cortisol-producing adrenal adenoma without physical symptoms or signs) *(94)* and preclinical Cushing's disease (absence of Cushingoid appearance, normal morning cortisol and ACTH, lack of diurnal rhythm, exaggerated ACTH response to CRH and desmopressin, and incomplete low-dose dexamethasone suppression) *(95)* have been reported. Consideration and recognition would prevent progression and complications *(95)*.

### Treatment

The prognosis of untreated Cushing's syndrome is poor, with a 50% 5-year survival *(36)*. Following successful treatment, morbidity and mortality remain elevated largely because of cardiovascular disease *(32,34)*. A recent Danish study *(35)* found that patients with nonmalignant disease had a standard mortality of 3.68, partly attributable to an increased mortality within the first year after diagnosis. This is strikingly similar to a Spanish figure of 3.8 *(32)*. The prognosis for malignant disease is very poor *(35)*. Long-term survivors of Cushing's disease also have impaired quality of health *(35)*. Alternatively, partial complete spontaneous remission of pituitary adenomas is well known, and spontaneous remission of Cushing's disease may not be very rare *(32)*.

Cushing's disease is the most common form of Cushing's syndrome. Bilateral adrenalectomy cures virtually all patients *(96)* but mandates permanent steroid replacement therapy, and some adrenalectomized patients ( ~20% ) develop Nelson's syndrome, with cutaneous pigmentation, secondary to a rapidly growing chromophobe adenoma, which may lead to visual field defects. The rapid growth is thought to reflect the lack of restraint from excess cortisol. Subtotal adrenalectomy is less satisfactory, and only about 60% of patients become symptom free *(97)*.

Laparoscopic adrenalectomy is now used as the preferred approach for benign disease where adrenalectomy is indicated *(98)*.

Selective excision of the pituitary adenoma by trans-sphenoidal microsurgery is the preferred treatment approach for Cushing's disease *(99)* and has a high response rate of more than 70% *(100)*. Around 10–30% of patients relapse *(35,100)*. This is less likely with trans-sphenoidal hypophysectomy, although hypopituitarism is not uncommon *(101)*. GC therapy is indicated postoperatively until the hypothalamic–pituitary–adrenal axis recovers *(16)*. Pituitary irradiation may be used following pituitary surgery to prevent recurrence or following adrenal surgery to prevent development of Nelson's syndrome. Pituitary irradiation has also been used as the primary treatment in younger patients *(102)* but has a lower response rate and may produce hypopituitarism. Internal irradiation with gold-198 or yttrium-90 needles produces good response but hypopituitarism is common *(101)*.

Medical management of Cushing's disease is varyingly successful. Drugs used include metyrapone, an inhibitor of 11 β-hydroxylase; cyproheptadine, a serotonin antagonist; bromocriptine and lisuride, both dopaminergic agonists; aminoglutethimide, an inhibitor of the cytochrome P450 side-chain cleavage enzyme; reserpine, mitotane (o,pDDD), which destroys fasciculata, and reticularis *(103)*; trilostane, an inhibitor of 3 β-hydroxysteroid dehydrogenase; sodium valproate, an inhibitor of γ-aminobutyric acid -transaminase; ketaconazole (which blocks steroid synthesis and itself may produce hypertension *(104)*), and the GC antagonist, RU486 *(105)*. Propranolol therapy was effective in a patient with Cushing's syndrome secondary to ectopic adrenal β-adrenergic receptors *(106)*. Most of these medications are used only as adjunctive therapy because they do not "cure" Cushing's syndrome and their use is often limited by side effects.

Adrenal tumors are treated surgically. Adrenal malignancy carries a poor prognosis, and medical therapy has been used in widespread disease—in particular, aminoglutethimide and mitotane (o,p-DDD). Ectopic ACTH-secreting tumors are usually malignant and often inoperable. Benign adrenal adenoma is treated by unilateral adrenalectomy, usually laparoscopic with excellent results *(97)*.

There is no good evidence to support the use of one particular class of antihypertensive drug over another in Cushing's syndrome, and conventional antihypertensive treatment is mostly ineffective *(107,108)*. Effective control of Cushing's syndrome may control BP, but as in other surgically remediable forms of secondary hypertension, a significant proportion of patients, particularly older patients *(73)*, have persistent hypertension and require ongoing antihypertensive medication. Experimental studies in humans (see below) suggest that sodium restriction is likely to be useful. The preoperative BP level in Cushing's syndrome is a predictor of persistent hypertension after surgery *(109)* and duration of hypertension, i.e., long-lasting exposure to cortisol, also correlates with postoperative BP *(107)*. These findings imply that early diagnosis and intensive BP control preoperatively are important therapeutic determinants of hypertensive outcome *(109)*. Furthermore, in patients successfully treated surgically who remain hypertensive, BP control by antihypertensive medication is usually satisfactory, further emphasizing the role of cortisol hypersecretion in the BP elevation *(107,108)*.

### Experimental Studies of ACTH and Cortisol Administration in Human Subjects

ACTH (Synacthen Depot [Novartis Pharmaceuticals, Sydney, Australia]) 1 mg/day increases BP by around 20 mmHg in normal subjects and patients with untreated mild essential hypertension but not patients with treated Addison's disease, indicating that the BP-raising effects of ACTH in humans are adrenally dependent. The BP rise is highly reproducible *(68)*, with invariable increases in systolic pressure and mean arterial pressure over 5 days and rises in diastolic pressure in some studies.

ACTH produced hypernatremia, hypokalemia, and increase in fasting blood glucose, body weight, and total white cell count, urine sodium retention, and a fall in hematocrit and eosinophil count. Plasma cortisol, deoxycortisol, corticosterone, and DOC concentrations increased. Plasma aldosterone concentrations rose initially, but then returned to the low-normal range *(67)*. Plasma renin, angiotensin, and noradrenaline concentrations fell, adrenaline and vasopressin concentrations were unchanged, and plasma atrial natriuretic peptide concentrations *(68)* and urinary kallikrein activity rose *(110)*. ACTH administration was associated with increased cardiac output, plasma volume, extracellular fluid volume, exchangeable sodium, inulin clearance, filtration fraction, fractional sodium reabsorption, and renal vascular resistance *(68)*. Creatinine and para-amino hippurate clearances were unchanged *(68)*.

The threshold dose of ACTH required to raise pressure was 50 μg/day by continuous intravenous infusion *(111)*. ACTH concentrations rose with infusion, but remained within the normal range.

At doses to achieve blood concentrations appropriate for conditions of ACTH stimulation *(112)*, the hemodynamic and metabolic effects of ACTH were mimicked by cortisol, whereas DOC and aldosterone produced mineralocorticoid effects but did not raise BP. The BP-raising effects of ACTH are caused by ACTH-induced increases in cortisol secretion.

The rise in BP with ACTH occurs even when dietary sodium is very low, but sodium intake determines the degree to which BP rises. On sodium intake of 100–150 mmol/day, ACTH increased systolic BP by around 20 mmHg *(67,68)*, on sodium 200–300 mmol/day BP rose 30 mmHg *(113)*, and on 15 mmol/day *(114)* only 10 mmHg. Cortisol administration does not modify salt preference in normal subjects *(115)*.

Plasma volume, extracellular fluid volume (ECFV), and exchangeable sodium are all increased by both ACTH and cortisol treatment *(68)*. Sodium restriction *(114)* profoundly reduced the rise in exchangeable sodium and completely prevented the increase in ECFV, but the increase in plasma volume was unchanged. Thus, a rise in ECFV is not necessary for ACTH-induced rises in BP. Spironolactone, at a dose that blocks mineralocorticoid effects of cortisol, has no effect on the rise in BP *(116)*.

The synthetic GCs, prednisolone, methylprednisolone, dexamethasone, and triamcinolone, all increased BP, without urinary sodium retention and with no increase in body weight or plasma volume *(28)*. Thus, volume expansion and/or urinary sodium retention are not essential for steroid-induced rises in BP in humans.

ACTH and cortisol administration are associated with increases in cardiac output and renal vascular resistance, but calculated total peripheral resistance is unchanged *(68,117)*. Prevention of the rise in cardiac output by β-blockade does not prevent the hypertension *(117)* and the calcium channel blocker, felodipine, which reduces peripheral resistance, similarly had no effect on the BP rise *(118)*.

Both ACTH and cortisol increased pressor responses to phenylephrine *(119)* and decreased the threshold dose for a pressure response. Increases with Ang II were less pronounced *(119,120)*, although sodium retention and reduced circulating plasma Ang II concentrations would be expected to increase pressor responses to exogenous angiotensin. The increased phenylephrine responsiveness following ACTH was also seen in subjects on low sodium intake *(121)* but was not modified by indomethacin in subjects on regular sodium intake *(120)*.

In cortisol-treated subjects *(122)*, we found increases in forearm vascular resistance both to cold pressor test and intra-arterial noradrenaline infusion. A shift to the left of the dose–response relation and fall in threshold suggested cortisol increased vascular sensitivity to noradrenaline. Sympathetic nervous system activity (assessed by measurement of resting noradrenaline spillover rate to plasma and noradrenaline uptake) was not increased *(123)*, nor was reflex sympathetic function *(124)* or neuroreptide Y concentrations *(125)*. Muscle sympathetic vasoconstrictor activity was decreased by cortisol *(126)* and the hypertension was amplified by autonomic blockade *(127)*. Thus, the sympathetic nervous system appears to modulate or damp down cortisol hypertension, and there is no evidence that it plays any role in causation.

Hypertension and mineralocorticoid effects were not directly related *(128)*, supporting the notion that steroids may raise pressure by a hypertensinogenic mechanism distinct from their classical mineralocorticoid or GC activities *(78,116,128)*.

Cortisol has significant effects on vascular endothelial function *(129)*. Cortisol inhibits cholinergic dilation in the human forearm. The inhibition is of similar magnitude to that produced by nitric oxide synthase inhibition *(129)*. Studies of nitric oxide metabolites, performed in cortisol-treated subjects on a low nitrate diet *(130)*, indicate that cortisol-induced hypertension is associated with a fall in plasma reactive nitrogen intermediates, but not L-arginine or asymmetric dimethyl arginine concentrations *(131)*. However, L-arginine administration at maximum tolerated doses does not prevent the rise in BP produced by cortisol *(132)*.

Cortisol administration also increases plasma erythropoeitin concentrations and the rise in BP correlates with the rise in erythropoeitin *(133)*. This is of interest given the association of erythropoeitin administration with nitric oxide resistance *(133)*.

### Studies in Animals

Naturally occurring Cushing's syndrome occurs in animals, including horses and dogs *(134,135)*, and hypertension and cardiovascular disease are prominent. Experimentally, ACTH increases BP in the sheep *(136)*, rat *(137)*, and mouse *(138)* but probably not the rabbit or the dog *(139)*. Effects of ACTH have been studied extensively in the sheep and rat but are beyond the scope of this chapter.

## CONCLUSION

Hypertension in Cushing's syndrome is common. Naturally occurring Cushing's syndrome is rare but it occurs commonly secondary to steroid therapy. Cortisol appears to be responsible for the hypertension of Cushing's syndrome. Cardiovascular morbidity and mortality are prominent.

## ACKNOWLEDGMENTS

Ms. Laura Vitler and Ms. Amanda Jacobsen prepared the manuscript. Dr. Tony O'Sullivan provided valuable advice, and he and Dr. Peter Rohl kindly provided the illustrations.

## REFERENCES


1. Firkin BG, Whitworth JA. Dictionary of medical eponyms. 2nd ed. New York: Parthenon Publishing; 1996;83–84.
2. Ross EJ. Cushing's syndrome: current status. Cardiology 1985;72(Suppl 1):64–69.
3. Danese RD, Aron DC. Cushing's syndrome and hypertension. Endocrinol Metab Clin N Am 1994;23:299–324.
4. Bishop PMF, Close GH. A case of basophil adenoma of the anterior lobe of the pituitary: "Cushing's Syndrome." Guy's Hosp Rep 1932;82:143–153.
5. Whitworth JA, Mangos GJ, Kelly JJ. Cushing, cortisol and cardiovascular disease. Hypertension 2000;36:912–916.
6. Gold EM. The Cushing syndromes: changing views of diagnosis and treatment. Ann Intern Med 1979;90:829–844.
7. Krieger DT, Liotta AS, Suda T, Goodgold A, Condon E. Human plasma immunoreactive lipotropin and adrenocorticotropin in normal subjects and in patients with pituitary adrenal disease. J Clin Endocrinol Metab 1979;48:566–571.
8. Gomez-Sanchez CE. Cushing's syndrome and hypertension. Hypertension 1986;8:258–264.
9. Schambelan M, Slaton PE, Biglieri EG. Mineralocorticoid production in hyperadrenocorticism: role in pathogenesis of hypokalemic alkalosis. Am J Med 1971;51:299–303.
10. Nagae A, Murakami E, Hiwada K, Kubota O, Takada Y, Ohmori T. Primary aldosteronism with cortisol overproduction from bilateral multiple adrenal adenomas. Jpn J Med 1991;30:26–31.
11. Kloos RT, Gross MD, Francis IR, Korobkin M, Shapiro B. Incidentally discovered adrenal masses. Endocr Res 1995;16:460–484.
12. Beuschlein F, Reincke M, Koniger M, D'Orazio D, Dobbie Z, Rump LC. Cortisol producing adrenal adenoma: a new manifestation of Gardner's syndrome. Endocr Res 2000;26:783–790.
13. Hiroi N, Chrousos GP, Kohn B, et al. Adrenocortical-pituitary hybrid tumor causing Cushing's syndrome. J Clin Endocrinol Metab 2001;86:2631–2637.
14. Hocher B, Bahr V, Dorfmuller S, Oelkers W. Hypercortisolism with non-pigmented micronodular adrenal hyperplasia: transition from pituitary-dependent to adrenal-dependent Cushing's syndrome. Acta Endocrinol 1993;128:120–125.
15. Luton JP, Cerdas S, Billaud L, et al. Clinical features of adrenocortical carcinoma, prognostic factors, and the effect of mitotane therapy. N Engl J Med 1990;322: 1195–1201.
16. Boscaro M, Barzon L, Fallo F, Sonino N. Cushing's syndrome. Lancet 2001;357: 783–791.
17. Bertagna X. New causes of Cushing's syndrome. N Engl J Med 1992;327: 1024–1025.
18. Khardon R. Considerations in diagnosis of Cushing syndrome. Arch Intern Med 2001;161:1780.
19. Takamura T, Nagai Y, Taniguchi M, et al. Adrenocorticotropin-independent unilateral adrenocortical hyperplasia with Cushing's syndrome: immunohistochemical studies of steroidogenic enzymes, ultrastructural examination and a review of the literature. Pathol Int 2001;51:118–122.
20. Uwaifo GI, Robey PG, Akintoye SO, Collins MT. Clinical picture: fuel on the fire. Lancet 2001;357:2011.
21. Hench PS, Kendall EC, Slocumb CH, Polley HF. The effect of a hormone of the adrenal cortex (17-OH, 11-dihydrocorticosterone: compound E) and of pituitary

adrenocorticotrophic hormone on rheumatoid arthritis. Proc Staff Meet Mayo Clin 1949;24:181–197.

22. Treadwell BLJ, Sever ED, Savage O, Copeman WSC. Side effects of long term treatment with corticosteroids and corticotrophin. Lancet 1964;i:1121–1123.
23. Hrachovy RA, Frost JD, Kellaway P, Zion T. A controlled study of ACTH therapy in infantile spasms. Epilepsia 1980;21:631–636.
24. Jackson RV, Nye EJ, Grice JE, et al. Early rise in blood pressure following administration of adrenocorticotropic hormone-[1-24) in humans. Clin Exp Pharmacol Physiol 2001;28:773–775.
25. Armbruster H, Vetter W, Reck G, Beckerhoff R, Segenthaler W. Severe arterial hypertension caused by chronical abuse of a topical mineralocorticoid. Int J Clin Pharmacol Biopharmacol 1975;12:170–173.
26. O'Sullivan MM, Rumfeld WR, Jones MK, Williams BD. Cushing's syndrome with suppression of the hypothalamic-pituitary-adrenal axis after intra-articular steroid injections. Ann Rheum Dis 1985;44:561–563.
27. Savage O, Copeman WSC, Chapman L, Wells MV, Treadwell BLJ. Pituitary and adrenal hormones in rheumatoid arthritis. Lancet 1962;i:232–234.
28. Whitworth JA, Gordon D, Andrews J, Scoggins BA. The hypertensive effect of synthetic glucocorticoids in man: role of sodium and volume. J Hypertens 1989;7:537–549.
29. Villanueva RB, Brett E, Gabrilove JL. A cluster of cases of factitious Cushing's syndrome. Endocr Pract 2000;6:143–147.
30. Smals AG, Kloppenborg PW, Njo KT, Knoben JM, Ruland CA. Alcohol induced Cushingoid syndrome. BMJ 1979;2:1298.
31. Marks V, Wright JW. Endocrinological and metabolic effects of alcohol. Proc R Soc Med 1977;70:337.
32. Etxabe J, Vazquez JA. Morbidity and mortality in Cushing's disease: an epidemiological approach. Clin Endo 1994;40:479–484.
33. Ross EJ, Marshall-Jones P, Friedman M. Cushing's syndrome, diagnostic criteria. QJM 1966;35:149–193.
34. Ross EJ, Linch DC. Cushing's syndrome—killing disease: discriminatory value of signs and symptoms aiding early diagnosis. Lancet 1982;ii:646–649.
35. Lindholm J, Juul S, Jorgensen JO, et al. Incidence and late prognosis of Cushing's syndrome: a population-based study. J Clin Endocrinol Metab 2001;86:117–123.
36. Plotz C, Knowlten A, Ragan C. The natural history of Cushing's syndrome. Am J Med 1952;13:597–614.
37. Sonino N, Fallo F, Opocher G, Boscaro M. Hypertension in Cushing's syndrome. Med Sci Res 1992;20:431–434.
38. Agrest A, Finkilman S, Elijovich F. Haemodinamica de la hipertension arterial en al sindrome de Cushing. Medicina (B Aires) 1974;34:457.
39. Ritchie CM, Sheridan B, Fraser R, et al. Studies on the pathogenesis of hypertension in Cushing's disease and acromegaly. QJM 1990;280:855–867.
40. Sugihara N, Shimizu M, Kita Y, et al. Cardiac characteristics and postoperative courses in Cushing's syndrome. Am J Cardiol 1992;69:1475–1480.
41. Fallo F, Budano S, Sonino N, Muiesen ML, Agabiti-Rosei E, Boscaro M. Left ventricular structural characteristics in Cushing' syndrome. J Hum Hypertens 1994;8:509–513.
42. Hersbach FMRJ, Bravenboer B, Doolen JJ. Hearty hormones. Lancet 2001; 358:468.
43. Nashel DJ. Is atherosclerosis a complication of long-term corticosteroid treatment? Am J Med 1986;80:925–929.

44. Padfield PL, Stewart MJ. Ambulatory blood pressure monitoring in secondary hypertension. J Hypertens 1991;9(Suppl 8):S69–S71.
45. Piovesan A, Panarelli M, Terzolo M, et al. 24 hour profiles of blood pressure and heart rate in Cushing's syndrome: relationship between cortisol and cardiovascular rhythmicities. Chronobiol Int 1990;7:263–265.
46. Turner SW, Fraser TB, Mangos CJ, Whitworth JA: Circadian blood pressure variability in adrenocorticotrophin-induced hypertension in the rat. Hypertens 2001;8:1411–1420.
47. Soffer L, Iannacore A, Gabrilove J. Cushing's syndrome. Am J Med 1961;30: 129–146.
48. Greminger P, Tenschert TW, Vetter W, Luscher T, Vetter H. Hypertension in Cushing's syndrome. In: Mantero F, Biglieri EG, Edwards CRW, eds. Endocrinology in hypertension. London and New York: Academic Press, 1982;50:103–110.
49. Welbourn RB, Montgomery DAD, Kennedy GL. The natural history of treated Cushing's syndrome. Br J Surg 1971;58:1–16.
50. Suzuki H, Shibata H, Muramaki M, Nakamoto H, Kondo K, Saruta T. Case report: hypertension in Cushing's syndrome. Am J Med Sci 1992;303:329–332.
51. Soszynski P, Slowinska-Srzednicka J, Kasperlik-Zaluska A, Zgliczynski S. Endogenous natriuretic factors: atrial natriuretic hormone and digitalis-like substance in Cushing's syndrome. J Endocrinol 1991;129:453–458.
52. Biglieri EG, Hane S, Slaton PE, Forsham PH. In vivo and in vitro studies of adrenal secretions in Cushing's syndrome and primary aldosteronism. J Clin Invest 1963;42:516–524.
53. Dyrenfurth I, Sybulski S, Notchev V, Beck JC, Venning EH. Urinary corticosteroid excretion patterns in patients with adrenocortical dysfunction. J Clin Endocrinol Metab 1958;18:391–408.
54. Guthrie GP, Kotchen TA. Hypertension and aldosterone over-production without renin suppression in Cushing's syndrome from an adrenal adenoma. Am J Med 1979;67:524–528.
55. Boscaro M, Scaroni C, Masarotto P, Ridolfi P, Benato M, Mantero F. Circadian secretion of ACTH, cortisol, and mineralocorticoids in Cushing's syndrome. Clin Exp Hypertens (A) 1982;4:1779–1794.
56. Oddie CJ, Coghlan JP, Scoggins BA. Plasma desoxycorticosterone levels in man with simultaneous measurement of aldosterone, corticosterone, cortisol and 11-deoxycortisol. J Clin Endocrinol Metab 1972;34:1039–1054.
57. Melby JC, Dale SL, Grekin RJ, Gaunt R, Wilson TE. 18-Hydroxy-11-deoxycorticosterone ((18-OH-DOC) secretion in experimental and human hypertension. Recent Prog Horm Res 1972;28:287–351.
58. Ehlers ME, Griffing GT, Wilson TE, Melby JC. Elevated urinary 19-nor-deoxycorticosterone glucuronide in Cushing's syndrome. J Clin Endocrinol Metab 1987;64:926–930.
59. Yamaji T, Ishibashi M, Teramoto A, Fukushima T. Hyperprolactinemia in Cushing's disease and Nelson's syndrome. J Endocrinol Metab 1984;58:790–795.
60. Hermus A, Hobma S, Pieters G, Benraad T, Smals A, Kloppenborg P. Do weak mineralocorticoids affect the pathogenesis of hypertension in Cushing's disease? J Hypertens 1989;7(Suppl6):S208–S209.
61. Mendlowitz M, Gitlow S, Naftchi N. Work of digital vasoconstriction produced by infused norephrine in Cushing's syndrome. J Appl Physiol 1958; 13:252–256.
62. Saruta T, Suzuki H, Handa M, Igarashi Y, Kondo K, Senda S. Multiple factors contribute to the pathogenesis of hypertension in Cushing's syndrome. J Clin Endocrinol Metab 1986;62:275–279.

63. Tabarin A, Minot AP, Dallochio M, et al. Plasma concentrations of neuropeptide Y in patients with adrenal hypertension. Regul Pept 1992;42:51–62.
64. Axelrod L. Inhibition of prostacyclin production mediates permissive effect of glucocorticoids on vascular tone. Lancet 1983;i:904–906.
65. Shimamoto K, Ura N, Nomura N, et al. Significance of renal kininases in patients with Cushing's syndrome. Clin Exp Hypertens 1995;17:1173–1182.
66. Saruta T. Mechanism of glucocorticoid-induced hypertension. Hypertens Res 1996;19:1–8.
67. Whitworth JA, Saines D, Thatcher R, Butkus A, Scoggins BA. Blood pressure and metabolic effects of ACTH in normotensive and hypertensive man. Clin Exp Hypertens (A) 1983;5:501–522.
68. Connell JMC, Whitworth JA, Davies DL, Lever AF, Richards AM, Fraser R. Effects of ACTH and cortisol administration on blood pressure, electrolyte metabolism, atrial natriuretic peptide and renal function in normal man. J Hypertens 1987;5:425–433.
69. Tenschert W, Baumgart P, Greminger P, Vetter W, Vetter H. Pathogenetic aspects of hypertension in Cushing's syndrome. Cardiology 1985;72(Suppl 1):84–90.
70. Ganguly A, Weinberger MH, Grim CE. The renin-angiotensin-aldosterone system in Cushing's syndrome and phaeochromocytoma. Hormone Res 1983; 17:1–10.
71. Dalakos TG, Elias AN, Anderson GH, Streeten DHP, Schroeder ET. Evidence for an angiotensinogenic mechanism of the hypertension of Cushing's syndrome. J Clin Endocrinol Metab 1978;46:114–118.
72. Vetter W, Vetter H, Beckerhoff R, Redlich B, Cottier P, Siegenthaler W. The effect of saralasin (1-sar-8-ala-angiotensin II) on blood pressure in patients with Cushing's syndrome. Klin Wochenschr 1976;54:661–663.
73. Streeten DHP, Anderson GH, Wagner S. Effect of age on response of secondary hypertension to specific treatment. Am J Hypertens 1990;3:360–365.
74. Yamaji T, Ishibashi M, Yamada A, et al. Plasma levels of atrial natriuretic hormone in Cushing's syndrome. J Clin Endocrinol Metab 1988;67:348–352.
75. Wambach G, Helber A, Allolio B, Winkelmann W, Kaufmann W. Increased activity of the Na-K ATPase in red cell ghosts of patients with Cushing's syndrome: possible significance of the pathogenesis of glucocorticoid induced hypertension. Klin Wochenschr 1980;58:485–487.
76. Hermus AR, Hobma S, Pieters G, et al. Are the hypokalaemia and hypertension in Cushing's disease caused by apparent mineralocorticoid excess? Horm Metab Res 1991;23:572–573.
77. Ulick S, Wang JZ, Blumenfeld JD, Pickering TG. Cortisol inactivation overload: a mechanism of mineralocorticoid hypertension in the ectopic adrenocorticotropin syndrome. J Clin Endocrinol Metab 1992;74:963–967.
78. Whitworth JA, Kelly JJ. Evidence that hydrocortisone induced sodium retention in man is not mediated by the mineralocorticoid receptors. J Endocrinol Invest 1995;18:586–591.
79. Newell-Price J, Grossman A. Diagnosis and management of Cushing's syndrome. Lancet 1999;353:2087–2088.
80. Newell-Price J, Grossman AB. The differential diagnosis of Cushing's syndrome. Ann Endocrinol 2001;62:173–179.
81. Kennedy L, Atkinson AB, Johnston H, Sheridan B, Hadden DR. Serum cortisol concentrations during low dose dexamethasone suppression test to screen for Cushing's syndrome. BMJ 1984;289:1188–1191.
82. Liddle GW. Tests of pituitary adrenal suppressibility in the diagnosis of Cushing's syndrome. J Clin Endocrinol 1960;20:1539–1545.

83. Berson SA, Yalow RS. Radioimmunoassay of ACTH in plasma. J Clin Invest 1968; 47:2725–2751.
84. Findling JW, Aron DC, Tyrrell JB, et al. Selective venous sampling for ACTH in Cushing's syndrome. Ann Intern Med 1981;94:647–652.
85. Drury PL, Ratter S, Tomlin S, et al. Experience with selective venous sampling in diagnosis of ACTH-dependent Cushing's syndrome. BMJ 1982;284:9–12.
86. Oldfield EH, Doppman JL, Nieman LK, et al. Petrosal sinus sampling with and without corticotropin-releasing hormone for the differential diagnosis of Cushing's syndrome. N Engl J Med 1991;325:897–905.
87. Orth DN, DeBold CR, DeCherney GS, et al. Pituitary microadenomas causing Cushings disease respond to corticotrophin-releasing factor. J Clin Endocrinol Metab 1982;55:1017–1019.
88. Torpy DJ, Jackson RV, Grice JE, Hockings GI, Strakosch CR, Topliss DJ. Naloxone stimulation of ACTH secretion during petrosal sinus sampling in Cushing's syndrome. Clin Exp Physiol Pharmacol 1993;20:299–302.
89. Catania A, Cantalamessa A, Orsatti A, et al. Plasma ACTH-response to the corticotropin releasing factor in patients with Cushing's disease: comparison with the lysine-vasopressin test. Metabolism 1984;33:478–481.
90. Hoffman L, Martin FIR, Buchanan MRC, Butkus A, Whitworth JA. Cushing's syndrome due to an ACTH-secreting adrenal medullary tumour. Aust NZ J Med 1980;10:654–656.
91. Sarkar SD, Cohen EL, Bier Waltes WH, Ice RD, Cooper R, Gold EN. A new and superior adrenal imaging agent 1310 - 6β iodimethyl-19-nor cholesterol (NP - 59): an evaluation in humans. J Clin Endocrinol Metab 1977;45:353–362.
92. Puig J, Wagner A, Caballero A, Rodriguez-Espinosa J, Webb SM. Cost-effectiveness and accuracy of the tests used in the differential diagnosis of Cushing's syndrome. Pituitary 1999;1:125–132.
93. Buescher MA, McClamrock HD, Adashi EY. Cushing syndrome in pregnancy. Obstet Gynecol 1992;79:130–137.
94. Reincke M, Nieke J, Krestin GP, Saeger W, Allolio B, Winkelmann W. Preclinical Cushing's syndrome in adrenal incidentalomas: comparison with adrenal Cushing syndrome. J Clin Endocrinol Metab 1992;75:826–832.
95. Takao T, Mimoto T, Yamomoto M, Hashimoto K. Pre-clinical Cushing disease. Arch Intern Med 2001;161:892–893.
96. Orth DN, Liddle GW. Results of treatment in 108 patients with Cushing's syndrome. N Engl J Med 1971;285:243–247.
97. Racker J, Cope O, Ackerman I. Surgical experience with the treatment of hypertension of Cushing's syndrome. Am J Surg 1964;107:153–158.
98. Gagner M, Lacroix A, Bolte E. Laparoscopic adrenalectomy in Cushing's syndrome and pheochromocytoma. N Engl J Med 1992;327:1033.
99. Burch WM. Cushing's disease. Arch Intern Med 1985;145:1106–1111.
100. Cavagnini F, Pecori Giraldi F. Epidemiology and follow-up of Cushing's disease. Ann Endocrinol 2001;62:168–172.
101. Jeffcoate WJ. Treating Cushing's disease. BMJ 1988;296:227–228.
102. McHardy KC. Suspected Cushing's syndrome. BMJ 1984;289:1519–1521.
103. Kawai S, Ichikawa Y, Kaburaki J, Yoshida T. 18 years mitotane therapy for intractable Cushing's disease. Lancet 1999;354:951.
104. Leal-Cerro A, Garcia-Luna PP, Villar J, et al. Arterial hypertension as a complication of prolonged ketoconazole treatment. J Hypertens 1989;7(Suppl 6): S212–S213.

105. Chu JW, Matthias DF, Belanoff J, Schatzberg A, Hoffman AR, Feldman D. Successful long-term treatment of refractory Cushing's disease with high-dose mifepristone (RU486). J Clin Endocrinol Metab 2001;86:3568–3573.
106. Lacroix A, Tremblay J, Rousseau G, Bouvier M, Hamet P. Propranolol therapy for ectopic β-adrenergic receptors in adrenal Cushing's syndrome. New Engl J Med 1997;337:1429–1434.
107. Fallo F, Sonino N, Barzon L, et al. Effect of surgical treatment on hypertension in Cushing's syndrome. Am J Hypertens 1996;9:77–80.
108. Fallo F, Paoletta A, Tona F, Boscaro M, Sonino N. Response of hypertension to conventional antihypertensive treatment and/or steroidogenesis inhibitors in Cushing's syndrome. J Int Med 1993;234:595–598.
109. Suzuki T, Shibata H, Ando T, et al. Risk factors associated with persistent postoperative hypertension in Cushing's syndrome. Endocr Res 2000;26:791–795.
110. Whitworth JA, van Leeuwen BH, Hannah MC, Scoggins BA, Thatcher R. Effect of ACTH administration on urinary kallikrein excretion in man. Clin Exp Pharmacol Physiol 1984;11:87–90.
111. Whitworth JA, Gordon D, Scoggins BA. Dose-response relationships for adrenocorticotrophin-induced hypertension in man. Clin Exp Pharmacol Physiol 1987;14:65–71.
112. Whitworth JA, Saines D, Scoggins BA. Blood pressure and metabolic effects of cortisol and deoxycorticosterone in man. Clin Exp Hypertens (A) 1984;6: 795–809.
113. Whitworth JA, Saines D, Scoggins BA. Potentiation of ACTH hypertension in man with salt loading. Clin Exp Pharmacol Physiol 1985;12:239–243.
114. Connell JMC, Whitworth JA, Davies DL, Richards AM, Fraser R. Haemodynamic, hormonal and renal effects of adrenocorticotrophic hormone in sodium-restricted man. J Hypertens 1988;6:17–23.
115. Wong KS, Williamson PM, Brown MA, Zammit VC, Denton DA, Whitworth JA. Effects of cortisol on blood pressure and salt preference in normal humans. Clin Exp Pharmacol Physiol 1993;20:121–126.
116. Williamson PM, Kelly JJ, Whitworth JA. Dose-response relationships and mineralocorticoid activity in cortisol-induced hypertension in humans. J Hypertens 1996;14(Suppl 5):S37–S41.
117. Pirpiris M, Yeung S, Dewar F, Jennings GL, Whitworth JA. Hydrocortisone-induced hypertension in men: the role of cardiac output. Am J Hypertens 1993;6:287–294.
118. Whitworth JA, Williamson PM, Ramsay D. Hemodynamic responses to cortisol in man: effects of felodipine. Hypertens Res 1994;137–142.
119. Whitworth JA, Connell JMC, Lever AF, Fraser R. Pressor responsiveness in steroid-induced hypertension in man. Clin Exp Pharmacol Physiol 1986;13:353–358.
120. Whitworth JA, Connell JMC, Gordon D, Scoggins BA. Effects of indomethacin on steroid-induced changes in pressor responsiveness in man. Clin Exp Pharmacol Physiol 1988;15:305–310.
121. Connell JMC, Fisher BM, Davidson G, Fraser R, Whitworth JA. Effect of sodium depletion on pressor responsiveness in ACTH-induced hypertension in man. Clin Exp Pharmacol Physiol 1987;14:237–242.
122. Sudhir K, Jennings GL, Esler MD, et al. Hydrocortisone-induced hypertension in humans: pressor responsiveness and sympathetic function. Hypertension 1989; 13:416–421.

123. Pirpiris M, Sudhir K, Yeung S, Jennings GL, Whitworth JA. Pressor responsiveness in corticosteroid-induced hypertension in humans. Hypertension 1992;19: 567–574.
124. Tam SH, Kelly JJ, Williamson PM, Whitworth JA. Reflex sympathetic function in cortisol-induced hypertension in humans. Clin Exp Hypertens 1997;19:479–493.
125. Whitworth JA, Williamson PM, Brown MA, Morris MJ. Neuropeptide Y in cortisol-induced hypertension in male volunteers. Clin Exp Pharmacol Physiol 1994;21:435–438.
126. Macefield VG, Williamson PM, Wilson LR, Kelly JJ, Gandevia SC, Whitworth JA. Muscle sympathetic vasoconstrictor activity in hydrocortisone-induced hypertension in humans. Blood Press 1998;7:215–222.
127. Tam SH, Williamson PM, Kelly JJ, Whitworth JA. Autonomic blockade amplifies cortisol-induced hypertension in man. Clin Exp Pharmacol Physiol 1997;31–33.
128. Whitworth JA, Scoggins BA. A "hypertensinogenic" class of steroid hormone activity in man? Clin Exp Pharmacol Physiol 1990;17:163–166.
129. Mangos GJ, Walker BR, Kelly JJ, Lawson JA, Webb DJ, Whitworth JA. Cortisol inhibits cholinergic vasodilation in the human forearm. Am J Hypertens 2000;13:1155–1160.
130. Wang J, Brown MA, Tam SH, Chan MC, Whitworth JA. Effects of diet on measurement of nitric oxide metabolites. Clin Exp Pharmacol Physiol 1997; 24:418–420.
131. Kelly JJ, Tam SH, Williamson PM, Lawson J, Whitworth JA. The nitric oxide system and cortisol-induced hypertension in humans. Clin Exp Pharmacol Physiol 1998;25:945–946.
132. Kelly JJ, Williamson P, Martin A, Whitworth JA. Effects of oral L-arginine on plasma nitrate and blood pressure in cortisol treated humans. J Hypertens 2001;19:263–268.
133. Kelly JJ, Whitworth JA. Role of erythropoietin in cortisol induced hypertension. J Hum Hypertens 2000;14:195–198.
134. Nichols R. Concurrent illness and complications associated with canine hyperadrenocorticism. Probl Vet Med 1990;2:565–572.
135. van der Kolk JH, Nachreiner RF, Schott HC, Refsal KR, Zanella AJ. Salivary and plasma concentration of cortisol in normal horses and horses with Cushing's disease. Equine Vet J 2001;33:211–213.
136. Scoggins BA, Denton DA, Whitworth JA, Coghlan JP. ACTH dependent hypertension. Clin Exp Hypertens (A) 1984;6:599–646.
137. Whitworth JA, Hewitson TD, Li M, et al. Adrenocorticotrophin-induced hypertension in the rat: haemodynamic, metabolic and morphological characteristics. J Hypertens 1990; 8:27–36.
138. Schyvens CG, Mangos GJ, Zhang Y, McKenzie KUS, Whitworth JA. Telemetric monitoring of adrenocorticotrophin-induced hypertension in mice. Clin Exp Pharmacol Physiol 2001;28:758–760.
139. Lohmeier TE, Kastner PR. Chronic effects of ACTH and cortisol excess on arterial pressure in normotensive and hypertensive dogs. Hypertension 1982;4:652–661.

# IV Adrenal Medulla and Hypertension

# 13 Biochemical Diagnosis and Localization of Pheochromocytoma

*Emmanuel L. Bravo,* MD

*CONTENTS*



## CLINICAL FEATURES OF PHEOCHROMOCYTOMA

Pheochromocytoma is a symptom complex that reflects excessive exposure to norepinephrine and/or epinephrine. Thus, in general, patients should be screened for catecholamine excess when they present with typical signs and symptoms of the disorder. Also, because clinical abnormalities reflect the amount and duration of catecholamine excess, patients with low (≤2000 pg/mL) circulating catecholamines have fewer features than those with circulating catecholamines in excess of 2000 pg/mL.

A complicating factor in the clinical assessment of possible excess catecholamine production is that few signs and symptoms are specific

From: *Secondary Hypertension: Clinical Presentation, Diagnosis, and Treatment*
Edited by: G. A. Mansoor © Humana Press Inc., Totowa, NJ

for pheochromocytoma, but they occur rather frequently in the general population. Labile hypertension or excessive sweating, tachycardia, or headaches illustrates this difficulty as each symptom is common in middle-aged or older adults but is caused by pheochromocytoma in very few of them. Additionally, about 13% of patients are normotensive and 8% are asymptomatic.

The fact that pheochromocytoma is rare but many of its clinical features are common in the general population raises the dilemma of who should be screened for the disorder. Because missing a pheochromocytoma can result in a catastrophic outcome, it is of utmost importance that the physician become acutely aware of the varied and bizarre manifestations that can occur in familial as well as sporadic pheochromocytoma. One must have a high index of suspicion when confronting any patient with a clinical history and/or the signs and symptoms mentioned in Table 1. Pheochromocytoma has been called the "great mimic" because of its remarkably varied manifestations, which closely simulate a variety of diseases (Table 2) *(1)*.

## BIOCHEMICAL SCREENING TESTS FOR PHEOCHROMOCYTOMA

Screening tests should be performed in the context of the clinical setting. For example, in overtly symptomatic patients, total plasma catecholamines (norepinenephrine [NE] and epinephrine [E]) more than or equal to 2000 pg/mL, 24-hour urinary total metanephrines more than or equal to 1.8 µg/24 hour and 24-hour urinary NE less than or equal to 156 µg/24 hour usually suggest the presence of pheochromocytoma *(1a)*. Lower biochemical values in similar patients usually suggest a neurogenic etiology for the clinical manifestations. Patients with large (>50 g) and cystic tumors are often asymptomatic and may have near normal plasma catecholamines but markedly elevated urinary catecholamine metabolites *(2)*. Patients with prominent tachycardia, tremors, and labile hypertension are likely to have either pure—or predominantly—E-producing tumors *(3)*. Patients with familial pheochromocytoma may be completely asymptomatic despite high circulating catecholamines. The pathophysiological reason for this finding is unclear.

### *Plasma Catecholamines and Urinary Catecholamine Metabolites*

When reliably carried out and performed in an appropriate setting, the measurement of plasma catecholamines and urinary catecholamine metabolites can establish the diagnosis in more than 95% of cases. Of the

Table 1
**Signs and Symptoms Requiring Evaluation for Pheochromocytoma**

| |
|---|
| Episodic symptoms of headaches, tachycardia, and diaphoresis (with or without hypertension) |
| Family history of pheochromocytoma or a multiple endocrine neoplasia syndrome |
| Incidental suprarenal or abdominal masses |
| Unexplained paroxysms of tachyarrhythmias, hypertension during intubation, induction of anesthesia, parturition, or prolonged unexplained hypotension after an operation |
| Adverse cardiovascular response to ingestion, inhalation, or injection of certain drugs; including anesthetic agents, histamine, glucagon, tyramine, thyrotrophin-releasing hormone, adrenocorticotropic hormone, antidopaminergic agents, naloxone, succinylcholine chloride, phenothiazine, β-blockers, guanethidine, tricyclic antidepressants, and methacholine |
| Spells or attacks during physical exertion, twisting and turning of the torso, straining (Valsalva's maneuver), coitus, or micturition |

Table 2
**Clinical Conditions Likely To Be Confused With Pheochromocytoma**

| |
|---|
| β-Adrenergic hyper-responsiveness |
| Acute state of anxiety |
| Angina pectoris |
| Acute infections |
| Autonomic epilepsy |
| Hyperthyroidism |
| Idiopathic orthostatic hypotension |
| Cerebellopontine angle tumors |
| Acute hypoglycemia |
| Acute drug withdrawal |
| Clonidine |
| β-Adrenergic blockade |
| α-Methyldopa |
| Alcohol |
| Vasodilator therapy |
| Hydralazine |
| Minoxidil |
| Factitious administration of sympathomimetic agents |
| Tyramine ingestion in patients on monoamine oxidase inhibitors |
| Menopausal syndrome with migraine headaches |

From ref. *1*.

various biochemical tests, resting plasma catecholamines (NE and E) and total urinary metanephrines have the lowest false-negative rate (7%), assays of urinary NE and E the next higher (14%), and assays of urinary vanillylmandelic acid the highest (41%). In 109 consecutive cases in whom all four biochemical tests were performed, the combination of resting plasma catecholamines and total urinary metanephrines gave a false-negative rate of only 2.7% (3/109). All three patients not diagnosed by this combination had multiple endocrine neoplasia syndrome *(1a)*.

### *Chromogranin A in Pheochromocytoma*

Chromogranin A (CgA) is an acid-soluble protein that is costored and coreleased with catecholamines from adrenal medullary and sympathetic neuronal vesicles during exocytosis *(4)*. CgA is markedly elevated in patients with pheochromocytoma and has been suggested as a diagnostic test in the differential diagnosis of suspected pheochromocytoma *(5)*.

The overall sensitivity, specificity, positive predictive value, and negative predictive value are 86, 74, 67, and 94%, respectively. However, its clinical utility decreases significantly even with mild degrees of renal impairment. At creatinine clearances less than 80 mL/minute, the sensitivity remains essentially unaltered (85%); however, specificity is reduced to 50%, the positive predictive value to 38%, and the negative predictive value to 90%.

Plasma catecholamines had slightly lower overall sensitivity (84% vs 86%) but much higher specificity than serum CgA (88% vs 74%). Combining the two tests provided the best overall specificity (95%), accuracy (88%), and positive predictive value (91%). In subjects with creatinine clearances greater than 80 mL/minute, these indices were even more impressive: 98, 89, and 97%, respectively *(6)*.

### *Plasma-Free Metanephrines*

The measurement of plasma-free metanephrines has been advocated as the best marker for the presence of pheochromocytoma. This conclusion is based on findings that plasma-free metanephrines are produced independently of catecholamine release by tumors and that some tumors do not secrete catecholamines but metabolize catecholamines to free metanephrines *(7)*. In a recent study *(8)*, the test has a reported sensitivity and specificity of 97 and 96%, respectively, in the diagnosis of hereditary pheochromocytomas. In sporadic pheochromocytoma, the test has a reported sensitivity of 99% but a specificity of only 82%. In the same study, the test specificity of urinary total metanephrines is highest at 89%. A preliminary study *(9)* in another laboratory has reported a false-positive rate of about 15% for the test. The test is currently available in only one facility (the Mayo Clinic laboratories); the normal values are less than 0.90 nmol/L for plasma free normetanephrine and less than 0.50 nmol/L for plasma-free metanephrine.

## PHARMACOLOGICAL TESTING

Pharmacological testing should be performed when clinical suspicion is high but catecholamine values are equivocal. In such cases, the goal is to separate pheochromocytoma patients with relatively low levels of biosynthetic activity from nonpheochromocytoma patients with increased sympathetic outflow. Tests may be suppressive (to inhibit central sympathetic outflow) or stimulatory (to provoke catecholamine secretion from a tumor with low activity).

Suppressive testing is used in patients with plasma catecholamines between 1000 to 2000 pg/mL with or without hypertension *(10)*. Clonidine is given as a single oral dose of 0.3 mg. Blood pressure (BP), heart rate, and objective signs of central effects (i.e., dry mouth, thirst, and sleepiness) should be recorded before and at 30-minute intervals for 3 hours after clonidine administration. A normal test consists of a fall in the basal values of plasma catecholamines below 500 pg/mL at 2 or 3 hours into the test. Clonidine has no effect on plasma concentrations of E. A fall in BP and heart rate, and objective signs of central effects, ensure adequate absorption of the drug. The following precautions should be exercised. Volume depletion should be avoided and β-adrenergic blocking agents should be discontinued 48 hours before testing. Both tend to enhance the hypotensive response to clonidine. In addition, β-adrenergic blocking agents interfere with hepatic clearance of NE *(11)* and attenuate the NE-lowering effect of clonidine in patients with increased neurogenic tone, resulting in a false-positive test.

The clonidine suppression test is based on the principle that normal increases in levels of circulating NE are mediated through activation of the sympathetic nervous system, whereas in patients with pheochromocytoma, the increases result from diffusion of excess catecholamines from a tumor into the circulation, bypassing normal storage and release mechanisms. Because clonidine suppresses neurogenically mediated catecholamine release *(12)*, it should not be expected to suppress the release of catecholamines in patients with pheochromocytoma. This expectation is borne out by studies showing that clonidine administration significantly decreases plasma catecholamines in essential hypertension, whereas the levels are unaltered in pheochromocytoma (Fig. 1)*(13)*.

A provocative test is employed when plasma catecholamines are between 500 and 1000 pg/mL but the clinical manifestations are highly

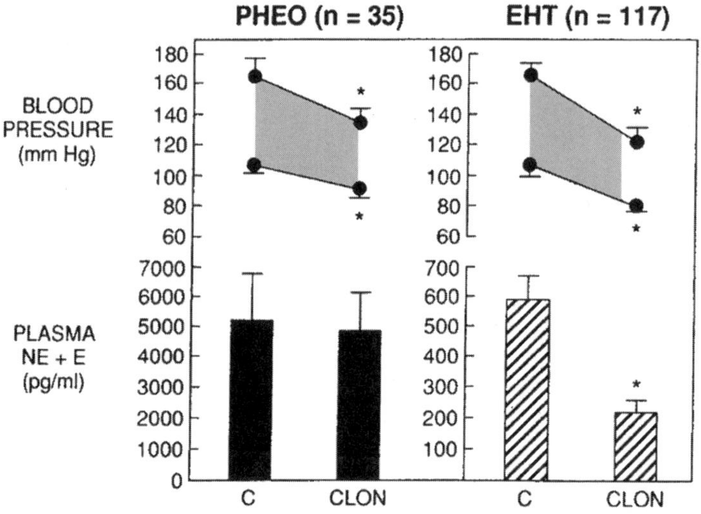


**Fig. 1.** Blood pressure and plasma catecholamine response to oral clonidine in patients with pheochromocytoma and essential hypertension. (From ref. *13a.*) C, control; Clon, 3 hours after single oral dose of 0.3 mg clonidine.

suspicious of pheochromocytoma. Glucagon is given as an intravenous (IV) bolus of 2.0 mg after an appropriate control. A positive glucagon test requires at least a threefold or greater than 2000 pg/mL increase in plasma catecholamines 1 to 3 minutes after drug administration. A simultaneous increase in BP is not essential *(14)*. BP should be recorded continuously. If values rise to or exceed 200/120 mmHg, then either phentolamine (5–10 mg IV bolus) or sodium nitroprusside by continuous drip should be initiated. For patients who may be at risk of sudden increases in BP, the test may be performed under cover of calcium channel blockers (CCBs) to prevent the rise in BP without interference with catecholamine release *(15)*.

## CLINICAL SITUATIONS THAT MAY ALTER THE LEVELS OF PLASMA CATECHOLAMINES AND URINARY CATECHOLAMINE METABOLITES

Certain clinical situations may increase both plasma catecholamines and urinary catecholamine metabolites to levels usually seen in pheochromocytoma. These include the following:

1. Acute clonidine withdrawal
2. Acute alcohol withdrawal
3. Vasodilator therapy with hydralazine or minoxidil

4. Acute myocardial ischemia or infarction
5. Acute cerebrovascular accident
6. Cocaine abuse
7. Severe congestive heart failure (Classes III–IV)

Intravenously administered dopamine (even in small doses), dopaminergic drugs, and acute hypoglycemia produce significant elevations in plasma E concentrations.

Drugs that inhibit central sympathetic outflow (e.g., clonidine, methyldopa, bromocriptine, and haloperidol) decrease levels of plasma catecholamine secretion in normal and hypertensive patients, but they have little effect on the excessive catecholamine secretion by pheochromocytoma. Drugs that tend to increase levels of plasma catecholamines (e.g., phenoxybenzamine, phentolamine, theophylline, β-blockers, and diuretics) do so only slightly, and levels rarely approach those usually encountered in pheochromocytoma. Labetalol significantly increases plasma catecholamines through biochemical interference *(16)*. Methylglucamine, a component of iodinated contrast media, may cause urinary metanephrine values to be falsely normal for as long as 72 hours when measured with the Pisano spectrophotometric method.

## SUGGESTED DIAGNOSTIC APPROACH

From the foregoing discussion, the following approach is suggested for patients clinically suspected of having pheochromocytoma (Fig. 2) *(1,13)*. Initially, resting plasma catecholamines, serum CgA, and serum creatinine levels (for calculation of the creatinine clearance by Cockcroft–Gault equation) should be determined. An increase in both plasma catecholamines (≥2000 pg/mL) and serum CgA (≥70 pg/m) and creatinine clearance of 80 mL/minute or more suggest the presence of pheochromocytoma. This combination has a positive predictive value of 97%. Patients with equivocal increases in plasma catecholamines (between 1000 and 2000 pg/mL) and normal serum CgA are likely to have neurogenically mediated catecholamine release and will require a clonidine suppression test for definitive diagnosis. Patients with plasma catecholamine values of 1000 pg/mL or more and serum CgA greater than 70 pg/mL are likely to have creatinine clearance values less than 80 mL/min; a glucagon-provocative test may be necessary in highly suspect patients. Patients with normal plasma catecholamine and serum CgA values are unlikely to have pheochromocytoma. Clinical judgment will dictate whether additional testing (i.e., use of plasma free metanephrines or urinary catecholamines and catecholamine metabolites) should be performed.

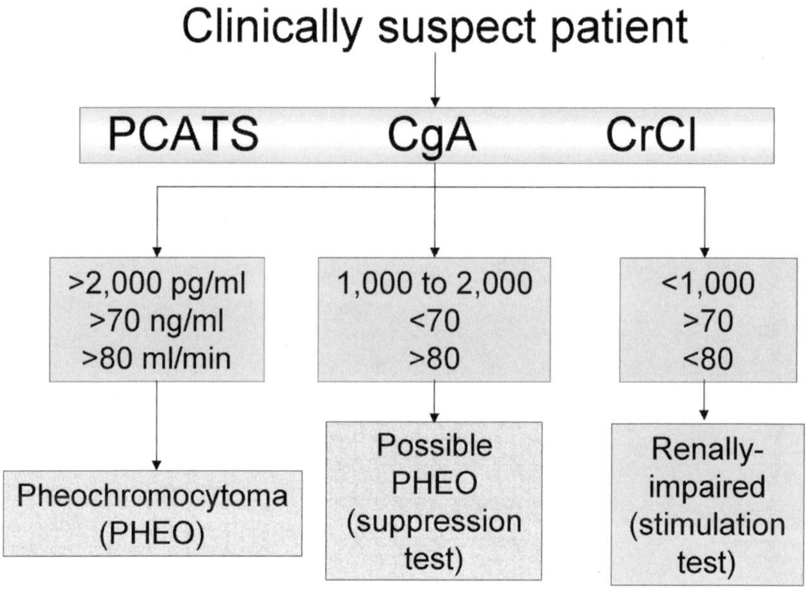


**Fig. 2.** Diagnosis of pheochromocytoma. CgA, chromogranin A; CrCl, creatinine clearance; PCATs, plasma catecholamines. (From ref. *13*.)

## LOCALIZATION

Radiologic evaluation should follow and not precede biochemical confirmation of the diagnosis. Anatomic localization is mandatory because of the variable location of these tumors: 97% are found in the abdominal region. The majority are found in the adrenal gland. Familial pheochromocytomas are frequently bilateral or arise from multiple sites. Pheochromocytoma occurring in children is commonly extra-adrenal and more frequently extra-adrenal than in adults. The most common extra-adrenal locations are the superior and inferior paraortic areas (75%), the bladder (10%), the thorax (10%), and the head, neck, and pelvis (5%).

Current experience suggests that computed tomography (CT) scanning and magnetic resonance imaging (MRI) provide the best sensitivities (98% and 100%, respectively) in the localization of pheochromocytoma. Metaiodobenzylguanidine (MIBG) has excellent specificity (100%) but a sensitivity of only 78%. Pheochromocytomas appear heterogeneous on CT and appear hyperintense to the liver on MRI $T_2$-weighted image. By contrast, benign tumors appear homogeneous,

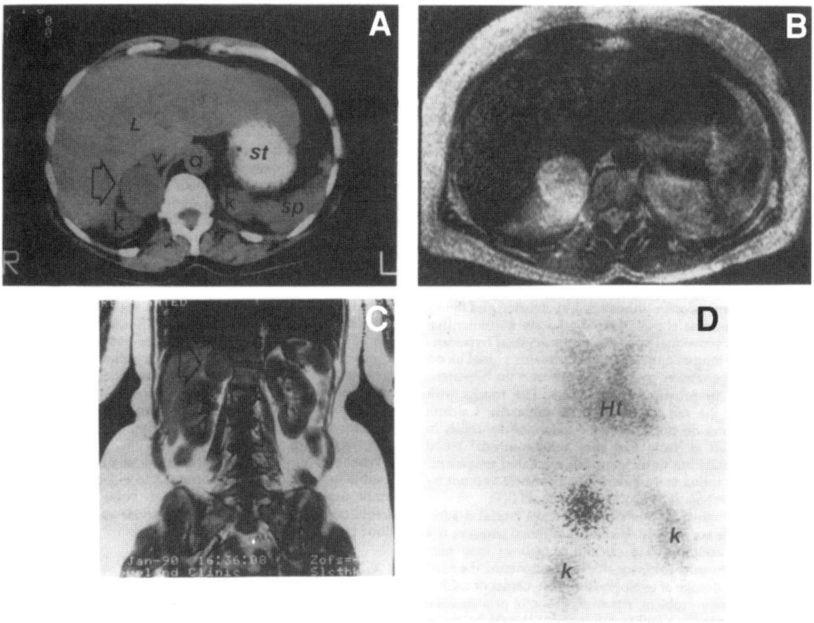


**Fig. 3. (A)** Abdominal computed tomography scan at the level of the adrenal glands. a, aorta; k, kidney; L, liver; sp, spleen; st, stomach; v, vena cava. Arrow points to a solid suprarenal mass in the area of the right adrenal gland and measures about 6.0 cm in greatest diameter. **(B)** Magnetic resonance imaging (MRI) scan with $T_2$-weighted partial saturation sequences demonstrates the high signal intensity typical of pheochromocytoma. **(C)** Coronal section of the MRI scan with $T_1$-weighted saturation sequences demonstrating the mass (arrow) above the kidney and medial to the liver. **(D)** [$^{131}$I]MIBG scan. Adrenal scintigraphic image at 48 hour after intravenously administered [$^{131}$I]metaiodobenzylguanidine. Focal increased right suprarenal $^{131}$I activity consistent with a right adrenal pheochromocytoma. Ht, heart; k, kidney. (From ref. *17a.*)

have low attenuation by CT, and are isointense by MRI $T_2$-weighted image (Fig. 3) *(1a)*. MIBG may be employed if more specific tissue characterization is required.

In more difficult cases, especially in the presence of a metastatic site, $^{123}$I-MIBG offers superior image quality compared to $^{131}$I-MIBG *(17)*. However, it is not routinely used and is available in only a few centers. Positron emission tomography with 6[$^{18}$F] fluorodopamine visualizes pheochromocytoma almost immediately with a high degree of sensitivity and specificity *(18)*. This test is still at its early evaluation.

## REFERENCES


1. Bravo EL. The syndrome of primary aldosteronism and pheochromocytoma. In: Schrier RW, Gottschalk CW, eds. Diseases of the Kidney, 5th ed. Boston: Little, Brown & Co, 1993, pp. 1475–1503.

1a. Bravo EL. Evolving concepts in the pathophysiology, diagnosis and treatment of pheochromocytoma. Endocr Rev 1994;15:356–368.

2. Crout JR, Sjoerdsma A. Turnover and metabolism of catecholamine in patients with pheochromocytoma. J Clin Invest 1964;43:94–102.

3. Page LB, Raker JW, Berberich FR. Pheochromocytoma with predominant epinephrine secretion. Am J Med 1969;47:648–652.

4. O'Connor DT, Frigon RP. Chromogranin A, the major catecholamine storage vesicle soluble protein: multiple size forms, subcellular storage, and regional distribution in chromaffin and nervous tissue elucidated by radioimmunoassay. J Biol Chem 1984;259:3237–3247.

5. O'Connor DT, Bernstein KN. Radioimmunoassay of chromogranin A in plasma as a measure of exocytotic sympathoadrenal activity in normal subjects and patients with pheochromocytoma. N Engl J Med 1984;311:764–770.

6. Canale MP, Bravo EL. Diagnostic specificity of serum chromogranin-A for pheochromocytoma in patients with renal dysfunction. J Clin Endo Metab 1994;78: 1139–1144.

7. Lenders JW, Keiser HR, Goldstein DS, et al. Plasma metanephrines in the diagnosis of pheochromocytoma. Ann Intern Med 1995;123:101–109.

8. Lenders JW, Pacak K, Walther MM, et al. Biochemical diagnosis of pheochromocytoma: which test is best? JAMA 2002;287:1427–1434.

9. Sawka AM, Singh RJ, and Young WF Jr. Fractionated plasma metanephrines are highly sensitive but less specific than urinary total metanephrines and catecholamines in detection of pheochromocytoma. Endocrinology [Abstract] 2002;PI-642,285.

10. Bravo EL, Tarazi RC, Fouad FM, Vidt DG, Gifford RW, Jr. Clonidine-suppression test: a useful aid in the diagnosis of pheochromocytoma. N Engl J Med 1981;305:623–626.

11. Maas JW, Landis DH. The metabolism of circulating norepinephrine by human subjects. J Pharmacol Exp Ther 1971;177:600–612.

12. Bravo EL, Fouad-Tarazi FM, Rossi G, et al. A reevaluation of the hemodynamics of pheochromocytoma. Hypertension 1990;15:I128–I131.

13. Bravo EL. Adrenal medullary function. In: Moore WT, Eastman RC, eds. Diagnostic Endocrinology. 2nd ed. St. Louis, MO: Mosby-Year Book, Inc., 1996, pp. 299–309.

13a. Bravo EL, Gifford RW Jr. Pheochromocytoma. In: Ober KP, ed. Endocrine Crises. Philadelphia: WB Saunders, 1993, pp. 329–341.

14. Bravo EL, Tarazi RC, Gifford RW, Jr., Stewart BH. Circulating and urinary catecholamines in pheochromocytoma: diagnostic and pathophysiological implications. N Engl J Med 1979;301:682–686.

15. Bravo EL. Pheochromocytoma: an approach to antihypertensive therapy. Ann NY Acad Sci 2002;970:1–10.

16. Feldman JM. Falsely elevated urinary excretion of catecholamines and metanephrines in patients receiving labetalol therapy. J Clin Pharmacol 1987;27:288–292.

17. Shulkin BL, Shapiro B, Francis IR, Dorr R, Shen SW, Sisson JC. Primary extra-adrenal pheochromocytoma: positive I-123 MIBG imaging with negative I-131 MIBG imaging. Clin Nucl Med 1986;11:851–854.

17a. Bravo EL, Gifford RW Jr, Manger WM. Adrenal medullary tumors: pheochromocytoma. In: Mazzaferri , and Seaman , eds. Endocrine Tumors. Cambridge, UK: Blackwell Scientific, 1993, pp. 1426–1438.
18. Pacak K, Eisenhofer G, Carrasquillo JA, Chen CC, Li ST, Goldstein DS. 6-[18F]fluorodopamine positron emission tomographic (PET) scanning for diagnostic localization of pheochromocytoma. Hypertension 2001;38:6–8.

# 14 Pheochromocytoma Treatment

*Carl D. Malchoff,* MD, PhD,
*Dougald MacGillivray,* MD,
*and Steven Shichman,* MD

*Contents*



## OVERVIEW

Surgical resection remains the cornerstone of pheochromocytoma therapy. Because most of these tumors are benign and unifocal, resection produces a permanent cure. Prior to 1950, the operative mortality was more than 25% . With a better understanding of the potential complications that contribute to perisurgical mortality and with the introduction of $\alpha$-adrenergic antagonists, the current surgical mortality is 2% or less. Surgical therapies continue to evolve and are supported by a greater choice of localizing techniques and treatment strategies both preoperatively and perioperatively. Combined surgical and medical therapy is required for the management of metastatic pheochromocytoma.

## PREPARATION FOR SURGERY

Patients should be stabilized prior to surgery with control of blood pressure (BP) and expansion of blood volume. The arguments for pre-

From: *Secondary Hypertension: Clinical Presentation, Diagnosis, and Treatment*
Edited by: G. A. Mansoor © Humana Press Inc., Totowa, NJ

Table 1
Agents Used to Prepare Patients for Pheochromocytoma Surgery

| *Pharmaceutical Agent* | *Dose* | *Description* | *Potential Complications* |
|---|---|---|---|
| Phenoxybenzamine (Dibenzyline) | 10 mg/day to 100 mg/day po | α-Adrenergic blockade<br>Irreversible<br>Lowers BP | Orthostatic hypotension<br>Postoperative hypotension |
| Prazosin (Minipress) | 6 mg/day to 20 mg/day po<br>Divided doses | α-Adrenergic blockade<br>Reversible<br>Half-life = 3 hours<br>Lowers BP | Inadequate blockade with catecholamine surges<br>Short half-life; deliver tid<br>Do not discontinue on day of surgery |
| Labetalol (Normodyne, Trandate) | 200 mg/d to 2400 mg/day<br>Divided doses | Combined α- and β-adrenergic blockade<br>Lowers BP | Inadequate blockade with catecholamine surges<br>May exacerbate hypertension<br>Ratio α:β blockade = 1:7<br>Interferes with HPLC catecholamine assays |
| Amlodipine (Norvasc) | 5 mg/day to 10 mg/day po<br>Divided doses | Calcium channel blockade<br>Lowers BP | Limited experience<br>Does not block α-adrenergic receptors |

| | | | |
|---|---|---|---|
| Metyrosine (Demser) | 500 mg/day to 2000 mg/day po<br>Divided doses | Blocks tyrosine hydroxylase<br>Depletes catecholamine stores<br>Lowers BP | Sleepiness often limits dose to 1 g/day |
| Propranolol (Inderal) | 40 mg/day to 320 mg/day po<br>Divided doses<br>or<br>0.1 mg/kg IV every 30 minutes | β-Adrenergic blockade<br>Reversible<br>Oral or parenteral<br>Treat tachyarrhythmias | May exacerbate hypertension |
| Phentolamine (Regitine) | 0.1 mg/kg IV every 30 minutes | α-Adrenergic blockade<br>Reversible<br>Rapid onset<br>Lowers BP | Only available intravenously |
| Sodium nitroprusside (Nipride) | 1.0 μg/kg/minute to 10 μg/kg/min uteIV<br>Constant infusion | Used intraoperatively<br>Rapid onset<br>Rapid end of effect<br>Vasodilator | Only available intravenously<br>Metabolized to cyanide |

operative preparation are theoretical. Although there are reports demonstrating the success of this approach, these studies are retrospective and experiential. Several different approaches have successfully controlled BP. Prospective controlled studies that compare different management regimens will have adequate statistical power to demonstrate the superiority of a given approach only if large numbers of patients are studied. Such large studies have not been performed. Blood volume expansion is uniformly implemented. This may also occur as a physiologic response to the vasodilating agents used for BP control in the preoperative period.

It is logical to control BP and to expand blood volume prior to surgery. Both the stress of intubation and the physical manipulation of the pheochromocytoma will precipitate catecholamine surges and predispose to complications from the ensuing hypertension. These BP excursions are likely to be less severe if BP has been well controlled. With the introduction of phentolamine, an α-adrenergic antagonist, to control BP, the perisurgical mortality fell from more than 20% to 2% *(1,2)*. More recently, in a large series of 156 surgeries for pheochromocytoma by a standard approach, serious complications were positively associated with preoperative systolic hypertension and urinary excretion of metanephrines *(3)*. Therefore, it is reasonable to expect that preoperative BP control will reduce the frequency of these complications. In contrast, some physicians have reported very good results without prolonged preoperative preparation *(4)*. However, in these reports they proceed without preparation in subjects with normal BP *(4,5)*, and they expand blood volume. In summary, there are cogent arguments for preoperative BP and volume expansion. This approach, which is associated with a low incidence of morbidity and mortality in the hands of experienced clinicians, should be continued even in the absence of prospective controlled studies.

The generally accepted approach is to prepare the patient for at least 7 to 14 days before surgery to control BP, deplete catecholamine stores, and expand blood volume. Options for antihypertensive therapy include short- and long-acting α-adrenergic antagonists and catecholamine synthesis inhibitors. When necessary, β-adrenergic blockade is instituted to treat tachyarrhythmias. These agents are summarized in Table 1. The optimum duration of preparation has not been investigated. We usually prepare patients for about 3 to 6 weeks. This is the amount of time required to lower BP to 120/70 mmHg and to negotiate a date for surgery that accommodates the patient, surgeon, endocrinologist, and operating room.

α-Adrenergic blockade is logical choice for lowering BP and is probably the most widely used approach. Several α-adrenergic blocking agents are available. There are advantages and disadvantages of each agent. Because phentolamine (Phentolamine, Regitine) is available only as an intravenous preparation, it is not appropriate for management in the days to weeks before surgery. Phenoxybenzamine (Dibenzyline) has been used widely for preoperative preparation. This irreversible α-adrenergic blocking agent may cause orthostatic hypotension and carries theoretical concerns of a slow onset of action and exacerbation of post-operative hypotension. Shorter acting reversible agents such as prazosin (Prazosin, Minipress) have theoretical advantages and disadvantages. In theory, reversible α-adrenergic blocking agents may not provide adequate BP control during surges of catecholamine release but are less likely to cause orthostatic hypotension in the preoperative period and are less likely to cause hypotension following resection. Intraoperative BP surges should be anticipated regardless of the preoperative preparation. There are no prospective controlled studies comparing different α-adrenergic antagonists. Irreversible antagonists and reversible antagonists have been used successfully as monotherapy or in combination with each other. There is one case report of the efficacy of phenoxybenzamine in the face of prazosin failure to control hypertension preoperatively *(6)*. In contrast, a retrospective review compared nine patients who were prepared for surgery with phenoxybenzamine with six patients who were prepared with prazosin. Intraoperative hemodynamic stability was the same in both groups *(7)*. Similarly, in a retrospective review of 156 surgeries for pheochromocytoma there was no difference in the complication rate in those patients prepared with phenoxybenzamine compared to those prepared with prazosin *(3)*. Prazosin usually is given in divided doses of 6 to 20 mg/day, and phenoxybenzamine usually is given as a single dose of 10 to 100 mg/day. Higher doses have been used when necessary. The usual preparative dose should be given the morning of surgery with small sips of water. Because the half-life of prazosin is about 3 hours, failure to take this agent on the morning before surgery, because the patient is "NPO (nothing by mouth) for surgery," is likely to render the patient susceptible to hypertensive complications perioperatively. The use of reversible and irreversible α-adrenergic blocking agents is not mutually exclusive. In summary, α-adrenergic blockade is a logical approach to preoperative BP control that is successfully employed by experienced clinicians. There are theoretical arguments for both reversible and irreversible α-adrenergic blockade, and the agents can be used in combination. We frequently use phenoxybenzamine and prazosin together in an effort to reduce postresection hypotensive complications and provide good BP control both before and during surgery. Our goal is to reduce the BP to 120/70 mmHg prior to surgery.

Metyrosine (Demser) blocks tyrosine hydroxylase, the rate-limiting step of catecholamine synthesis. This agent decreases circulating catecholamine concentrations and catecholamine stores within the pheochromocytoma. Therefore, it is expected to reduce catecholamine surges and subsequent BP excursions. However, because some catecholamine stores persist, it probably should not be used alone for preoperative management. One hypertensive crisis was reported during surgery when this agent was used without α blockade but with β-adrenergic blockade *(8)*. Although this case is complicated by unopposed β-adrenergic blockade that can predispose to vasoconstriction, metyrosine is usually administered in combination with α-adrenergic blockade and not as a single agent. One retrospective study of 33 pheochromocytoma patients that compared metyrosine combined with α-adrenergic blockade to α-adrenergic blockade alone did not find statistically significant differences *(9)*. However, there was a tendency for combined therapy to reduce peak intraoperative systolic BPs, the frequency of phentolamine administration to control intraoperative BP elevations, and the need for vasopressor agents to treat hypotension following removal of the pheochromocytoma *(9)*. Similar trends were observed in another study of 25 pheochromocytoma patients *(10)*. The usual dose is 500 to 2000 mg/day given in divided doses, and the most common side effect is sleepiness. Other less common side effects are frightening dreams, depression, impaired memory, diarrhea, and extrapyramidal symptoms. In summary, metyrosine is a logical agent to use with α-adrenergic blockade to prepare patients for surgery. Retrospective studies do suggest some modest benefits to adding this agent to α-adrenergic blockade. Our approach is to use metyrosine at the maximum dose that is tolerated by the patient in addition to α-adrenergic blockade. This is usually about 1000 mg/day, and patients often find that higher doses produce intolerable sleepiness. We treat for 3 weeks before surgery to maximally deplete catecholamine stores.

In theory, β-adrenergic blockade for tachyarrhythmias should be initiated only after α-adrenergic blockade has been established. Because most patients do not have clinically significant tachyarrhythmias, β-adrenergic blockade is not routinely used. Stimulation of α-adrenergic receptors promotes vasoconstriction. In contrast, stimulation of β-adrenergic receptors promotes vasodilatation. Although norepinephrine, the catecholamine released by most pheochromocytomas, is known as an α-adrenergic agonist, it is not completely selective and will stimulate both α- and β-adrenergic receptors. Similarly, epinephrine is also a combined α- and β-adrenergic agonist. Therefore, institution of isolated β-adrenergic blockade may potentiate vasoconstriction. Case reports of pulmonary edema following institution of isolated β-adrenergic blockade in pheochromocytoma patients support this reasoning *(11,12)*. Labetalol (Labetalol, Normodyne, Trandate), a combined β- and α-adrenergic receptor antagonist, has been used successfully to prepare patients for surgery *(13)*. However, the potency ratio of β-adrenergic antagonism to β-adrenergic antagonism of this agent is about 7 to 1 *(14)*, giving rise to concerns that it may exacerbate hypertension, as has been reported *(15)*. In addition, this agent gives false positive results in urinary catecholamine assays and may interfere with metaiodobenzylguanidine (MIBG) scanning *(16,17)*. In summary, β-adrenergic blockade is used to treat tachyarrhythmias and should be instituted following α-adrenergic blockade in pheochromocytoma patients. Labetalol is a more potent β-adrenergic antagonist than it is an α-adrenergic antagonist. If labetalol is used as a β-adrenergic blocking agent, then its interfering effects should be known. We strictly adhere to the recommendation to avoid β-adrenergic blockade until after α-adrenergic blockade has been instituted and find that it is rarely required, because tachyarrhythmias are unusual. We do not use labetalol when preparing patients with pheochromocytoma for surgical resection.

Calcium channel blockers (CCBs) have been used successfully to prepare patients for surgery *(5)*. As anticipated, these vasodilating agents lower BP in pheochromocytoma patients. As with the use of other agents, BP surges should be anticipated at surgery and treated appropriately. Our approach is to add CCBs only if adequate BP control cannot be attained with α-adrenergic blockade plus metyrosine. This is a rare event.

Volume expansion with normal saline during the hours prior to surgery may help prevent hypotension following surgical resection. This is reasonable, because hypotension following adrenalectomy is related to volume contraction caused by vasoconstriction *(18)*. However, there are no prospective controlled studies that specifically demonstrate the benefit of this procedure. As discussed above, there is reason to believe that postsurgical hypotension may be exacerbated by pretreatment with phenoxybenzamine, an irreversible α-adrenergic blocker. Therefore, hypotension following surgical resection may be multifactorial. Probably, treatment of hypertension during the weeks before surgery with α-adrenergic agonists allows volume to expand before surgical resection.

In summary, theoretical, experiential, and retrospective evidence supports the decision to pretreat patients with both antihypertensive agents and catecholamine synthesis inhibitors for at least 1 to 2 weeks before resection of the pheochromocytoma. Arguments can be made in favor of either reversible or irreversible α-adrenergic blockade to lower BP. It is reasonable to combine the two. β-Adrenergic blockade is generally not routinely necessary and should be used only for tachyarrhythmias after α-adrenergic blockade has been instituted. Regardless of the preoperative preparation, there will be some patients with significant intraoperative BP elevations that require the rapid acting vasodilators described below.

## INTRAOPERATIVE MEDICAL THERAPY

As noted previously, the improved outcome of surgical resection in the 1950s is attributed to the institution of intravenous phentolamine for control of BP excursions before and during the surgical procedure. Before the 1950s, the surgical mortality of pheochromocytoma was more than 25% *(1)*. Since that time, the mortality has decreased to about 2% or less. In 1956, Kvale et al. reported no mortality in a series of 56 patients in whom 61 pheochromocytomas were resected *(2)*. The markedly improved survival was attributed to the use of intravenous phentolamine for α-adrenergic blockade and to the use of norepinephrine for the treatment of postresection hypotension *(2)*. Regardless of the medications used for preoperative preparation, episodic BP elevations should be anticipated particularly during intubation and manipulation of the pheochromocytoma. Blockade that is sufficient for baseline control is unlikely to be sufficient to control BP surges caused by the release of large quantities of stored catecholamines. Arterial BP should be monitored continuously. The anesthesiologist must be prepared to administer rapid acting agents to lower BP, and the surgeon must be prepared to discontinue manipulation of the tumor while awaiting BP surges to resolve.

Phentolamine (Regitine) and sodium nitroprusside (Nipride) are the two most commonly used intravenous agents for rapid reduction of BP during surgery. Both agents are very effective, and there are no comparison studies. Historically, phentolamine was available first. However, many anesthesiologists are more familiar with sodium nitroprusside and prefer to use this agent. The effect of sodium nitroprusside dissipates more rapidly than that of phentolamine. Therefore, there are theoretical advantages to using this agent when the pheochromocytoma is being manipulated and the BP excursions may last for only a few minutes because of the short half-life of the catecholamines. Phentolamine is given as a bolus of 0.1 mg/kg intravenously and is repeated as necessary, usually every 30 to 60 minutes. Sodium nitroprusside is infused at a rate of 1.0 to 10 μg/kg/minute to control BP. Toxic metabolites of cyanide and thiocyanate may accumulate if high doses are used for prolonged periods or in the setting of renal or hepatic insufficiency. In summary, sodium nitroprusside and phentolamine or both together can be used effectively to control BP excursions during surgery.

Hypotension immediately following resection of the pheochromocytoma should be anticipated. Support with normal saline and norepinephrine infusion are effective therapies *(18)*. There are at least three possible etiologies for the hypotension. Resection of the pheochromocytoma may produce a rapid decrease in circulating catecholamines accompanied by hypotension. As discussed, hypotension may be more profound if the patient is prepared with phenoxybenzamine because α-adrenergic blockade with the agent is irreversible. Finally, adrenal insufficiency may contribute to the hypotension. Because the contralateral adrenal gland produces adequate amounts of glucocorticoids (GCs) even during stress, adrenal insufficiency is not a common consequence of unilateral adrenalectomy. However, rarely a pheochromocytoma produces adrenocorticotropic hormone (ACTH), which drives cortisol production by the adrenal cortex *(19)*. Following prolonged hypercortisolism, the hypothalamic–pituitary axis will not respond to falling cortisol levels with increased ACTH production. Therefore, when an ACTH-secreting pheochromocytoma is resected, cortisol production is temporarily terminated. If this rare situation is suspected, then stress doses of GCs (2 mg of intravenous dexamethasone every 12 hours) should accompany fluid resuscitation. If this problem is anticipated, then GC administration should precede adrenalectomy. In summary, significant hypotension with multiple causes may occur as a complication of adrenalectomy. This complication should be anticipated and appropriate therapies initiated promptly.

## SURGICAL APPROACH

The laparoscopic approach to adrenalectomy is now the favored surgical approach for resection of pheochromocytomas at many tertiary centers. This represents a relatively recent change in thinking that has evolved in response to advances in imaging techniques, genetic analysis, and surgical expertise.

The traditional surgical approach to pheochromocytomas has been an anterior transperitoneal approach that allows for examination of both adrenal glands, the organ of Zuckerkandl, the urinary bladder, and periaortic and pericaval lymphatic chains. Those supporting this approach argue that the frequency of malignancy and bilateral tumors is about

10% and that re-explorations will be more difficult than the first surgery. Therefore, it is logical to perform the most complete operation the first time. Two recent series describe excellent results with this approach in 181 patients *(3,10)*. However, with the development of genetic analysis, more refined imaging techniques, and less invasive surgical approaches, the anterior transperitoneal approach is no longer in routine use in most centers. Currently, many physicians feel that a combination of computed tomography (CT) scanning, magnetic resonance imaging (MRI), and scanning with $^{131}I$ MIBG will identify metastatic disease, extra-adrenal pheochromocytomas, and bilateral pheochromocytomas in most subjects. Characteristics suggesting a high risk of malignancy include invasion into surrounding structures, obvious metastases to the liver or other organs, adenopathy, and very large size. In the absence of these features, the pheochromocytoma will be benign and amenable to a more limited approach. Bilateral pheochromocytomas will almost always occur in familial tumor syndromes such as multiple endocrine neoplasia type 2A (MEN2A), MEN type 2B (MEN2B), and the von Hippel-Lindau (VHL) syndrome. Therefore, a combination of family history, personal history, and, if necessary, genetic testing predicts those individuals most likely to have bilateral disease. Finally, with the laparoscopic adrenalectomy, it is possible to resect the contralateral adrenal gland at a later date without increased risk to the patient. Therefore, subjects at risk for developing bilateral pheochromocytoma need not undergo removal of the second adrenal gland until the pheochromocytoma develops, so that adrenocortical insufficiency and its associated risks can be avoided for as long as possible. We reserve the open transperitoneal approach for tumors that are judged to be at high risk for malignancy and for most extra-adrenal pheochromocytomas.

More limited surgical approaches include the open posterior approach and laparoscopic adrenalectomy. The latter has become the favored approach at most tertiary centers. The open posterior approach was the first of the limited procedures to be used to remove adrenal pheochromocytomas. Compared to the open transabdominal approach, the posterior approach may reduce morbidity and duration of hospitalization. Unfortunately, the posterior extraperitoneal approach is most appropriate for resection of small tumors. Additionally, the limited exposure usually requires significant manipulation of the gland to expose and control the adrenal vein. Early control of the adrenal vein with limited manipulation of the pheochromocytoma reduces intraoperative BP surges. Given these difficulties, it is not surprising that a series of 105 open posterior adrenalectomies excluded pheochromocytomas *(20)*. In

1992, Gagner first reported the use of laparoscopic adrenalectomy to remove a pheochromocytoma *(21)*. Since that time, this has become the procedure of choice at most large tertiary surgical centers *(1,22–25)*. Laparoscopic adrenalectomy can be technically difficult. However, when performed by experienced surgeons, patient morbidity is minimal and recovery is rapid. Both transperitoneal *(22,24,25)* and retroperitoneal *(26)* laparoscopic approaches have been reported. We prefer the transperitoneal approach. We believe that it allows for better exposure of the adrenal gland and surrounding organs and requires less manipulation of the tumor. As in open surgical approaches, early control of the adrenal vein with minimal tumor manipulation decreases the release of catecholamines into the circulation and limits intraoperative hypertension and tachyarrhythmias. The contralateral adrenal gland is left untouched. If a second pheochromocytoma develops in the future, it can be removed without encountering adhesions from a previous surgery. Therefore, it is no longer necessary to perform a bilateral adrenalectomy in MEN2A and MEN2B patients with a unilateral pheochromocytoma as has been done with the anterior transperitoneal approach. Although there are no prospective studies comparing the traditional transabdominal and thoracoabdominal incision to laparoscopic surgery, it seems likely that the laparoscopic technique shortens the periods of hospitalization and recovery *(1,25)*. No increase in hypertensive events has been noted *(27)*. One report describes three cases of recurrent pheochromocytomatosis that was apparently caused by seeding the adrenal bed with tumor tissue during laparoscopic resection. The entire neoplasm must be resected carefully without disruption of the contents within the tumor capsule *(28)*. The size of the pheochromocytoma may prohibit a localized approach. However, pheochromocytomas as large as 14 cm have been resected by the laparoscopic approach *(27)*. In summary, there is considerable experience with laparoscopic resection of pheochromocytomas, and this has become the favored approach at many tertiary centers. We have had considerable success with resection of more than 30 pheochromocytomas using a lateral transperitoneal approach for laparoscopic adrenalectomy. All tumors were removed in their entirety without disruption of the capsule, with the largest having an 8.7 cm diameter *(29)*. No procedure was converted from the laparoscopic approach to an open approach.

There is no agreement as to which structural or genetic studies should be performed before localized resection. Genetic studies for MEN2A and MEN2B are commercially available. We do not hesitate to obtain both CT and MRI scans if the surgeon considers more anatomical information to be necessary before proceeding with a laparoscopic approach. We obtain an MIBG scan even if there is no suspicion of malignancy or familial syndrome. When we introduced laparoscopic adrenalectomy at our center, we were aggressive about obtaining multiple structural studies by different modalities. However, the yield is very low. In the future, it may be appropriate to limit multimodality structural studies to those subjects in whom there is some suspicion of an extra-adrenal pheochromocytoma, a metastatic pheochromocytoma, or a familial tumor syndrome with bilateral pheochromocytomas.

In summary, laparoscopic adrenalectomy is appropriate for removal of most unilateral and bilateral pheochromocytomas, provided that the surgeon has the experience and skill to remove the tumor without violation of the tumor capsule. If the pheochromocytoma is felt to be malignant, then an open approach is recommended.

## THERAPY OF MALIGNANT PHEOCHROMOCYTOMA

Malignant pheochromocytoma is quite rare. Treatment requires a combination of medical and surgical therapy. These tumors are relatively slow growing, with a 5-year survival of metastatic pheochromocytoma being about 44% *(30)*. Therefore, surgical reduction of the tumor burden is a reasonable approach. Although there are no data to demonstrate that this prolongs life, a smaller tumor burden may be better tolerated, diminish substrate with potential for future metastases, and reduce the requirement for toxic medical therapies. More recently, radiofrequency ablation has been used to destroy metastases *(31)*, and radioisotope-guided surgery has been used to identify small metastases for resection *(32)*. The role of these modalities remains to be determined in future studies.

Control of the effects of increased catecholamines is performed in a manner similar to that of presurgical control. Combinations of α-adrenergic blocking agents and catecholamine synthesis inhibitors may be required. The relative risks and benefits of these agents have been discussed.

Both chemotherapy and targeted radiotherapy with high dose $^{131}$I MIBG are effective in managing this disorder. Chemotherapy is based on responses of childhood neuroblastoma, a similar tumor. MIBG structurally resembles catecholamines, is recognized by catecholamine reuptake mechanisms, and can be labeled with radioactive iodine isotopes. Most frequently, these modalities produce remissions but not cures.

Chemotherapy with cyclophosphamide, vincristine, and dacarbazine given at about 21-day intervals was considered because childhood neuroblastoma responds to this regimen. There are biochemical responses in about 80% of subjects with metastatic pheochromocytoma. About 50% of subjects will have diminished tumor burden (tumor response). Complete biochemical and tumor responses occur only in about 10 to 15% of subjects *(30,33)*. Because the pheochromocytomas lose sensitivity to these agents, it is generally recommended that chemotherapy be reserved for those subjects who have advanced disease, for whom debulking and control of catecholaminergic signs and symptoms is no longer adequate, or for those subjects in whom the tumor load is causing fatigue and weight loss.

High dose $^{131}$I MIBG is more difficult to obtain, and the results of this agent are not as good as they are with traditional chemotherapy *(34,35)*. In a review of 116 treated subjects, Loh et al. concluded that the expected hormonal response is 45%, and the expected tumor response is 30%. Complete and long-lasting remissions are rare, and most subjects escape from the therapeutic effect of this agent. As expected, responses are greatest when the metastatic pheochromocytoma avidly concentrates the radioactive ligand. Soft tissue metastases respond better than bony metastases, and there is a tendency of responders to live longer than nonresponders *(34,35)*.

Combined sequential therapy with $^{131}$I MIBG followed by 21-day cycles of cytoxan, vincristine, and dacarbazine has been tried in six patients *(36)*. This order of therapies was selected so that routine chemotherapy would not reduce MIBG uptake into tumors. The responses were not dramatically better than expected for either agent alone. There was a suggestion that the effects might be additive, but the bone marrow toxicities also appeared additive, limiting the doses of chemotherapy that subjects could tolerate.

In summary, $^{131}$I MIBG and chemotherapy with cytoxan, vincristine, and dacarbazine produce hormone and tumor responses in metastatic pheochromocytoma and may prolong life. Cure is unusual.

## REFERENCES


1. Duh Q-Y. Evolving surgical management for patients with pheochromocytoma. J Clin Endocrinol Metab 2001: 86; 1477–1479.
2. Kvale W, Roth G, Manger W, Priestley T. Pheochromocytoma. Circulation 1956:14;622–630.
3. Plouin P-F, Duclos J-M, Soppelsa F, Boublil G, Chatellier G. Factors associated with perioperative morbidity and mortality in patients with pheochromocytoma: analysis of 165 operations at a single center. J Clin Endocrinol Metab 2001:86;1480–1486.
4. Boutros A, Bravo E, Zanettin G, Straffon R. Perioperative management of 63 patients with pheochromocytoma. Cleve Clin J Med 1990:57;613–617.

5. Ulchaer J, Goldfarb D, Bravo E, Novick A. Successful outcomes of pheochromocytoma surgery in the modern era. J Urol 1999:61;764–767.
6. Knapp H, Fitzgerald G. Hypertensive crisis in prazosin-treated pheochromocytoma. S Med J 1984:77;535–536.
7. Havkujm R, Cahow C, Kindre B. Advances in the diagnosis and treatment of pheochromocytoma. Arch Surg 1988:123;626–630.
8. Ram C, Meese R, Hill S. Failure of alpha-methyltyrosine to prevent hypertensive crisis in pheochromocytoma. Arch Intern Med 1985:145;2114–2115.
9. Steinsapir J, Carr A, Prisant L, Bransome E. Metyrosine and pheochromocytoma. Arch Intern Med 1997:157;901–906.
10. Perry R, Keiser H, Norton J, et al. Surgical management of pheochromocytoma with the use of metyrosine. Ann Surg 1990:212;621–628.
11. Pogson G, Sharma J, Crouch T. Pulmonary edema with low-dose propranolol in pheochromocytoma. S Med J 1980:73;795–796.
12. Wark J, Larkins R. Pulmonary oedema after propranolol therapy in two cases of phaeochromocytoma. BMJ 1978:1;1395–1396.
13. Pearce CJ, Wallin JD. Labetalol and other agents that block both alpha- and beta-adrenergic receptors. Cleve Clin J Med 1994:61;59–69.
14. Kanto J. Current status of labetalol, the first alpha- and beta-blocking agent. Int J Clin Pharmacol Ther Toxicol 1985:23;617–628.
15. Briggs R, Birtwell A, Pohl J. Hypertensive response to labetalol in phaeochromocytoma. Lancet 1978:13;1045–1046.
16. Crawford GA, Gyory AZ, Gallery ED, Kelley D. HPLC of urinary catecholamines in the presence of labetalol, captopril, and alpha-methyldopa. J Clin Chem 1990:36;1849.
17. Khafagi FA, Shapiro B, Fig LM, Mallette S, Sisson JC. Labetalol reduces iodine-131 MIBG uptake by pheochromocytoma and normal tissues. J Nucl Med 1989:30;481–489.
18. Brunjes S, Johns V, Crane M. Pheochromocytoma: postoperative shock. N Engl J Med 1960:262;393–396.
19. Spark R, Connolly P, Gluckin D, White R, Sacks B, Landsberg L. ACTH secretion from a functioning pheochromocytoma. N Engl J Med 1979:23;416–418.
20. Proye C, Huart J, Cuvillier X, Assez M, Gambardella B, Carnaille B. Safety of the posterior approach in adrenal surgery. Surgery 1993:114;1126–1131.
21. Gagner M, Lacroix A, Bolte E. Laparoscopic adrenalectomy in Cushing's syndrome and pheochromocytoma. N Engl J Med 1992:327;1033.
22. Brunt L, Moley J, Doherty G, Lairmore T, Debenedetti M, Quasebarth M. Outcome analysis in patients undergoing laparoscopic adrenalectomy for hormonally active adrenal tumors. Surgery 2001:130;629–635.
23. Col V, Canniere L, Collard E, Michel L, Donckier J. Laparoscopic adrenalectomy for phaeochromocytoma: endocrinological and surgical aspects of a new therapeutic approach. Clin Endocrinol 1999:50;121–125.
24. Janetschek G, Neumann H. Laparoscopic surgery for pheochromocytoma. Urol Clin N Am 2001:28;97–105.
25. Shichman S, Herndon C, Sosa R, et al. Lateral transperitoneal laparoscopic adrenalectomy. World J Urol 1999:17;48–53.
26. Salomon L, Rabii R, Soulie M, et al. Experience with retroperitoneal laparoscopic adrenalectomy for pheochromocytoma. J Urol 2001:165;1871–1874.
27. Gagner M, Breton G, Pharand D, Pomp A. Is laparoscopic adrenalectomy indicated for pheochromocytomas? Surgery 1996:120;1076–1080.

28. Li M. Fitzgerald P, Price D, Norton J. Iatrogenic pheochromocytomatosis: a previously unreported result of pheochromocytoma. Surgery 2001;1072–1077.
29. MacGillivray D, Whalen GF, Malchoff CD, Oppenheim DS, Shichman SJ. Laparoscopic resection of large adrenal tumors. Ann Surg Oncol 2002;130: 480–485.
30. Averbuch S, Steakley C, Young R, et al. Malignant pheochromocytoma: effective treatment with a combination of cyclophosphamide, vincristine, and dacarbazine. Ann Int Med 1988:102;267–273.
31. Pacak K, Fojok T, Goldstein D, et al. Radiofrequency ablation: a novel approach for treatment of metastatic pheochromocytoma. J Natl Cancer Institute 2001:2001; 648–649.
32. Adams S, Acker P, Lorenz M, Staib-Sebler E, Hor G. Radioisotope-guided surgery in patients with pheochromocytoma and intraoperative tumor localization with histopathologic findings. Cancer 2001:92;263–270.
33. Keiser HR, Goldstein DS, Wade JL, Douglas FL, Averbuch SD. Treatment of malignant pheochromocytoma with combination chemotherapy. Hypertension 1985:7(Suppl I);18–24.
34. Loh K, Fitzgerald P, Matthay K, Yeo P, Price D. The treatment of malignant pheochromocytoma with iodine-131 metaiodobenzylguanidine (131I-MIBG): a comprehensive review of 116 reported patients. J Endocrinol Invest 1997:11;648–658.
35. Sisson J, Shapiro B, Beierwaltes W, et al. Radiopharmaceutical treatment of malignant pheochromocytoma. J Nucl Med 1984:24;197–206.
36. Sisson JC, Shapiro B, Shulkin BL, Urba S, Zempel S, Spaulding S. Treatment of malignant pheochromocytomas with 131-I metaiodobenzylguanidine and chemotherapy. Am J Clin Oncol 1999:22;364–370.

# 15 New Insights Into Pseudopheochromocytoma and Emotionally Provoked Hypertension

*Otto Kuchel*, MD, DSc

*CONTENTS*



## DEFINITION

Paroxysmal hypertension represents a frequent clinical dilemma, particularly when these bouts are of abrupt onset and severe (usually defined as blood pressure [BP] exceeding 200/110 mmHg). Although severe paroxysmal hypertension should always raise suspicions of a catecholamine-secreting pheochromocytoma *(1)*, pheochromocytoma and adrenal medullary hyperplasia, its controversial variant, are exceedingly rare. Pseudopheochromocytoma refers to the large majority of

From: *Secondary Hypertension: Clinical Presentation, Diagnosis, and Treatment*
Edited by: G. A. Mansoor © Humana Press Inc., Totowa, NJ

individuals with severe paroxysmal hypertension, whether normotensive or hypertensive between episodes, in whom pheochromocytoma has been ruled out *(2)*.

Recent evidence indicates that pseudopheochromocytoma is a clinically heterogenous condition, requiring its subdivision into a primary and a secondary form. Although the secondary form may be attributed to various pathologies, medications, or drug abuse, only essential hypertension is associated with the primary form.

## INCIDENCE

Despite improvements in diagnostic tools, pheochromocytoma remains an uncommon problem. For example, the incidence based on the Mayo Clinic statistics has been estimated at 0.14% of all hypertensive patients *(1)*. Our own substantial experience confirms these findings. During a 10-year period (1986–1996), we evaluated 7480 patients referred to the Clinical Research Institute and Hôtel Dieu Hospital of Montreal for hypertension. Of this total, only 8 patients (0.1%) were confirmed to have a pheochromocytoma. Approximately 9% (688) of all referrals had evidence of paroxysmal hypertension, with many being evaluated for a suspected pheochromocytoma based on clinical presentation and/or the presence of an adrenal mass. Remarkably, pheochromocytoma was eventually ruled out in all but 5 (0.72 %) of these 688 individuals.

Although still very low, this incidence of pheochromocytoma is higher than the 0.33% present in individuals being worked up for this problem in the setting of paroxysmal hypertension with a more restrictive clinical suspicion based on anxiety disorders *(3)*.

Analyzing further the subgroup of 688 patients with suspected but unconfirmed pheochromocytoma, we identified 63 patients (9%) whose clinical presentation included a number of unusual symptoms and clinical signs that may have contributed to their secondary hypertension. These 63 individuals (mean age 51.6 years) were hospitalized and studied in our clinical investigation unit. This allowed us to closely study their environment-dependent paroxysms and also to sample blood at the height of the paroxysm. BP and pulse rates were recorded hourly in both the recumbent and upright positions during the day. Diet remained controlled and stable (135 mmol $Na^+$). Peripheral catecholamines were determined both under basal conditions and at the height of the paroxysmal episodes *(4)*. As a result of these investigations, 38 (60%) of 63 patients fit the diagnosis of secondary pseudopheochromocytoma, whereas the remainder (40%) were felt to exhibit unexplained primary pseudopheochromocytoma. As a result of a selection bias, this ratio probably overestimates the natural occurrence of secondary pseudopheochromocytoma. Nevertheless, results of our screening study *(4)* highlight several important points. First of all, distinguishing the primary and secondary form of pseudopheochromocytoma requires fairly extensive investigations that must address multiple mechanisms.

Individuals in the primary pseudopheochromocytoma group who are normotensive between paroxysms require particular attention. Do they suffer from borderline hypertension *(5)*, a precursor stage of hypertension or are their paroxysms simply linked to emotions that, as recently shown *(6)*, may often may be repressed and not demonstrated?

## CLINICAL PRESENTATION

The most common clinical characteristics of this syndrome are attributable to a short-term activation of the sympathetic nervous system in response to more or less stressful stimuli. This is usually considered to be either newly developed hypertension or already established hypertension that is aggravated by episodic paroxysms. Paroxysmal hypertension is usually associated with tachycardia (mostly >100/min), clinical evidence of sympathetic discharge (palpitations, nervousness, tremor, weakness, excessive sweating, pounding headaches, feeling hot, paleness, or redness) probably dependent on the dominant biological activity of the released catecholamine. These episodes take place in hypertensive patients and are usually preventable by α-/β-adrenergic blockade, an approach that is generally less well tolerated in normotensive subjects. The abrupt elevations in BP should be documented by a trained health care professional. Unfortunately, some automatic BP measurement devices occasionally produce false BP peaks following an anxiety reaction, further perpetuating hypertension. Occasionally, claims of elevated BP have also been made by patients who seek to obtain a diagnostic label of hypertension for some secondary gain. Often accompanying the abrupt increases in BP increase is the equally abrupt onset of distressful physical symptoms such as headaches, chest pain, dizziness, palpitations, and sweating.

In terms of a clinical presentation, our data indicate that among our 38 patients who were labeled as having the secondary form (Table 1) *(4)*, the classical triad of pheochromocytoma-associated symptoms is not uncommon, with headaches, palpitations, and sweating in 76, 74, and 42%, respectively. In contrast, other symptoms such as flushing (74%) and panic attacks (47%) were quite frequent in the secondary form, yet these symptoms are quite rare in the setting of classical pheochromocytoma. The clinical presentation of primary unexplained pseudopheochromocytoma patients included flushing, anxiety, nausea, and polyuria, symptoms that do not appear to be manifestations of pheochro-

Table 1
Clinical Presentation Basal (B) and Episodic (E)
in Pheochromocytoma-Suspected Patients With Alternative Outcome

| | *Idiopathic Hypovolemia N = 4* | *Mastocytosis N = 9* | *Incidentaloma N = 9* | *Barorecptor Dysfunction N = 2* | *Pulsatile Medullary Compression N =1* | *Spinal Mechanisms N = 1* | *Cocain Abuse N = 1* | *Reninoma N = 1* |
|---|---|---|---|---|---|---|---|---|
| Mean age, years | 46.5 | 43 | 61 | 40 | 36 | 58 | 31 | 20 |
| High-low range of BP variation | B 107–78<br>E 201–116 | 91–63<br>141–88 | 126–71<br>200–107 | 110–73<br>225–150 | 130–80<br>200–130 | 70–50<br>220–120 | 110–60<br>230–160 | 120–90<br>240–180 |
| Clinical symptoms | | | | | | | | |
| Headache | 10/14 | 4/9 | 9/9 | 2/2 | + | + | + | + |
| Palpitations | 12/14 | 4/9 | 9/9 | 2/2 | + | + | + | |
| Sweating | 6/14 | 5/9 | 3/9 | 1/2 | + | – | – | – |
| Flushing | 8/14 | 9/9 | 5/9 | 2/2 | + | + | + | + |
| Nausea | 1/4 | 1/9 | 1/9 | 1/2 | +/– | – | – | – |
| Polyuria | 1/4 | 1/9 | 1/9 | 1/2 | – | – | – | – |
| Anxiety | 7/14 | 5/9 | 1/9 | 2/2 | – | – | – | – |
| Hyperventilation | | | | | | | | |

Values are mean of blood pressure. (From ref. *4* with permission.)

mocytoma. In fact, these four symptoms not only distinguish this disorder from pheochromocytoma, but also greatly resemble a syndrome described by Page nearly 66 years ago *(7)*, only 7 years after the first description of a pheochromocytoma (Table 2). In contrast to the absence of paleness seen in pheochromocytoma, Page instead observed "a blush over the face, neck and trunk as well as nausea during the paroxysm." Equally interesting was his observation that "an attack is brought on by excitement" and that the syndrome has a clear predominance in women. In fact, many more women than men undergo investigation for the possibility of pheochromocytoma, with the percentage of women ranging from 68% *(8)* and 70% *(4)* to 75% *(6)* in different series.

Among the common features of pseudopheochromocytoma are psychological symptoms such as fear, anxiety, and other symptoms fulfilling the criteria of panic disorder (particularly during the first attacks), which are together observed in up to 40% of patients with episodic hypertension *(9)*. Another important feature distinctive from pheochromocytoma are the circumstances under which episodes occur. In pheochromocytoma, symptoms are usually unprovoked, sometimes occurring even during sleep, while in pseudopheochromocytoma they usually follow some identifiable events. It is important, therefore, in questioning these patients, to search for specific provocative factors that may have precipitated these episodes. Such central nervous stimuli usually remain unreported and, as has been recently recognized *(6)*, may often be related to repressed emotions. Other more easily identifiable proprioceptive chemical, nutritional, or pharmacological stimuli (Fig. 1) in previous studies *(4,8,10)* were those reported by the patient or specifically asked about. Episodes may last from a half hour to several hours and may occur from once or twice a day to once every few months. Between episodes the BP is normal or may be mildly elevated.

## PATHOGENETIC DISTINCTION FROM PHEOCHROMOCYTOMA

BP variability is the undisputed intrinsic feature of pseudopheochromocytoma both in normotensive and hypertensive individuals. In individuals who are not receiving autonomic inhibitors, such BP variability often exceeds standard upward limits. Such increases associated with specific symptoms and signs point to the possibility of a sudden sympathetic discharge. The acute predominantly systolic BP increase and tachycardia in response to mental stress are caused by an increased cardiac output. Although total peripheral resistance is unaffected by stress, Brod *(12)* has shown that regional blood flows are modified in divergent ways. As would be expected in a typical "defense reaction"

Table 2

Clinical Distincition of Episodic Hypertension Caused by Pheochromocytoma and Page's Syndrome *(7)* Pseudopheochromocytomas Caused by Irritation of Diencephalic Autonomic Centers

| *Feature* | *Pheochromocytoma* | *Page's syndrome (pseudopheochromocytoma)* |
|---|---|---|
| Hot red flushes and sweating precipitated by emotion | 0[a] | +++ |
| Nausea, vomiting, epigastric discomfort | ± | ++ |
| Polyuria during and following the paroxysms | 0 | + |
| Sex distribution | Equal | Mainly women |

Common features include headaches, palpitations, sweating, anxiety, and dyspnea.

[a]Almost always pallor and sweating.

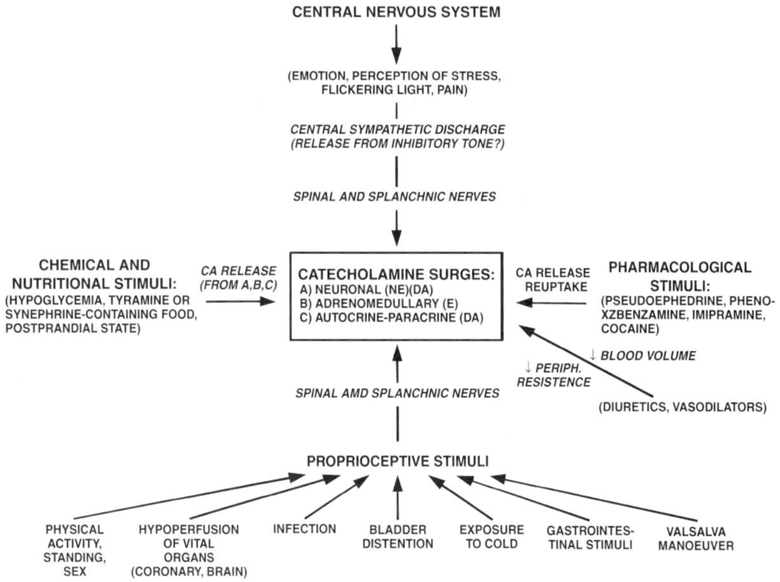


**Fig. 1.** The multiplicity of observed *(4,8,10)* stimuli triggering catecholamine surges in hyperadrenergic *(46)* borderline *(5)* hypertensive patients in whom pheochromocytoma had been excluded. The supposed pathways of their provocative action are indicated in italics. The ratio of NE, E, and dopamine discharge depends on multiple factors including genetics *(20,25)* and time dependence following the stimuli *(23)*.

blood flow to muscle, heart, and brain increases, whereas blood flow to the splanchnic and renal vascular bed decreases.

Detection of this sudden short-lasting sympathetic discharge, attributed experimentally to C 1 neuron stimulation by fibers from the nucleus tractus solitarius *(13)*, is technically difficult. Because catecholamines have very short half-lives (3–5 min), blood sampling has to be done immediately to detect any increase of the respective catecholamine. As a result, blood catecholamine determinations are often negative because blood samples are not obtained during episodes of acute discharge. In contrast, in the setting of pheochromocytoma, catecholamine release may be somewhat more tonic because of diffusion from tumor cells.

The need to draw blood samples as soon as possible during or following the episode of paroxysmal discharge is most important when measuring norepinephrine (NE) and epinephrine (E) and their metabolites, yet these considerations were taken into account somewhat less when dealing with the third catecholamine, dopamine.

Urinary measurements of levels of catecholamines or their metabolites are most useful when detecting hypersecretion, which is more sustained or tonic, as in the case of pheochromocytoma.

Efferent sympathetic nerve traffic measurements *(14)* are much more reliable indicators of sudden increases in neuronal traffic, yet these detection methods are difficult to use because short-lasting neuronal peaks usually disappear before instrumentation can be put into place following an unexpected paroxysm.

Our ability to perform blood sampling almost immediately following a paroxysm in our 63 hospitalized patients *(4)* was a crucial determinant of diagnosis, one generally not possible in the outpatient setting. As a result, we were able to detect catecholamines shortly after their release. This ability was particularly helpful in our efforts to eliminate pheochromocytoma, because, unlike in the setting of pheochromocytoma, levels of NE and E tended to remain normal.

In a typical sympathetic discharge, blood levels of NE and E may not increase, and if they do, they tend to increase less than does dopamine. Thus, when sampling is performed immediately following the attack, it is likely to represent a true reflection of the early catecholamine discharge and is probably relevant to some of the clinical manifestations. The predominance of dopamine probably accounts for the four clinical elements in the original description of Page's syndrome *(7)*. The most frequent and distinctive among these symptoms are flushing, anxiety (occasionally to the point of panic), nausea, and polyuria. Dopamine-receptor mediated central and peripheral mechanisms have been shown to play a role in each of these four symptoms *(4,8,15)*. Moreover, studies published more than 25 years ago suggested that dopamine may play an important role by a mechanism, outlined on Fig. 2, in stress-induced sympathetic discharge, one that may be superior to that of NE and E *(16,17)*. These findings are in accordance with the concept that there is no unitary stress response and that each stressor has its own neurochemical signature *(18)*.

The stress-induced extracellular dopamine increase was demonstrated to be provoked by excitatory amino acids in the brain *(19)* and that genetic factors may also modify this response *(20)*. In the case of children born to mothers who abuse cocaine (a dopamine reuptake inhibitor) during pregnancy, the children's stress responsiveness may be modified *(21)*. Thus, dopamine appears to also have intrauterine effects. As demonstrated in Fig. 3, spontaneous hypertensive paroxysms are associated with a significant increase in levels of free dopamine and dopamine sulfate, whereas levels of both dopamine and its longer lasting metabo-

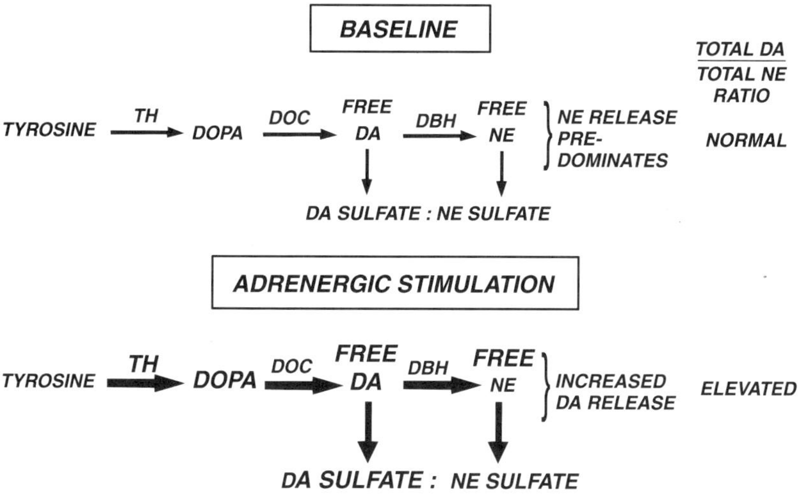


**Fig. 2.** Normal catecholamine synthetic pathways (above) and adrenergic stimulation-induced changes (below) in a temporarily increased peripheral dopamine release. The short-term effect of the adrenergic stimulation is a temporary increase in the rate of tyrosine hydroxylase (TH) as shown by Kopin threefold *(17)* and carried over by dopa decarboxylase (DDC) action. At the same time, the dopamine-β-hydroxylase (DbH) activity only doubles (represented by thick and intermediate arrows respectively). This disproportion may be one of the mechanisms temporarily transforming an adrenergic into a dopaminergic terminal and increasing dopamine relative to NE release in response to stress *(16)*. Dopamine is the most highly, rapidly sulfoconjugated catecholamine; the predominant dopamine release is thus more easily recognizable with separate free and sulfated dopamine determinations *(8,94)*.

lite are normal at baseline. At the same time, both baseline and episodic values of NE and E remained unchanged *(8)*.

Thus, acute peri- and postparoxysmal dopamine increases represent the basic pathogenetic distinction of this condition from pheochromocytoma. In contrast, NE and E release from pheochromocytoma cells occurs more continuously by their diffusion initiated by a still obscure trigger *(1)*. The increase in NE and E release is suppressible by a tyrosine hydroxylase inhibitor α-methyl-para-tyrosine *(22)*, unlike the sudden dopamine that results from a multistep process activated in response to stress *(17)*. In response to sympathetic activation, dopamine synthesis may exceed that of NE. As a result, prior to entering the vesicles of sympathetic nerve terminals to be hydroxylated by the dopamine-β-hydroxylase to norepinephrine, neuronal dopamine may accumulate.

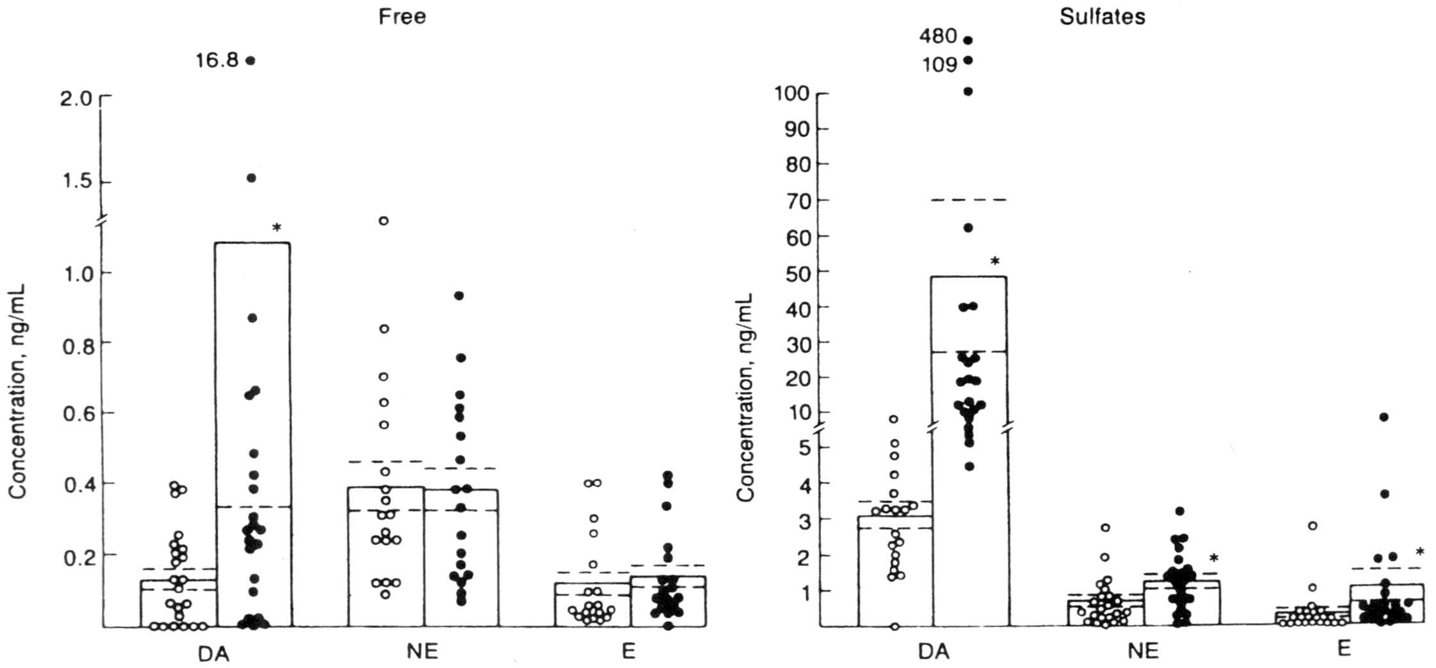


**Fig. 3.** Individual values and mean + SEs of plasma dopamine (DA), norepinephrine (NE), and epinephrine (E) free (left) and sulfoconjugated (right) baseline (open circles) and following hypertensive paroxysms in primary pseudopheochromocytoma patients (closed circles). Asterisks indicate $p < 0.05$ baseline vs immediately following paroxysm. (From ref. *8* with permission. )

Moreover, its release in response to sympathetic nervous activation may temporarily precede the exocytosis by which NE (and dopamine-β-hydroxylase) is extruded into the circulation. This phenomenon probably explains the immediate dopamine predominance in response to acute stress *(23)*, whereas exocytosis-mediated responses follow after the critical 3 to 5 minutes postparoxysmal period. Even the second-phase sympathetic responses are distinct in pseudopheochromocytoma. Whereas the NE increase remains as a cell diffusion process unaccompanied by dopamine-β-hydroxylase increase in pheochromocytoma, autonomic hyper-reflexia, a typical pseudopheochromocytoma condition with exocytosis-mediated NE increase is accompanied by a parallel rise in dopamine-β-hydroxylase *(24)*.

Genetics may modify the dopaminergic response to stress *(20)* at the level of a number of different steps *(25)*. One of these is the dopamine-β-hydroxylase enzyme, which appears to be the main determinant of the dopamine/NE ratio *(26)*. Dopamine discharge tends to decrease BP. Thus, in terms of BP increases, this dopamine discharge should be considered to be a noncausal epiphenomenon, a defensive initial arousal event that may play a role in determining longer term stress coping mechanisms *(23)*.

Thus, the relationship between dopamine and stress may be complex, because stress increases dopamine as part of the catecholamine response to stress *(27)*, while also playing a role in coping with stress *(23)*.

Although dopamine counterbalances some elements of the crucial hypertension-related defense reactions (e.g., splanchnic and renal vasoconstriction) *(12)*, it may also provoke some of the clinical signs and symptoms of Page's syndrome *(7)*, resulting in anxiety *(27)* during the process. A closer insight into the emotional backgrounds of pseudopheochromocytoma patients has shown that hypertension is predominantly related to emotions that are apparent, yet repressed *(6)*. Interestingly, these emotions are closest to those of panic syndrome, a condition in which increased dopaminergic activity has been shown to play a role *(15)*.

All of the above considerations demonstrate the shortcomings of evaluating sympathetic nervous system activation by the conventional NE determinations. The absence of NE increase is apparently still compatible with hypertension caused by increased neuronal traffic, as could have been demonstrated by increased muscle (and, by implication, vascular) sympathetic nerve traffic measurements in stroke-related paroxysmal hypertension *(28)*.

Other pathophysiological interpretations of pseudopheochromocytoma, such as primary hyperepinephrinemia *(29)* possibly related to an E conjugation defect that leaves more E free *(10)* in pseudopheochromocytoma, will require further studies. An adrenergic receptor hyper-reactivity was also considered in pseudopheochromocytoma patients on the basis of circulatory and second messenger plasma cyclic adenosine monophosphate (cAMP) hyper-reactivity to isoproterenol in hyperadrenergic hypertensive patients *(30 )*, their β hyperadrenergic state *(31)*, increased urinary excretion of cAMP *(32)*, and BP hyper-reactivity to the Valsalva maneuver when compared to pheochromocytoma *(33)*. Autonomic hyper-reflexia with hypertensive episodes was also associated with a headache-causing increase in prostaglandin E2 during the episodes *(34)*. The syndrome of baroreflex failure *(35)* exhibits its hypertensive crises that are extremely dependent on emotion and posture, with catecholamine discharge dominated by the previously unrecognized dopamine increase *(36)*.

Proprioceptive stimuli provoking hypertension are multiple (Fig. 1). Best known among such stimuli are reactions to surgery, demonstrated during and after coronary bypass *(37)*, coronary insufficiency *(38)*, or stroke *(28)*.

The reactive sympathetic discharge in response to hypovolemia in its unexplained idiopathic form *(39 )* was also found to have BP peaks associated with increased dopamine levels in the absence of any elevations in NE or E *(40 )*. Hypertensive reactions also occur in response to hypovolemia induced by salt and/or water depletion as a reflex vasoconstrictor response.

A genetic predisposition for dopamine excess without NE and E increase in initial forms of essential hypertension cannot be excluded. These patients were found to have a defect in β-hydroxylation, the final step of conversion of dopamine to NE, caused by a defective control of their dopamine-β-hydroxylase transcription *(41)*. A decreased tissue dopamine-β-hydroxylase activity content was also found in several tissues of prehypertensive spontaneously hypertensive rats *(42)*, probably explaining by decreased dopamine to NE conversion their increased urinary dopamine excretion in early hypertension *(43)*, a phenomenon similar to that observed in young hypertensive patients*(44)*.

## DIFFERENTIAL DIAGNOSIS

The most important consideration is the recognition of a pheochromocytoma because, unrecognized and untreated, it remains, almost without exception, a lethal disease *(1)*. Conversely, the clinical similarity of episodes falsely associated with nonfunctional adrenal adenoma (incidentaloma) occasionally leads to an unnecessary surgical exploration. In our initial series, 3 out of 31 such patients had undergone a negative surgical exploration prior to investigations *(8 )*. Between these two extremes, each with a real potential for a serious diagnostic error, there are a variety of pseudopheochromocytoma presentations, most comparable to the Page's syndrome description *(7)*. "White-coat hypertension" is the mildest form of an emotionally provoked paroxysmal hypertension and is estimated to be present in about 20% of untreated patients investigated for hypertension *(45)*. Within evolutionary stages of essential hypertension, hypertensive paroxysms occur most frequently in the hyperadrenergic form, on the basis of clinical and catecholamine criteria *(46)*. This form is closest to that also labeled as labile or borderline and was found to have a higher dopamine generation from administered dopa and more indirect evidence (by increased urinary 3-methoxy-tyramine excretion) of higher exocytotic dopamine release than control and stable hypertensive subjects *(47)*.

In many normo- or hypertensive subjects, their hyper-reactivity to any stressful stimuli may reflect differences in coping mechanisms and/or panic attacks. In a very recent study, 40% of all patients suspected of pheochromocytoma on clinical grounds fulfilled the criteria of panic disorder *(9)*. Mann commented on some clinical clues *(48)* that may distinguish paroxysms of labile hypertension from those seen in panic disorders. Patients with labile hypertension have a clear relationship between BP peaks and emotional distress (sometimes secondary to fear from symptoms). They know that they are upset and blame the episodes on emotional stress. In contrast, patients with panic disorders insist that the disorder is unrelated to psychological factors, and a subsequent deeper analysis indicates that they suffer from repressed emotions *(6)*. Unresponsiveness to psychotherapy with or without pharmacotherapy speaks against the presence of a panic disorder.

Secondary pseudopheochromocytoma patients associated with well-defined syndromes are rare, but the various possible associated conditions are numerous. Postural hypertension *(49)* alone or a suggested complication of type 2 diabetes *(50)* may be caused by an overreactive sympathetic response, possibly as an early irritative stage of diabetic neuropathy.

Within the central autonomic network, medullary disorders are associated with paroxysmal hypertension and orthostatic abnormalities *(51)*. Severe paroxysmal hypertension was found following sinoaortic baroreceptor denervation, after bilateral carotid bypass surgery *(52)* and glossopharyngeal nerve section *(53)*. Surprisingly, severe short episodic hypertensive bouts in baroreceptor failure followed up to 40 years were not complicated by left ventricular hypertrophy *(36,52,53)*. The heart is thus apparently less affected by short hypertensive peaks than is the brain. Brain tumors and central vascular abnormalities affecting pressure-regulating centers (e.g., redundant carotid artery buckle with pulsatile pounding on the lateral hypothalamus *[54]*) appear to be occasionally surgically correctable *(4)*. The primary clinical problem of these patients is trigeminal neuralgia, hemifacial spasm, or glossopharyngeal neuralgia.

Patients with mastocytosis exhibit episodes very similar to pseudopheochromocytoma. Flushing is accompanied by an initial hypotension caused by histamine and possibly autocrine-paracrine dopamine *(4)* release. It is followed by an "overshoot" reflex vasoconstriction resulting in compensatory hypertension. Mastocytosis patients masquerading as pheochromocytoma were quite common (9 out of 63 patients in our series *[4]*) as previously observed by Manger *(1)*. Their attacks are invariably associated with flushing. They can be diagnosed by skin or organ biopsy or tryptase determination. There are numerous other, mostly anecdotal, descriptions of paroxysmal hypertension imitating pheochromocytoma such as eclampsia, autonomic epilepsy *(55)*, tabes dorsalis crisis, head injury, sciatic neuritis, Friedreich's ataxia, cluster or migraine headaches, Guillain-Barre syndrome, spinal medulla compression *(4)* or spinal cord injury *(56)*, perioperative hypertension during anesthesia and/or surgery, burns, menopause, autonomic hyper-reflexia, hypertensive encephalopathy, renovascular hypertension, carcinoid, thyroid storm, baroreceptor dysfunction in Takayatsu aortitis, nervus vagus or Gasserian ganglion compression, meningitis, acute infectious encephalitis (e.g., tetanus), systemic diseases (periarteritis nodosa, acute intermittent porphyria), mitral valve prolapse, and allergic reaction (pork hypersensitivity) *(1)*.

Some degree of clinical overlap has been rarely seen between pseudopheochromocytoma and the controversial "chronic fatigue syndrome," both claiming extreme fatigue. The latter most widely known syndrome of autonomic dysfunction *(11)* epitomizes the multiplicity of mechanisms by which autonomic dysfunction can link hyper- or hypotensive episodes to many accompanying symptoms.

One form of secondary pseudopheochromocytoma that is sometimes difficult to detect is the factitious episodic hypertension from alimentary or drug causes. This may be the result of the ingestion of monoamine oxidase inhibitors (MAOIs) *(57)* in lead poisoning, as well as the abuse of cocaine *(4)*, lysergic acid diethylamide or amphetamine. Phenylpropanolamine is one of the most recently recognized causes of some cerebrovascular accidents secondary to hypertensive episodes *(58)*. Other toxic effects were recorded, such as those from prolonged skin application of mineralocorticoid ointment, lead poisoning, Parkinson's patients treated with MAOIs (e.g., selegiline) combined with a serotonin receptor inhibitor (fluoxetine) *(59)*, abrupt cessation of centrally acting α-2 agonists (e.g., clonidine) or alcohol withdrawal, ingestion of foods containing certain substances (e.g., tyramine in wine), kanamycin overdoses, or hypertensive episodes induced by gold treatment *(60)*. Also described were severe hypertensive episodes provoked by sympathomimetics administered with criminal *(61)* or self-damaging (Münchhausen syndrome) intent *(1)*. Some diagnostic procedures such as adrenal venography can also provoke a hypertensive attack *(62)*. Hypertensive episodes were also described in rare fatal familial insomnia and sickle cell anemia *(1)*.

The widely used home measurements of BP sometimes result in reporting extremely elevated BP (for technical or other reason) that cannot be reproduced by professionals. A physician expressing doubts to a susceptible subject may not always be appropriate because anticipation and anxiety may have a great impact on BP. We have observed extreme variability of BP even if professionally taken during hospitalization. For example, in a woman with baroreceptor dysfunction *(36)*, the BP taken in the right hand as she was visually fixated on one nurse (toward whom she had negative feelings) was consistently high. In contrast, when BP was taken in the same arm by a nurse whom she liked, it was perfectly normal. Both measurements were controlled by having a third nurse take simultaneous readings on the covered left hand. Similarly, merely mentioning the name of a physician was sufficient to provoke a severe hypertensive peak in this patient. Those effects are easier to detect in a quiet hospital environment, creating a more stable normotensive baseline. We have observed that out of 43 patients with a credible outpatient history of almost daily severe hypertensive paroxysms who were admitted to a quiet investigation unit for an average of 6 days, we could confirm the hypertension only in 31 patients *(8)*. Examining 12 of the 43 patients with unreproducible episodes revealed that they were younger (38 + 2 vs 49 + 2.5 years; $p < 0.05$). They also tended to feel much more secure in the hospital and were confident that the cause of these episodes would be found.

Feelings of insecurity, as well as higher age, may make those episodes more repetitive. Noradrenergic activity increases with age, whereas many dopamine-related functions, including dopamine-influenced cognitive performance *(63)*, dopamine brain circuits involved in coping with stress *(64)*, and peripheral dopaminergic functions *(65)*, all decrease with age. All of these factors may contribute to an increased vulnerability to stressful stimuli with age.

## DIAGNOSTIC APPROACHES

A thorough clinical history and physical examination are the most important elements in providing clues to the etiology of paroxysmal hypertension. Additional biochemical testing should be done under standardized conditions that control dietary and pharmacological interactions. Measurements of catecholamines and their metabolites in urine (metanephrines and vanyllilmandelic acid) should be accompanied by plasma catecholamine baselines ideally (but rarely possible) at the height of the hypertensive paroxysm. Plasma normetanephrines (the longer half-life metabolite of NE and E) became recently more sensitive diagnostic tools for detecting pheochromocytoma *(66)*. Almost no additional expenses are incurred in most available techniques if, in addition to NE and E, dopamine values are also requested. Dopamine elevation, if properly sampled, in combination with NE and E, provides strong diagnostic evidence for various forms of pseudopheochromocytoma and generally excludes pheochromocytoma, because dopamine-producing pheochromocytomas are exceedingly rare. Localizing procedures and functional tests (such as $^{123}$I-metaiodobenzylguanidine [MIBG] scintigraphy and 6-[$^{18}$F]fluorodopamine positron emission tomography [PET] *[66]*) should follow if suspicion persists.

## MANAGEMENT

Pseudopheochromocytoma is usually successfully treatable by antihypertensive agents, and/or psychotherapy with or without pharmacotherapy.

### *Antihypertensive Agents*

The sympathetic hyper-reactivity justifies the first-choice use of adrenergic blockade including β-blockers alone (e.g., atenolol 12.5 and 50 mg daily) or in combination with α-blockers (e.g., terazosine 1–10 mg daily). This treatment has been most effective in preventing hypertensive episodes but occasionally causes excessive fatigue and bradycardia. Combined α- and β-blockers (e.g., labetalol) rarely provide the very variable individual doses and combination ratio of both blockers. Central α-2 agonists (such as clonidine) may occasionally be effective, particularly in short-lasting headaches associated with paroxysmal hypertension *(67)*. Increasing doses, however, causes somnolence and fatigue.

The main limiting factor in using any of these medications is their excessive decrease in BP in patients having normotensive values between the paroxysms. Acute (oral or intravenous) intervention may be necessary during severe prolonged hypertensive episodes. The sublingual use of nifedipine has recently been discouraged because its violent hypotensive effect can result in adverse coronary events.

### *Psychotherapeutic Interventions*

Psychotherapeutic interventions are rarely considered in this syndrome because physical and emotional distress is seen as a consequence rather than a cause of this disorder. This is apparently not always the case, particularly in patients with detectable psychosomatic problems who react with anxiety and panic to many stimuli. A recent description *(68)* of the effects of different treatment modalities in 21 pseudopheochromocytoma patients found a 62% successful outcome mostly in patients without concomitant adrenergic blockade, but sometimes combined with antidepressants. Only milder forms benefit from psychotherapy without pharmacotherapeutic intervention.

### *Psychopharmacologic Agents*

In patients not responding to adrenergic blockade or psychotherapy alone, psychopharmacologic agents proved to be effective even if the patients did not admit an emotional basis for their episodes *(6)*. Tricyclic antidepressants (desipramine 10–25 mg/day) or the selective serotonin reuptake inhibitor paroxetine (10–20 mg/day) may be combined with anxiolytic agents and eliminate attacks. Another combination, sertraline with clonazepam, during the early stages of treatment provided a safe and rapid stabilization of panic attacks *(69)*. Similar combinations were also found to attenuate the dopaminergic neuronal response to stress, thus contributing to their anxiolytic effect *(70)*. Psychiatric consultation is rarely necessary. It may be even counterproductive in some patients who may see it as suggesting that they are being labeled as psychopathic. In fact, we have seen such to increase their anxiety, as well as augment the frequency of their hypertensive paroxysms.

## CONCLUSION AND RESEARCH PERSPECTIVES OF THE DISTINCTIVE PAROXYSMAL AUTONOMIC DISCHARGE

The inclusive diagnosis of pseudopheochromocytoma contains a heterogenous group of conditions that, by their clinical presentation, mimic many features seen in pheochromocytoma. Their common feature is a paroxysmal hypertension associated mostly with flushing and driven by increased sympathetic outflow, often in response to identifiable stimuli. This contrasts with mostly pale pheochromocytoma crises usually unaccounted for by environmental influences and caused by NE and/or E diffusion from tumor cells. The sympathetic outflow is in the short term dominated by the blush-inducing dopamine increase, usually without NE increase. In contrast, pheochromocytoma crises are almost exclusively associated with a vasoconstricting, paleness-inducing NE (and/or E ) increase. This unique catecholamine constellation conveys to elevated dopamine (in the presence of normal NE and E) the position of a novel unifying sympathetic marker of acute stress *(19,23)* for most pseudopheochromocytoma crises, providing that blood is sampled within the short half-life of circulating catecholamines (3–5 minutes) following the paroxysm. Dopamine increase does not cause hypertension, because infusing dopamine to similar levels failed to significantly raise BP *(71)*. Rather, dopamine increase reacts *(23)* and copes with *(72)* the stress and its hemodynamic impact. It also explains by its actions some clinical features that are distinct from pheochromocytoma crises (flushing, anxiety, nausea, and polyuria) *(73)*. This may become a positive diagnostic identification of pseudopheochromocytoma in addition to the negative connotation of the absence of NE and E increase. If unaccounted for by an associated pathology other than essential hypertension, the condition is primary pseudopheochromocytoma; otherwise, the minority of conditions with an identifiable cause are secondary pseudopheochromocytoma.

A new potential link between the dopamine increase-associated hypertension and personality disorders is recently emerging at the dopamine 2 receptor site, known to be a synaptic modulator of NE release *(74)*. A defect (polymorphism in the exon 6 coding region) of the dopamine 2 receptor gene (the potential cause of the selective compensatory dopamine increase in primary pseudopheochromocytoma) was found to be a feature common to cluster (schizoid, paranoid) personality disorders and BP elevation *(75)*. Such an association with a dopamine 2 receptor defect could result in acute-reactive increased circulating dopamine, which could contribute to dopamine's potential role as an "antistress molecule" *(76)*.

Whenever dopamine is released into the synapse, its stimulation of dopamine receptors is known to result in better performance of cognitive tasks *(77)*, an increased feeling of well-being, and stress reduction, considered a "reward response." Dopamine is the master modulator of "locomotion, mood, cognition, motivation, appetite and pleasure" *(78)*. A polygenic genetic defect in the "dopamine reward cascade" (best defined in the dopamine 2 receptor and associated with addictive, impulsive, and compulsive behavior) is proposed to be a drug-seeking "reward deficiency syndrome" and behavior that activates neuronal dopamine release, healing the abnormal craving *(76)*. What makes this model, centered on a dopamine 2 receptor defect (which already had been found to be associated with hypertension *(79)* and plasma dopamine increase relevant to acute hypertension is that dopamine increase is not only related to drug use but also occurs as "an antistress defense mechanism" beyond immediate drug use and in response to acute behavioral stressors. It occurs also independently of drugs in association with acute hemodynamic responses resembling those induced by cocaine *(80)*, both acutely elevating BP *(81)*. Psychosocial stress was found in monkeys to induce such a drug-independent "feel good" dopamine rise, probably initiated by a decreased dopamine 2 receptor availability traced by a potent new tool *(63,82)*, brain PET imaging *(66)*. When these animals were moved from a subordinate to a dominant status, their brain dopamine 2 receptor availability increased by 22%, thus upgrading their "dopamine reward cascade." Those remaining subordinate did not improve their dopamine 2 receptor availability and thus needed to be rewarded by more extraneuronal dopamine increase. They were consequently more likely to be vulnerable to cocaine addiction *(83)*, a means recognized easily even by the monkey, to increase dopamine artificially by blocking its synaptic reuptake.

Excessive dopamine increase-mediated coping with psychological stress *(23,70,72)* in response to a genetic or stress-induced defect of the dopamine 2 receptor function is thus associated with acute hypertension without taking drugs or being drug addicted. Even within this reaction model, cocaine-induced acute BP increases do not result in chronic hypertension *(84)*. This suggests that cocaine-like short-lived hemodynamic patterns of hypertension *(81)* associated with plasma dopamine surges *(80)* do not result in sustained hypertension even if angiotensis-converting enzyme inhibitor therapy had been suggested *(85)*, as a modulation of dopamine increase and cocaine abuse rather than simply as an antihypertensive agent. Thus, the above novel short-term sympathetic discharge model does not explain the cause of sustained hypertension that is today recognized to be predominantly caused by vascular structural changes unrelated to stress *(86)*. Paroxysmal hypertension exemplifies, however, the single most frequent neural aggravation of hypertension.

As to monitoring the overall role of sympathetic activity in essential hypertension, the absence of episodic NE increase in hyperadrenergic patients (where it would be most expected) devaluates NE as a sympathetic marker in hypertensive patients who were found to have as a group, despite their frequent hyperadrenergic presentation, normal age-adjusted plasma NE values *(87)*. Plasma NE did not increase in response to mental stress, one of the reasons for skepticism about its value in assessing neurogenic contribution to human hypertension *(88)*. This was mostly ignored *(89)* because no better marker of nonnoradrenergic neurotransmission (such as the usually undetectable baseline values of dopamine, neuropeptides, and purines) was available, in addition to difficulties of human sympathetic traffic measurements themselves *(14)*. It was tempting to associate hypertension with increased plasma NE because of its hypertensive action. This should not exclude, however, other short-lived markers pointing to an episodic hypertension-causing neural mechanisms even if NE does not increase.

Occurrence of a clear-cut sympathetic discharge, even if short-lived, without NE increase becomes not only a diagnostic marker of the absence of pheochromocytoma, but also a novel footprint of a short-term neuropsychologically induced episodic neural traffic increase, as rarely demonstrated in stroke-related hypertension *(28)*. Novel pathways in which dopamine does not cause hypertension but is a vintage point of stress responsiveness are also emerging. Sudden dopamine rise may indicate mental and nervous environmental stimuli suddenly increasing BP in subjects genetically predisposed at the very crucial dopamine 2 receptor site. This site was linked not only to hypertension *(74,79)*, but also linked hypertension to obesity *(90)*. Mental factors aggravate episodic hypertension in modern societies *(91)*, which is no stranger to its "sister disease," obesity. The dopamine 2 receptor subsensitivity with dopamine hypersecretion has been related not only to appetite but also, to paraphrase "paroxysmal hypertension," to "binge eating" *(92)*.

Short-lived episodic dopamine increase accompanying paroxysmal hypertension appears thus to be an exceptional marker of mental and neural effects on BP in the framework of acute stress responses *(19,20)* and longer term behavioral coping with stress *(20,21)*. The very low or even undetectable baseline free dopamine enhances the detection of episodic dopamine surges. Dopamine sulfate only partly reflects neural free dopamine, and its concentrations are overshadowed by its huge autocrine-paracrine and nutritional sources *(93)*. It can be useful only if those sources are properly controlled *(94,95)*, not an easy task in an acute postattack setting.

Difficulties in identifying markers of peripheral dopamine functions probably explain why, in relation to hypertension, we know today more about its receptors, the site of dopamine action, than about dopamine itself. There are two families of dopamine receptors in the central and peripheral nervous systems, the DA 1-like (DA 1 and DA 5) and DA 2-like (DA 2, DA 3, and DA 5), the latter being predominant in the central nervous system regulation of BP (postsynaptic increasing and predominant presynaptic receptors decreasing BP *(74)*). A candidate gene (chromosome 8 locus) encodes a brain dopamine receptor *(96)* central to the role of dopamine in the pathogenesis of hypertension *(97)*, its paroxysmal form in particular. A subsensitivity of presynaptic dopamine 2 receptors resulting in a disinhibitory BP increase *(74)* in parallel with a compensatory dopamine increase *(64,76,77,80)* was related to compulsive, impulsive, and addictive behaviors *(75,76)*. Expressed in other terms, this corresponds to the high incidence of personality disorders associated with pseudopheochromocytoma as emotional *(6)*, panic *(9,15)*, and anxiety disorders *(3)*. The key to the otherwise difficult plasma dopamine peaks' detectability is the blood sampling immediately following the usually acute event. This offers a window of opportunity to recognize an otherwise elusive behavioral impact on a hypertensive peak and exploit it for diagnosis and therapy.

## REFERENCES


1. Manger WM,Gifford RW. Clinical and experimental pheochromocytoma, 2nd ed. Cambridge, MA: Blackwell Science, 1996.
2. Kuchel O. Pseudopheochromocytoma, Harvard Clinical Conference Hypertension 1985;7:151–158.
3. Fogarty J, Engel C, Russo J, et al. Hypertension and pheochromocytoma testing: the association with anxiety disorders. Arch Fam Med 1994;3:55–59.
4. Kuchel O. Increased plasma dopamine in patients presenting with the pseudopheochromocytoma quandary: retrospective analysis of 10 years' experience. J Hypertens 1998;16:1531–1537.
5. Kaplan NM, Rose BD. Natural history of borderline hypertension, UpToDate @,Inc.,Copyright 2000,text/hyperten/10546
6. Mann SJ. Severe paroxysmal hypertension: an autonomic syndrome and its relationship to repressed emotions. Psychosomatics 1996;37:444–450.
7. Page IH. A syndrome simulating diencephalic stimulation occurring in patients with essential hypertension Am J Med Sci 1935;190;9–14.
8. Kuchel O, Buu NT, Larochelle P, Hamet P, Genest J Jr. Episodic dopamine discharge in paroxysmal hypertension: Page's syndrome revisited. Arch Intern Med 1986;146;1315–1320.
9. White WB, Baker LH. Episodic hypertension secondary to panic disorder. Arch Intern Med 1986;146:1129–1131.
10. Kuchel O, Buu NT, Hamet P,. Larochelle P, Bourque M, Genest J. Unconjugated hyperepinephrinemia: a hallmark of hypertension imitating pheochromocytoma? Hypertension 1981;3:II129–II133.
11. Streeten DHP,, Thomas D, Bell DS. The role of orthostatic hypotension, orthostatic tachycardia and subnormal erythrocyte volume in the pathogenesis of chronic fatigue syndrome. Am J Med Sci 2000;102:294–299.

12. Brod J, Fencl V, Hejl K , Jirka J. Circulatory changes underlying blood pressure elevation during acute emotional stress in normotensive and hypertensive subjects. Clin Sci 1959;18:269–279.
13. Reis DJ, LeDoux JE. Some central neural mechanisms governing resting and behaviorally coupled control of blood pressure. Circulation 1987:76(suppl.I):12–19.
14. Mathias CJ. Role of sympathetic efferent nerves in blood pressure regulation and in hypertension. Hypertension 1991;18(5 Suppl):III 22–30.
15. Pitchot W, Ansseau M, Gonzales Moreno A, Hansessne M, von Frenckell R. Dopaminergic function in panic disorder: comparison with major and minor depression. Biol Psychiatry 1992:32(11);1004–1011.
16. Carlsson A, Snider SR, Almgren O, Lindquist M. The neurogenic short-term control of catecholamine synthesis and release in the sympathoadrenal system, as reflected in the levels of endogenous and beta-hydroxylated catecholamines. In: Usdin E, Snyder S. eds. Frontiers in Catecholamine Research, Pergamon Press, New York:, 1973, p. 551.
17. Kopin IJ. Catecholamines, adrenal hormones and stress. In Krieger D, Hughes JC, eds. Neuroendocrinology. H.P. Publishing , New York, 1980 pp. 159–166.
18. Pacak K, Palkovits M, Yadid G,, Kvetnansky R, Kopin IJ, Goldstein DS. Heterogeneous neurochemical responses to different stressors: a test of Selye's doctrine of nonspecificity. Am J Physiol 1998;275:R1247–R1255.
19. Castro SL, Zigmond HI. Stress-induced increase in extracellular dopamine in striatum: role of glutamatergic action via *N*-methyl-D-aspartate receptors in substantia nigra. Brain Res 2001:901:47–54.
20. Puglisi-Allegra S, Kempf E, Cabib S. Role of genotype in the adaptation of the brain dopamine system to stress. Neurosci Biobehav Rev 1990;14(4):523–528.
21. Elsworth JD, Morrow BA, Roth RH. Prenatal cocaine exposure increases mesoprefrontal dopamine neuron responsivity to mild stress. Synapse 2001; 42(2):80–83.
22. Kuchel O, Buu NT, Edwards DJ. Alternative catecholamine pathways after tyrosine hydroxylase inhibition in malignant pheochromocytoma. J Lab Clin Med 1990; 115:449–453.
23. Puglisi-Allegra S, Imperato A, Angelucci L, Cabib S. Acute stress induces time-dependent responses in dopamine mesolimbic system. Brain Res 1991;19:217–222.
24. Manger WM, Davis SW, Chu DS. Autonomic hyperreflexia and its differentiation from pheochromocytoma Arch Phys Med Rehabil 1979;60(4):159–161.
25. Kuchel O. Genetic determinants of dopaminergic activity: potential role in blood pressure regulation. Hypertens Res 1995;18 suppl.I:S1–S10.
26. Weinshilbaum RM Biochemical genetics of catecholamines in humans. Mayo Clin Proc. 1983;58:319–330.
27. Horger BA, Roth RH. The role of mesoprefrontal dopamine neurons in stress. Crit Rev Neurobiol 1996;10(3–4):395–418.
28. Phillips AM, Jardine DL, Parkin PJ, Hughes T, Ikram H. Brain stem stroke causing baroreflex failure and paroxysmal hypertension. Stroke 2000;31:1997–2001.
29. Streeten DHP. Primary hyperepinephremia in patients without pheochromocytoma. Arch Int Med 1990;150:1528–1533.
30. Messerli FH, Kuchel O, Hamet P, et al. Plasma cyclic adenosine 3':5' monophosphate response to isoproterenol and glucagon in hyperkinetic borderline (labile) hypertension. Circ Res 1976;38 supp.II:42–47.
31. Frohlich ED, Dustan HP, Page IH. Hyperdynamic beta-adrenergic circulatory state. Arch Int Med 1966;117:614–619.

32. Blum I, Weinstein R, Sztern M, Lahav M. Adrenergic receptor hyperactivity: a cause for pseudopheochromocytoma? Med Hypotheses 1987;22(1):89–96.
33. Hamada M, Shigematsu Y, Mukai M, Kazatani Y, Kokobu T, Hiwada K. Blood pressure response to the Valsalva maneuver in pheochromocytoma and pseudopheochromocytoma. Hypertension 1995;25(2):266–271.
34. Naftchi NE, Demeny M, Lowman EW, Tuckman J. Hypertensive crises in quadriplegic patients. Circulation 1978;57(2):336–341.
35. Robertson D, Hollister AS, Biaggioni I, Netterville JL, Mosqueda-Garcia R, Robertson RM. The diagnosis and treatment of baroreflex failure. N.Engl J Med 1993;339:1449–1455.
36. Kuchel O, Cusson JR, Larochelle P, Buu N.T, Genest J. Posture and emotion-induced severe hypertensive paroxysms with baroreceptor dysfunction. J Hypertension 1987;5:277–283.
37. Wallach R , Karp RFB, Reves JG, Oparil S, Smith LR, James TN. Pathogenesis of paroxysmal hypertension developing during and after coronary bypass surgery: a study of hemodynamic and humoral factors. Am J Cardiol 1980;46(4):559–565.
38. Horwitz D, Sjoerdsma A. Some interrelationships between elevation of blood pressure and angina pectoris. Circ Res 1964;13:39–48.
39. Cohn JN. Paroxysmal hypertension and hypovolemia. N Engl J Med 1966;275: 643–646.
40. Kuchel O, Leveille J. Idiopathic hypovolemia: a self-perpetuating autonomic dysfunction? Clin Autonomic Res 1998;8:341–346.
41. Higashimori K, Higaki J, Kamitani A, Zhao Y, Mikami H, Ogihara T. Significant relationship between dopamine beta hydroxylase(dbH) gene polymorphism at the 3'terminal region and the plasma dbH activity in normotensive subjects, but not in hypertensives. Hypertension 1992;18:9(36).
42. Kuchel O, Racz K, Debinski W, Buu NT. A defective beta hydroxylation of dopamine may precede the full development of hypertension in spontaneously hypertensive rats. Can J Cardiol 1989;5:327–331.
43. Racz K, Kuchel O, Buu NT, Tenneson S. Peripheral dopamine synthesis and metabolism in spontaneously hypertensive rats. Circ Res 1986:58;889–897.
44. Saito I. Increased urinary dopamine excretion in young patients with essential hypertension. Clin Exp Hypertension. 1994;16:29–39.
45. Pickering TG, James GD, Boddie C, et al. How common is white coat hypertension? JAMA 1988;259:225–228.
46. Cuche JL, Kuchel O, Barbeau A, Langlois Y, Boucher R, Genest J. Autonomic nervous system and benign essential hypertension in man: usual blood pressure, catecholamines, renin and their interrelationships. Circ Res 1974;35:281–289.
47. Shigetomi S, Buu NT, Kuchel O. Dopaminergic abnormalities in borderline essential hypertensive patients. Hypertension 1991;17:997–1002.
48. Mann SJ. Severe paroxysmal hypertension (pseudopheochromocytoma): understanding the cause and treatment. Arch Intern Med 1999;159:2091–2002.
49. Streeten DHP, Auchincloss JH, Anderson GH et al. Orthostatic hypertension: pathogenetic studies. Hypertension 1985;7:196–203.
50. Yoshinari M, Wakisaka N, et al. Orthostatic hypertension as a complication of type 2 diabetes. Diabetes Care 2001;24:1783–1786.
51. Benarroch EE. The central autonomic network: functional organization, dysfunction and perspectives. Mayo Clin Proc 1993;68:988–1001.
52. Aksamit TR, Floras JS, Victor RG, Aylward PE. Paroxysmal hypertension due to sinoaortic baroreceptor denervation in humans. Hypertension 1987;9:309–314.

53. Ripley RC, Hollifield JW, Nies AS. Sustained hypertension after section of the glossopharyngeal nerve. Am J Med 1977;62:297–302.
54. Janetta PJ, Segal R, Wolfson SK. Neurogenic hypertension: etiology and surgical treatment. Ann Surg 1985;201:391–398.
55. Metz SA, Halter JB, Porte D, Robertson RP. Autonomic epilepsy: clonidine blockade of paroxysmal catecholamine release and flushing. Ann Intern Med 1978; 88:189–193.
56. Chua KS, Kong KH, Tan ES. Paroxysmal hypertension in a C4 spinal cord injury: a case report. Ann Acad Med Singapore 1995;24:470–472.
57. Golwyn DH, Sevlie CP. Monoamine oxidase inhibitor, hypertensive crisis headache and orthostatic hypotension. J Clin Psychopharmacol 1993;13:77–78.
58. Kuchel O. Phenylpropanolamine , stroke and hypertension. Can Med Ass J 2001;164:621.
59. Lefebvre H, Noblet C , Moore N , Wolf LM. Pseudophaeochromocytoma after multiple drug interactions involving the selective mono-amino-oxidase inhibitor selegiline. Clin Endocrinol 1995;42:95–99.
60. Mendlovitz DB, Bravo EL. Gold myokymia syndrome mimicking pheochromocytoma, 75th Endocrine Society annual meeting, 1998:46.
61. Lurvey A, Yussin A, DeQuattro V. Pseudopheochromocytoma after self-administered isoproterenol. J Clin Endocrinol Metab 1973;36766–36769.
62. DeQuattro V , Margolin AH, Stocks LO. Pseudopheochromocytoma. J Clin Endocrinol Metab 1970;30:138–140.
63. Backman L, Farde L. Dopamine and cognitive functioning: brain imaging findings in Huntington's disease and normal aging. Scand J Psychol 2001:42:287–296.
64. Del Arco A, Segovia G, Mora F. Dopamine release during stress in the prefrontal cortex of the rat decreases with age. Neuroreport 2001;12:4019–4022.
65. Fukagawa NK, Bandini LG, Lee MA, Young JB. Effect of age on dopaminergic responses to protein feeding. Am J Physiol 1995;268:F613–F625.
66. Pacak K, Linehan WM, Eisenhofer G, Walther MM, Goldstein DS. Recent advances in genetics, diagnosis, localization, and treatment of pheochromocytoma. Ann Intern Med 2001;134:315–329.
67. Dodick DW. Recurrent short-lasting headache associated with paroxysmal hypertension: a clonidine-responsive syndrome. Cephalalgia 2000;20:509–514.
68. Mann SJ. Paroxysmal hypertension (pseudopheochromocytoma), UpToDate @,hyperten/24720,Copyright 2000.
69. Goddard AW, Brouette T, Almai A, Jetty P, Woods SW, Charney D. Early coadministration of clonazepam with sertraline for panic disorder. Arch Gen Psychiatry 2001;58:681–686.
70. Dazzi L, Serra M, Spiga F, Pisu MG, Jentsch JD, Biggio G. Prevention of the stress-induced increase in frontal cortical dopamine efflux of freely moving rats by long-term treatment with anti-depressant drugs. Eur Neuropsychopharmacol 2001; 11:343–349.
71. Kuchel O, Buu NT. Role of peripheral dopamine in essential hypertension. In Usdin E, et al, eds. Catecholamines: Basic and Peripheral Mechanisms. Allan R. Liss ., New York, 1984, pp. 345–357.
72. Pani L, Porcella A, Gessa GL. The role of stress in the pathophysiology of the dopaminergic system. Mol Psychiatry 2000;5:14–21.
73. Chapman JN., French AT, Poulter NR, Sever PS. Page's syndrome: a case of pseudophaeochromocytoma. J Hum Hypertens 2000;14:149–150.
74. Mannelli M, Ianni L, Lazzeri C, et al. In vivo evidence that endogenous dopamine modulates sympathetic activity in man. Hypertension 1999;34:398–402.

75. Rosmond R, Rankinen T, Chagnon M, et al. Polymorphism in exon 6 of the dopamine D2 receptor gene is associated with elevated blood pressure and personality disorders in man. J Hum Hypertens 2001;15:553–558.
76. Blum K, Braverman ER, Holder JM, et al. Reward deficiency syndrome: a biogenetic model for the diagnosis and treatment of impulsive, addictive and compulsive behaviors. J Psychoactive Drugs 2000;32(Suppl.i–iv):1–112.
77. Fried I, Wilson CL, Morrow JW, et al. Increased dopamine release in the human amygdala during performance of cognitive tasks. Nature Neuroscience 2001; 4:201–206.
78. Pani L, Gessa GL. Evolution of the dopaminergic system and its relationships with the psychopathology of pleasure. Int J Clin Pharmacol Res 1997;17:55–58.
79. Linthorst AC, De Lang H, De Jong W, Versteeg DH. Effect of the dopamine 2 receptor agonist quinpirole on the in vivo release of dopamine in the caudate nucleus of hypertensive rats. Eur J Pharmacology 1991;201:125–133.
80. Faraj BA, Camp VM, Davis DC, Kutner M, Cotsonis GA, Holloway T. Elevated concentrations of dopamine sulfate in plasma of cocaine abusers. Biochem Pharmacol 1993;46:1453–1457.
81. Knuepfer MM, Purcell RM, Gan Q, Le KM. Hemodynamic response patterns to acute behavioral stressors resemble those to cocaine. Am J Physiol 2001;281: R1778–R1786.
82. Volkow ND, Fowler JS, Wang GJ, et al. Decreased dopamine D2 receptor availability is associated with reduced frontal metabolism in cocaine abusers. Synapse 1993;14:169–177.
83. Morgan D, Grant KA, Gage HD, et al. Social dominance in monkeys: dopamine D2 receptors and cocaine self administration. Nat Neurosci 2002;5:169–174.
84. Brecklin CS, Gopaniuk-Folga A, Kravetz T , et al. Prevalence of hypertension in chronic cocaine users. Am J Hypertens 1998;11:1279–1283.
85. Margolin A , Avants SK, Setaro JF, Rinder HM, Grupp L. Cocaine, HIV and their cardiovascular effects: is there a role for ACE-inhibitor therapy? Drug Alcohol Depend 2000;61:35–45.
86. Genest J. Progress in hypertension research 1900–2000. Hypertension 2001; 38:e13–e18.
87. Lake CR, Ziegler MG, Coleman MD, Kopin IJ. Age-adjusted plasma norepinephrine levels are similar in normotensive and hypertensive subjects. N Engl J Med 1977;296;208–209.
88. Folkow B, Di Bona GF, Hjemdahl P, Thoren P, Wallin BG. Measurements of plasma norepinephrine concentrations in human primary hypertension: a word of caution on their applicability for assessing neurogenic contribution. Hypertension 1983;5:399–403.
89. Mancia G, Grassi G, Giannattasio C, Seravalle G. Sympathetic activation in the pathogenesis of hypertension and progression of organ damage. Hypertension 1999;34:724–728.
90. Thomas GN, Tomlinson B, Critchley JA. Modulation of blood pressure and obesity with the dopamine D2 receptor gene TaqI polymorphism. Hypertension 2000; 36:177–182.
91. Charvat J, Dell P, Folkow B. Mental factors and cardiovascular diseases. Cardiologia 1964;44:124–141.
92. Brambilla F, Bellodi L, Arancio C, Ronchi P, Limonta D. Central dopaminergic function in anorexia and bulimia nervosa: a psychoneuroendocrine approach. Psychoneuroendocrinology 2001;26:393–409.

93. Goldstein DS, Swoboda KJ, Miles JM, et al. Sources and physiological significance of plasma dopamine sulfate. J Clin Endocrinol Metab 1999 84:2523–2531.
94. Kuchel O, Buu NT, Racz K, DeLean A, Serri O, Kyncl J. Role of sulfate conjugation of catecholamines in blood pressure regulation. Federation Proc 1986;45: 2254–2259.
95. Yoshizumi M, Kitagawa T, Hori T, et al. Physiological significance of plasma sulfoconjugated dopamine in patients with hypertension: clinical and experimental studies. Life Science 1996;59:323–330.
96. Kren V, Pravenec M, Lu S, et al. Genetic isolation of a region of chromosome 8 that exerts major effects on blood pressure and cardiac mass in the spontaneously hypertensive rat. J Clin Invest 1997;99:577–581.
97. Jose PA, Eisner GM, Felder RA. Role of dopamine in the pathogenesis of hypertension. Clin Exp Pharmacol Physiol, 1999;26:S10–S13.

# V Children and Secondary Hypertension

# 16 Secondary Hypertension in Children and Adolescents

*Empar Lurbe,* MD *and Josep Redon,* MD

***Contents***



## INTRODUCTION

Although not all books on hypertension have a section on children and adolescents, there should be one for a number of reasons. To begin with, the diagnosis of hypertension is different from that for adults. Hypertension in children, as defined by casual blood pressure (BP) values, is not well correlated to any particular form of hypertensive target organ damage. No single cutoff point defines hypertension in a pediatric patient, making identification of childhood hypertension difficult. Physicians have traditionally used population-based percentiles to define pediatric hypertension. Next, pediatric hypertension is associated with a broad spectrum of diseases that changes from childhood through adolescence. Definable causes of hypertension are the rule in the early years of life, whereas essential hypertension is more common in adolescence. Conse-

From: *Secondary Hypertension: Clinical Presentation, Diagnosis, and Treatment*
Edited by: G. A. Mansoor © Humana Press Inc., Totowa, NJ

quently, techniques for the evaluation and diagnosis of hypertension differ, at least in part, from those that are used with adult patients.

## DEFINITION OF HYPERTENSION

Of all that is known about the levels and distribution of casual BP in childhood and adolescents, two facts are well accepted: BP increases during growth and maturation, and adolescence is a fast growth period during which body mass and BP change rapidly *(1)*. These are the main reasons for why reference BP values over the last few decades have been referred to as ones specific to sex, age, and/or height in children and adolescents up to 18 years of age.

In 1977, the first age-related norms for BP in children were developed by the Task Force for Blood Pressure in Children, a group sponsored by the National Heart, Lung and Blood Institute and by the National Institutes of Health *(2)*. In 1987, a revision of the standards evaluated data from more than 70,000 white, African American, and Mexican American children *(3)*. Age-specific percentile curves of BP measurements for boys and girls ranging in age from birth to 18 years were created. These revised standards also defined the proper techniques for measuring BP in infants, children, and adolescents. All measurements used in constructing the Task Force's tables were made with a standard mercury sphygmomanometer placed on the child's right arm, using a cuff size that covered 80 to 100% of the circumference of the arm. In 1996, the Task Force became aware of the importance of considering age and height together when defining reference values *(4)*. This approach avoids misclassifying children at the extremes of normal growth because tall children will not be misclassified as hypertensive, and very short children with high normal BP or even hypertension will not be missed. In children of the same age, the upper limit of systolic BP (SBP) normality for the third percentile of height is 8 mmHg to 9 mmHg lower than those values for the 90th percentile. At the same time, the Task Force redefined diastolic BP (DBP) as the fifth rather than the fourth Korotkoff sound for children in all age groups. No changes to the standards for SBP and Ddiastolic BP for infants younger than 1 year were reported in the 1996 update.

Using the Task Force data table *(4)*, normal BP is defined as SBP and DBP less than the 90th percentile for age, sex, and height. Borderline, or high normal, BP is defined as an average systolic and/or average DBP between the 90th and 95th percentiles for age, sex, and height. Hypertension consequently is defined as an average systolic and/or average DBP greater than or equal to the 95th percentile for age, sex, and height, measured on at least three separate occasions.

The objective of detecting high BP in children is to identify those who are at risk for the morbidity and mortality associated with hypertension. The detection of childhood hypertension is important because hypertension is frequently related to an identifiable and potentially treatable disease process *(5)*, whereas untreated severe hypertension in childhood is associated with significant morbidity and mortality *(6)*. Elevated BP in childhood may be identified during the evaluation of a child with chronic illness or in subpopulations of children at increased risk for hypertension.

Although it is generally agreed that early essential hypertension poses little immediate risk to most children, it carries the potential for future end-organ damage. In children, accurate identification of hypertension at the earliest possible age would, therefore, give health care providers the opportunity to initiate preventive measures, thereby reducing the chance of developing end-organ damage and its attendant morbidity and mortality. Consequently, repeated BP measurements over time would become a routine part of pediatric well-child care.

Two studies by the Task Force in 1987 *(3)* and by Sinaiko in 1989 *(7)* found the prevalence of hypertension in a general population to be only 1%. In a study published in 2001 *(8)*, using the new Task Force standards *(4)*, the combined prevalence of systolic and diastolic hypertension in junior high school-aged children did not substantially change from the previously reported level. Statistically, 5% of children had a BP measurement higher than the 95th percentile during a single office visit. BP, however, tended to normalize on subsequent measurements because of the accommodation of the child to the measurement procedure and to the statistical phenomenon of regression toward the mean *(9)*. Consequently, the prevalence of hypertension decreased to 1% after only one repeated examination. (The diagnostic algorithm of hypertension is found in Fig. 1.)

Persistent, high office BP combined with a normal BP outside of the medical setting, referred to as "white-coat" or "office" hypertension, has not been studied in this segment of the population, and ambulatory BP monitoring could shed light on the topic *(10)*. Despite the diagnosis of hypertension being one of the main indications for the use of ambulatory BP monitoring in children, this type of monitoring does not appear to add substantially to the accurate identification of children with severe hypertension, although it may help in the proper assessment of mild hypertension *(11)*.

Aside from the ability of ambulatory BP monitoring to obtain more accurate and reproducible BP values *(12)*, two more advantages of this method are the assessment of BP during sleep and the estimation of circadian variability *(13)*. There is a physiological nocturnal fall of BP during sleep subsequent to the reduction in sympathetic driving. Patients

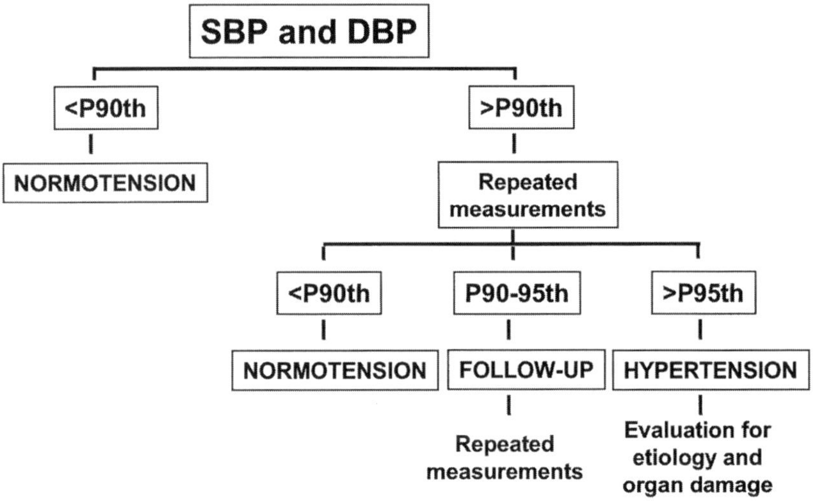


**Fig. 1.** Algorithm diagnostic of hypertension in children and adolescents.

with renal disease and/or volume expansion are consistently found to have abnormalities in circadian BP variability with a high prevalence of the so-called nondipping pattern—namely, a blunted decline in the physiological nocturnal fall. Although this may be related to the severity of the hypertension, as in subjects with renovascular hypertension, in the majority of the other causes of hypertension, the severity of BP values does not preclude the abnormal circadian variability pattern observed *(14,15)*.

## ETIOLOGY OF CHILDHOOD HYPERTENSION

Usually, sustained hypertension in children and adolescents is classified as secondary with a specific cause that may be correctable or as essential and without an identifiable cause *(3)*. The most common causes of hypertension can change during childhood. Essential hypertension is rarely seen in infants and young children, but its prevalence increases significantly in adolescence *(16)*. A good general rule to follow is that the likelihood of identifying a secondary cause of hypertension is inversely related to the age of the child and directly related to the degree of BP elevation. Consequently, the evaluation of children with hypertension, especially young children and those with severe hypertension, should be comprehensive and aimed at identifying known causes of the disease.

Definable causes of hypertension are associated with a broad spectrum of diseases. The distribution of causes clearly varies with age.

Renal parenchymal disorders predominate, accounting for a majority of secondary causes *(17)*. Renal parenchymal disorders with renovascular disease, and coarctation of the aorta, account for 70 *(18)* to 90% *(19)* of all cases. These figures vary depending not only on the age group, but also on referral center and referral bias. Additionally, hypertension is often related to prescribed drugs with hypertensive potential. Other infrequent causes of sustained hypertension, tumors and central nervous and endocrine disorders, must be considered once more common causes of secondary hypertension have been eliminated. An emerging cause of secondary hypertension is a single gene mutation that produces large changes in BP *(20)*.

Hypertension in term or preterm neonates may be seen in up to 2% of all infants in modern neonatal intensive care units. Although the definition of hypertension in this age group has not been completely standardized, useful data to this regard have been published recently *(21)* and may be used to facilitate the identification of such infants. As in older children, the causes of hypertension in neonates are numerous, with the two largest categories being renovascular and parenchymal diseases. More specifically, thromboembolism associated with an umbilical artery catheter affecting either the aorta and/or the renal arteries probably accounts for the majority of cases of hypertension seen in the typical neonatal intensive care unit *(22)*. A careful history and physical examination will usually identify the cause in most cases, without the need for extensive laboratory or radiological testing.

In very young children (<6 years), hypertension is most often the result of such renal parenchymal disease as glomerulonephritis, renal scarring, polycystic kidney diseases, and renal dysplasia. Renal artery stenosis and cardiovascular disorders such as coarctation of the aorta—less frequent causes of hypertension in this age group—are usually detected within the first decade of life. Late in the first decade and throughout the second, essential hypertension is the most common cause of sustained hypertension, particularly in those children with mild asymptomatic disease *(23)*.

## CLUES TO THE INITIAL APPROACH TO DIAGNOSIS OF SECONDARY HYPERTENSION

When confronted with an infant, child, or adolescent with hypertension, the first question to be asked concerns the chronicity of the problem. Clearly, the most helpful information to have when one is attempting to establish the hypertension chronicity is past BP readings. Unfortunately, these are by no means always available because routine BP

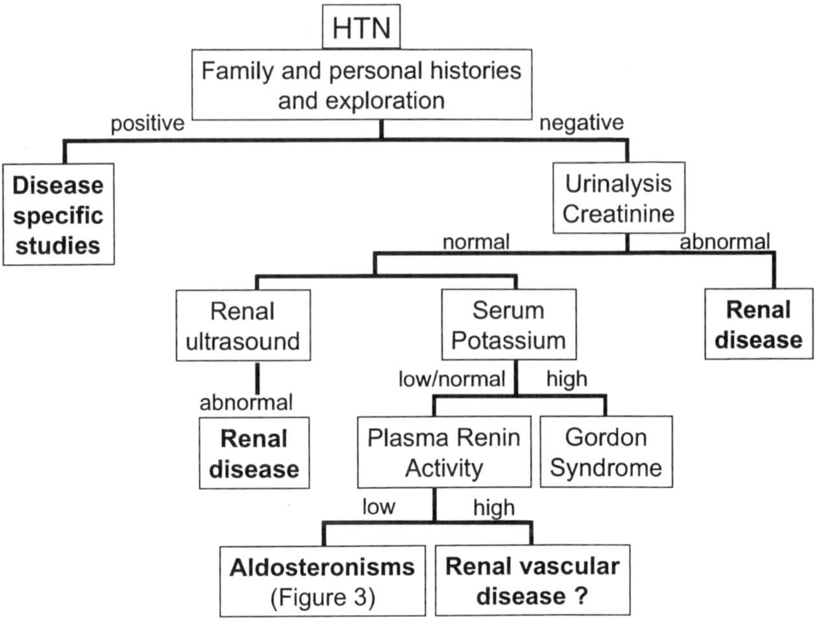


**Fig. 2.** Initial approach to the diagnosis of secondary causes of hypertension (HTN).

measurements in children over 3 years of age are not yet uniformly obtained. In the absence of previous readings, one needs to look for the evidence of target organ damage: left ventricular hypertrophy or an increase in urinary albumin excretion.

Faced with a child with chronic hypertension of unknown etiology, a diagnostic evaluation is based to some degree on the level of BP, age, sex, clinical findings, and family history. A significant number of children with secondary forms of hypertension, often renal ones, can be identified using a selective approach (Fig. 2). Afterward, a careful selection of the necessary test often shortens the diagnostic process.

## *History and Physical Examination*

The initial approach to uncovering the cause of hypertension requires a careful clinical evaluation that, in many cases, can provide clues not only to a specific diagnosis, but also to the most successful diagnostic procedure.

When recording family histories, it is not sufficient simply to ask which relatives have high BP; one needs to know the age at which hypertension was detected in these relatives. A strong familial history of hypertension or hemorrhagic stroke in young members points to the presence of specific hereditary conditions (polycystic kidney disease *[24]*, familial pheochromocytoma in multiple endocrine adenomatosis [multiple endocrine neoplasia {MEN type II}, von Hippel-Lindau disease, or neurofibromatosis *[25]*) or to one of the familial syndromes (glucocorticoid [GC]-remediable aldosteronism, apparent mineralocorticoid excess [AME], Liddle's syndrome, Gordon's syndrome, and mineralocorticoid receptor [MR] hypersensitivity syndrome) and in some of the latter, there is a specific responsible mutation with a Mendelian trait *(26)*.

Episodic hypertension indicates the presence of pulsatil secretion of hypertensive substances, mainly chatecolamines, and indicates the necessity to look for a secreting tumor of neural or adrenal origin. Exposure to pressor substances (recreational drugs, licorice, vasoconstrictor drops, and GCs) or neurologic processes (dysautonomia, increased intracranial pressure, and Guillaine-Barré syndrome) need to be excluded. Other situations such as orthopedic traction, stress, cyclic vomiting, and burns also temporarily increase BP.

Among the additional information that needs to be recorded are birth weight, development data, recent changes in weight, headaches, visual problems, weakness, muscle cramps, sexual development, abdominal pain, dysuria, nicturia, and enuresis. Any of these may raise the suspicion of disease.

Things to seek out during physical examination include the presence of edema, cutaneous stigmata of facomatosis, Cushing morphological changes, virilization or thyroid enlargement, heart murmurs, bruits over the great vessels or in the epigastrium, absent or delayed femoral pulses, and unilateral or bilateral abdominal masses. All are indicative of specific diseases.

### *Laboratory Studies*

In the absence of any telltale data obtained from the family and personal histories or from the physical exploration, there are several analytical procedures that should then be performed. Assessments of glomerular filtration rate (GFR) by serum creatinine, of potassium levels, and of urinalysis are mandatory. High creatinine levels or abnormal urinalysis herald a renal cause of hypertension, although the renal impact of an otherwise secondary hypertension needs to be considered.

Hypokalemia, in the absence of diuretic intake, is a low sensitive but high specific marker for diseases that lead to urine potassium wasting. An algorithm diagnostic (Fig. 2) is used if hypokalemia is present. Hyperkalemia, in conjunction with metabolic acidosis, may suggest

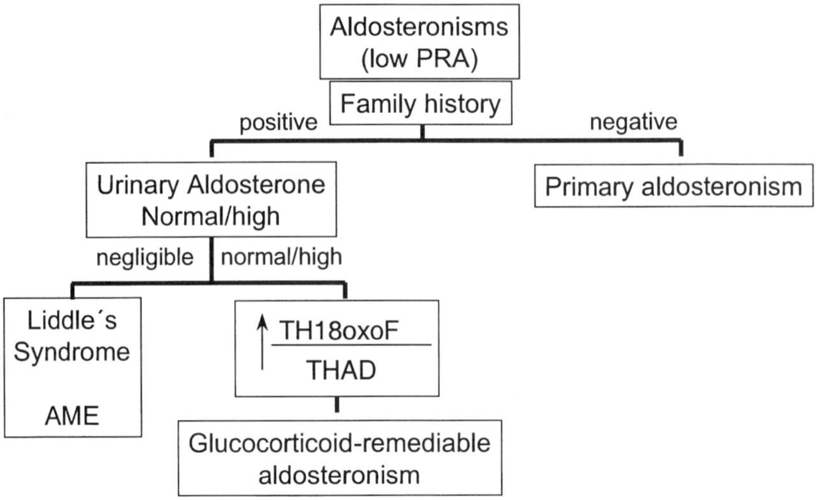


**Fig. 3.** Algorithm diagnostic of low renin aldosteronisms.

chronic renal disease, which is confirmed by elevated serum creatinine. A more uncommon situation is hyperkalemia with a normal GFR, suggesting the presence of Gordon's syndrome.

The next step includes an assessment of the renin-aldosterone axis. High peripheral plasma renin activity (PRA) may suggest a renal, parenchymal, or renovascular cause for hypertension, and other studies then need to be performed to delineate these lesions. Low PRA points to several of the monogenic syndromes that lead to volume expansion. The algorithm diagnostic is shown in Fig. 3.

### *Image-Diagnostic Techniques*

If the previously mentioned procedures do not point to a specific cause of the hypertension, and considering that renal causes are the most frequent, a renal ultrasound is appropriate early in the evaluation. Masses, cortical scars, or asymmetry of the kidneys prompt the performance of more specific procedures to better delineate the nature of the disease.

## MOST FREQUENT CAUSES OF SECONDARY HYPERTENSION

Based on these data, the evaluation of the hypertensive child in current clinical practice generally focuses on the search for an underlying renal parenchymal lesion, vascular anomaly, catecholamine-secreting tumor, or surreptitious pharmacological agents. In addition to these eti-

Table 1
Most Common Causes of Hypertension by Age Group

| | |
|---|---|
| < 1 Month | > 6 years to 10 years |
| • Renal arterial thrombosis | • Renal parenchymal disease |
| • Coarctation of the aorta | • Renovascular disease |
| • Congenital renal disease | • Essential hypertension |
| > 1 Month to < 6 years | > 10 years to 18 years |
| • Renal parenchymal disease | • Essential hypertension |
| • Coarctation of the aorta | • Renal parenchymal disease |
| • Renovascular disease | • Renovascular disease |

ologies, clinicians should be aware of several hypertensive syndromes that are inherited as single Mendelian traits. The most common causes of hypertension, according to age group, are shown in Table 1. A description of causes, included below, focuses on the most important evidence, diagnostic keys, and specific treatment, if any exists.

## *Renal Parenchymal Diseases*

In secondary hypertension, renal parenchymal nonvascular disorders predominate, accounting for a majority of secondary causes, 73–78% *(27,28)*. Despite this, there is a relative lack of investigation and a paucity of long-term follow-up studies when compared to the abundance of literature on the less common renovascular disorders. Morbidity and mortality associated with renal parenchymal hypertension are determined by the nature of the underlying disease and the severity of the hypertension. Because hypertension is a common problem in many different types of renal parenchymal disease, BP should be taken carefully at each evaluation.

Hypertension is frequent in both glomerular *(29)* and autosomal recessive polycystic kidney disease *(30)*. Glomerular and small artery diseases, which are generally thought to be associated with a high prevalence of hypertension, are acute postinfectious glomerulonephritis, glomerulonephritis secondary to systemic vasculitis, poliarteritis involving the kidney, crescenting glomerulonephritis, focal and segmental glomerulosclerosis, cortical necrosis, and hemolitic-uremic syndrome. In contrast, a moderate prevalence of hypertension is found in such glomerular diseases as membranous glomerulopathy, membranoproliferative glomerulonephritis, and Alport's syndrome *(31)*. When hypertension does occur in these diseases, it often does not develop until serious impairment of kidney function is present.

Hypertension occurs less often in obstructive uropathy and in chronic pyelonephritis with reflux. In children with primary interstitial disease, it is an unusual occurrence until end-stage renal disease develops.

### *Reflux Nephropathy*

Vesicoureteric reflux is the term used to describe the retrograde flow of urine from the bladder back into the ureter(s) and kidney(s). The more severe the reflux, the higher the grade. With severe reflux, the ureters become dilated and tortuous, the pelvocalycine outline becomes distorted by pelvic dilatation, and often renal scarring coexists. This constellation of features is known as reflux nephropathy. Between 30 and 60% of patients with vesicoureteral reflux will develop reflux nephropathy, with 5 to 10% progressing to end-stage renal failure. Thus, reflux nephropathy is responsible for end-stage renal disease in 16% of children who have end-stage renal failure *(32)*.

Hypertension affects at least 10% of patients with reflux nephropathy and can accelerate the deterioration of renal function, making early diagnosis and treatment very important. Hypertension caused by reflux nephropathy is unlikely to develop during early childhood, and normotensive adolescents with this disease require long-term followup. Factors associated with the early onset of hypertension are likely to be operative during the first two decades of life. It is, therefore, reasonable to initiate studies during childhood with longitudinal evaluation into adulthood.

There has been some investigation into the mechanisms responsible for hypertension associated with reflux nephropathy and renal scarring. A study by Goonasekera et al. *(33)* reports the results of a 15-year prospective study of hypertension in patients diagnosed at age 2–15 with reflux nephropathy. This study showed a rise of SBP as the years passed, together with concurrent rise in plasma renin activity, suggesting an association among BP, renin in reflux nephropathy, and age, especially during the teenage years. Although this supports a renin-BP link in the etiology of hypertension in reflux nephropathy, individual PRA values do not reliably predict the later onset of hypertension. Although the renin-angiotensin system (RAS) plays an important role, its action in the contribution of other physiological systems of prominent distribution and action within the kidney remains difficult to establish.

In patients with reflux nephropathy, proteinuria may be the most important indicator of a poor prognosis, and microalbuminuria the most sensitive and specific test for early identification of renal injury *(34)*. In patients with reflux nephropathy, the microalbuminuria is thought to be mediated by changes in glomerular hemodynamics secondary to hyperfiltration and compensatory hypertrophy in both the affected and the contralateral kidney. This adaptive mechanism results in an elevated glomerular permeability. This is postulated to be the major determinant for the progression of glomerular injury. Microalbuminuria appears to be correlated with the severity of reflux nephropathy but not with its duration. Treatment with angiotensin-converting enzyme inhibitors (ACEIs) can reduce microalbuminuria and slow the progression of renal damage in patients with reflux nephropathy.

### *End-Stage Renal Disease and Kidney Transplantation*

Hypertension is highly prevalent in pediatric patients undergoing chronic dialysis *(35)* or after renal transplantation *(36,37)*. A better understanding of the factors that cause this hypertension in children with end-stage renal disease is important for several reasons. To begin with, hypertension in these patients is often particularly difficult to control, not only because of the multifactorial nature of the BP elevation, but also because of the necessity of maintaining a high level of control in order to achieve the maximum preservation of renal function. Furthermore, because the risk of BP-induced renal disease is continuous, the BP target needs to be much lower than that normally used in other diseases. In proteinuric subjects, further BP decreases are needed *(38)*.

There are several mechanisms by which hypertension is produced in parenchymatous chronic renal failure *(39)*. Undoubtedly, it has been demonstrated that salt plays a fundamental role by causing an increase in interchangeable sodium and vascular wall sodium as well as an expansion in the extracellular volume, principally an intravascular one. This results in a volume-dependent hypertension that leads to an increase in cardiac output. The RAS is generally stimulated in moderate renal insufficiency, especially when it is considered that the intravascular volume is decreased. In response to renal insufficiency, plasma noradrenaline increases as an expression of the increased activity of the sympathetic nervous system and is associated with increases in the peripheral resistance and in cardiac output.

Studies in subjects with chronic renal disease, and in those undergoing renal replacement therapy, show that BP control is suboptimal in many patients even though office BP is below the recommended threshold *(40)*. The maintenance of high BP values throughout the day may contribute to further damaging of renal structures. The use of ambulatory BP monitoring may help to uncover patients with an insufficient level of control. Several studies have focused on ambulatory BP abnormalities in patients with end-stage renal disease. Patients with a decrease in the GFR, whatever the etiology, frequently show an increase in nocturnal vs diurnal BP levels when compared with BP profiles from normotensives or hypertensives with a normal GFR *(41)*. Blunted nocturnal BP fall is frequent during both hemodialysis *(42)* and continuous ambulatory peritoneal dialysis *(43)*. No significant differences between therapy modalities are observed in terms of waking or sleeping BP values and frequency of nondipping pattern.

The prevalence of hypertension in children who have undergone renal transplantation has been reported to be high *(36,37)*. Its causes are many and are often related to the time elapsed since transplantation. In the early posttransplant period, hypertension is almost universal and secondary to a variety of factors including volume overload, poor perfusion of the transplanted kidney, release of pressor substances by the transplanted kidney, acute rejection, high-dosage corticosteroid therapy, stenosis of the renal artery, and hypercalcemia.

It has been reported by Sorof et al that antihypertensive medications are required in 79% of pediatric patients at 1 month posttransplant and in 58% at 5 years posttransplant *(44)*. The results from this study, using the largest data set available for pediatric renal transplantation, raise important questions regarding the risk factors for posttransplant hypertension in children and the effect of this hypertension on long-term graft survival.

Multiple factors that may contribute to sustained hypertension include preexisting hypertension caused by the primary renal disease, treatment with corticosteroids and cyclosporine, renal artery stenosis in the transplanted kidney, chronic rejection, and decreased functional renal mass. Patients with prior glomerulonephritis are at a greater risk of developing hypertension. The most common etiologies of posttransplant hypertension are rejection and medication-related hypertension from steroids and cyclosporine A. The contribution of cyclosporine A to elevations in BP after renal transplantation has been reported in several studies *(45)*. It is possible that the increase in the routine use of cyclosporine A over time may contribute to the greater need for antihypertensive medications. Patients with stable renal functions have less hypertension than those with chronic rejection. As a corollary, recipients of cadaveric kidneys, who generally experience more rejection than do recipients of kidneys from living, related donors, also experience more severe hypertension.

### *Renovascular*

Hypertension in children and adolescents caused by lesion of the renal vessels accounts for 8–10% of patients referred for evaluation and treatment of hypertension *(46)*. Potentially curable, it is second only to coarctation of the aorta as a cause of surgically remediable hypertension in children. Primary diseases of the renal arteries, such as fibromuscular dysplasia that often involves the large renal arteries, account for about 70% of the cases, whereas secondary diseases are characterized by small-vessel and intrarenal vascular disease. Renovascular hypertension has also been reported in children with renal artery aneurysms, arteriovenous fistula, traumatic rupture, thrombosis (following umbilical artery catheterization, embolism from a ductus arteriosus, or Takayasu's disease) or external compression by tumors.

Fibromuscular dysplasia is a collection of vascular diseases that affects the intima, media, and adventitia. The cause of this disorder is unknown, although genetic predisposition, hormonal factors, and disorders of the vasa vasorum may be risk factors. It has been associated with neurofibromatosis (intimal only), Marfan's syndrome, Klippel-Trenaunay syndrome, and idiopathic hypercalcemia. Fibromuscular dysplasia tends to affect girls, frequently involves the distal two-thirds of the renal artery and its branches, and is characterized by a beaded, aneurysmal appearance on angiography. Intimal and periarterial dysplasia are commonly associated with progressive dissection and thrombosis, whereas medial dysplasia is rarely associated with these complications. Nonetheless, medial dysplasia progresses to stenosis in 30% of all cases.

A large percentage of children with renovascular disease have bilateral lesions, and the association of renovascular disease with abdominal coarctation (middle aortic syndrome) was present in 20% of the cases studied in the Hospital for Sick Children, London *(46)*. Other accompanying abnormalities involving the mesenteric, splenic, and hepatic vessels are present in patients with neurofibromatosis *(47)*.

Renovascular disease produces hypertension through a renin-dependent mechanism. A decrease in renal perfusion pressure activates the RAS, leading to the release of renin and to the production of angiotensin II (Ang II), which has direct effects on sodium excretion, sympathetic nerve activity, intrarenal prostaglandin concentrations, and nitric oxide production *(48)*. When hypertension is sustained, PRA can decrease. This phenomenon is often referred to as reverse tachyphylaxis.

The clinical presentation of renovascular disease in children is quite variable, from asymptomatic children to those presenting severe forms of hypertension with neurologic, cardiac, or renal end-organ damage. No symptoms are pathognomonic of renovascular disease, but associated findings on examination might suggest it. The presence of stigmata of syndromes in which renal artery diseases are frequent, such as abdominal bruit or aortic or intracerebral vascular disease, are suggestive of renal artery lesions.

Diagnosis of renovascular disease includes logical explorations, those that produce morphological images and those that assess differential renal blood flow. One should look for high PRA, small unilateral kidney, or asymmetry of the kidneys with ultrasonography. Recording the magnitude of the hypotensive response to administered captopril to identify children with renal artery stenosis among subjects with hypereninemic hypertension has been abandoned because it is associated with uncertainties and the results can be influenced by many other conditions *(49)*.

Methods displaying morphological representation of the vascular renal tree have improved during the last few years. The classic study is invasive angiography, still the gold standard for the diagnosis and as part of a therapeutic maneuver through angioplasty. In an attempt to avoid the performance of an invasive test, other methods have been developed. Duplex ultrasonography shows the renal arteries and measures flow velocity and resistance index as a means of assessing the severity of stenosis. It is an inexpensive and widely available technique but requires a high level of expertise. Computed tomography (CT) angiography shows the renal arteries and perirenal aorta and provides excellent images even when an intravascular prosthesis is present. Because this method requires a large volume of potentially nephrotoxic contrast medium, use is limited in young children. Magnetic resonance angiography has the same potential as CT angiography with absence of toxicity, but it is expensive and is not effective in the presence of intravascular stents *(50)*.

Assessing differential blood flow between the kidneys has the potential to uncover renal blood flow abnormalities produced by renal artery diseases *(50)*. Nuclear images with technetium-99 diethylenetriamine pentaacetic acid ($^{99m}$Tc-DTPA) estimates fractional flow to each kidney, although the results may be influenced by the presence of an obstructive uropathy. Captopril renography explores the captopril-mediated fall in filtration pressure, which amplifies differences in renal perfusion, and normal results exclude renovascular hypertension. In the presence of renal insufficiency, however, this method has limitations. Finally, selective renal vein renin sampling provides valuable information as to the kidney from which the renin release is occurring.

The choice of the appropriate pathway to diagnosing renal artery disease and/or its functional impact depends on the availability of the method chosen and the experience of the staff. Treatment of renovascular disease requires both a careful evaluation of the lesion or lesions responsible for the BP rise and a capacity to correct the rise. At the same time, or in the case that BP correction proves insufficient, a symptomatic treatment with antihypertensive drugs needs to be started. A combination of several drugs may well be necessary to successfully control BP *(51)*.

A possible association between renal and extrarenal arterial diseases has been described, and vascular cerebral imaging techniques are required at times, mainly for children in whom there have been cerebral symptoms or signs suggestive of features of cerebral arterial involvement.

## *Coarctation of the Aorta*

Today, coarctation of the aorta is largely a disorder of infants and young children. In diagnosing hypertension, palpation of the pulses should be attempted in both upper and lower extremities. If BP values are not obtained in all four extremities or if the BP values for the upper ones differ greatly from those of the lower ones, coarctation is the probable cause. The anatomical lesions in the aorta that produce secondary hypertension differ from those that produce symptoms early in life, such as infantile coarctation complex, and those that manifest themselves during childhood and adolescence, such as isolated structure lesions. Most isolated structure lesions are located in the thoracic aorta, although in a few cases the location may be in the abdominal aorta *(52)*. In both cases, the mechanisms for hypertension involve hyperactivity of the RAS, an increase in the activity of renal sympathetic nerves, and baroreceptor resetting *(53)*.

Among infants presenting coarctation, associated cardiovascular anomalies are the rule, with isolated coarctation occurring in only 10% of these cases. The most commonly associated abnormalities include proximal aortic arch hypoplasia in three fourths of the patients and patent ductus arteriosus in two-thirds of them. Clinically, the complex most frequently manifests itself as congestive heart failure. In contrast, coarctation present in an older child may be a clinically isolated lesion. In about two thirds of these patients, however, a bicuspid aortic valve is present, the proximal aorta is generally normal or dilated, and the ductus is normally closed *(53)*. Unlike infants presenting a symptomatic coarctation complex, older children and adolescents are generally asymptomatic, although increased fatigability and leg weakness may be present. Congestive heart failure is rare.

The diagnosis in all older children and a majority of infants with coarctation is based on clinical criteria. These include differential SBP with upper extremity BP greater than that in the lower extremities; delayed, decreased, or absent femoral pulses relative to normal or full upper extremity pulses; and the presence of collaterals detected by thoracic murmurs or palpation. Chest X rays revealing an hourglass configuration of the thoracic aorta or rib notching, indicating collaterals through bronchial arteries, confirm the clinical suspicion. Echocardiography and magnetic resonance imaging (MRI) confirm the diagnosis. Cardiac catheterization is reserved for patients with complex diseases.

Surgical correction or balloon angioplasty are the necessary treatments, but postoperative problems are not unusual. Approximately two-thirds of patients who undergo corrective surgery manifest paradoxical hypertension. In early paradoxical hypertension, within the first 12–24 hours, a moderate to severe hypertensive state presents itself. Late paradoxical hypertension, 2–5 days postoperative, is generally preceded by early paradoxical hypertension. Approximately one out of five patients with late paradoxical hypertension will suffer persistent postoperative hypertension *(54)*.

## *Tumors*

Tumors account for about 3–4% of the causes of secondary hypertension. The majority of them—neuroblastoma, pheochromocytoma, ganglioneuroblastoma, and ganglioneuroma—are tumors of neuroectodermal origin. Neuroblastoma arises from neural crest elements, including the thoracolumbar sympathetic ganglia and adrenal medulla. These are intra-abdominal in three-fourths of the cases and one-half are of the adrenal gland, whereas only one-fourth are intrathoracic. Hypertension is not a common finding, but oversecretion of cathecolamines is not always the mechanism causing the hypertension. Distortion and/or stretching of the renal arteries can be implicated in cases with normal catecholamine levels *(55)*.

Pheochromocytoma that arises from the cromaffin cells of the sympathoadrenal system is a much less common cause of hypertension in children than is neuroblastoma. Localized in any place where sympathetic tissue has occurred during development, from the neck to the urinary bladder, the most common location is the adrenal glands. Bilateral tumors are frequent in familial pheochromocytoma with MEN II, von Hippel-Lindau disease, or neurofibromatosis *(25)*. Catecholamine secretion is responsible for the hypertension, although these tumors can produce substances such as cortisol and others. Hypertension, either episodic or continuous, is accompanied by prominent sweating and other, less frequent symptoms such as vision change, polyuria, polidipsia, and weight loss. Episodic hypertension may be precipitated by drugs, angiography, or other physical stimuli.

The diagnostic steps for pheochromocytoma are the measurement of catecholamines or their metabolites, and tumor localization *(56)*. Because catecholamines are normally produced by sympathetic nerves and by the adrenal medulla, high catecholamine levels in urine are not specific to pheochromocytoma and may accompany other conditions or disease states. Moreover, secretion is episodical, and between episodes, levels of catecholamines may be normal. Measurements of plasma levels of normetanephrine and metanephrine have higher sensitivities than do other biochemical tests for diagnosis. Additionally, they have a high level of specificity: 80 and 94% for sporadic and familial pheochromocytoma, respectively.

A tumor is localized through radiological imaging and/or radionuclide studies with substances that are specifically trapped by the tumor. CT scans have good sensitivity when the tumor is in the adrenal gland, but the level of sensitivity decreases if the tumor is located extra-adrenally, which is frequent. Magnetic nuclear resonance (MNR) offers advantages over the CT scan in the extra-adrenal case. Body scanning with metaiodobenzylguanidine (MIBG) or positron emission tomography (PET) with $^{18}$F-fluorodeoxyglucose, $^{11}$C-hydroxyephedrine, or 6[$^{18}$F]fluordopamine offer specific images of the tumor *(25)*.

A recommended procedure pathway for the localization of a highly suspected pheochromocytoma is to start with a CT scan or an MNR, and if a mass is uncovered, a MIBG scan should be performed to confirm the diagnosis. A negative scan does not exclude a tumor, and a more specific PET may be necessary *(57)*.

On diagnosis, and only after a complete blockade of the sympathetic system is achieved with the adrenoceptor blocker phenoxybenzamine, with or without β-blockers, surgery must be performed.

Other tumors that produce hypertension are Wilms' tumor, renal tumors secreting renin, or adrenal tumors secreting aldosterone. Additionally, tumors invading renal structures or the central nervous system may lead to hypertension in some cases.

### *Drugs*

Because many drugs have the potential to raise BP, a careful evaluation of prescribed, over-the-counter, and recreational substances should be conducted during the initial approach to the diagnosis. Drug- or alcohol-related hypertension in children and adolescents increases in frequency as age increases, and much of this increase is caused by exposure to recreational drugs or alcohol. There are several mechanisms involved in most drug-induced hypertension. They interfere with the vasodilatory systems or enhance the vasoconstrictor systems. Some drugs, however, have a direct impact on arterial pressure.

Among the prescribed drugs, anti-inflammatories, immunosuppresors, GCs, cylosporine, and tacrolimus are the most common contributors to BP increases *(58)*. When these kinds of treatment are required, the prevalence of hypertension associated with primary diseases or after transplantation increases. Immunosuppresive therapy, with the addition of prednisone, may contribute to the nondipper pattern frequently observed in transplanted patients *(59)*. Taler et al. *(60)*, in a comparison of 24-hour ambulatory BP profiles before and after orthotopic liver transplantation in patients with end-stage liver disease, find that the normal circadian variability observed before transplantation is reversed afterward, regardless of whether cyclosporine or tacrolimus is used.

In teenage girls, oral contraceptives may induce BP elevation, in those prone to developing it, by increasing angiotensinogen synthesis and salt retention. Oral contraceptive-induced hypertension remains for as long as 2 to 3 months after use ceases.

The most common over-the-counter drugs that produce hypertension are the sympathomimetic agents, ephedrine, pseudoephedrine, phenylpropanolamine, and oxymatazoline, used as decongestants. They activate the α-receptors, inducing vasoconstriction. Licorice, used in cough drops or as candy, increases the bioavailability of cortisone by blocking the activity of the 11-β-hydroxysteroid dehydrogenase, leading to the activation of the MRs, thereby increasing sodium reabsorption.

Use of one specific common recreational drug, cocaine, can lead to a higher risk of triggering hypertensive crises *(61)*. Cocaine acts by inhibiting the reuptake of norepinephrine (NE) and dopamine at presynaptic sites, leading to an excess of neurotransmitters and an activation of the sympathetic nervous system, vasoconstriction, and tachycardia.

### *Monogenic Disorders*

Much of the current research effort is focused on identifying the specific genes responsible for hypertension. While these disorders are thought to be rare, their precise prevalence is unknown and their specific diagnosis requires a high level of clinical suspicion.

A major focus of such studies has been the epithelial sodium channel (ENaC), which can be activated by mutations in the channel subunits or MR, and changes in the response to or production of mineralocorticoids *(26)*. As a result, there are now clearly defined Mendelian syndromes in which ENaC activity is dysregulated, with the subsequent development of systemic hypertension with suppressed PRA that can be attributed to a primary renal mechanism. There are several monogenic forms of human hypertension, including Liddle's syndrome *(62,63)*, glucocorticoid-remediable aldosteronism *(64)*, mineralocorticoid apparent excess *(65)*, Gordon's syndrome *(66,67)*, and MR hypersensitivity syndrome *(68)*.

Liddle's syndrome can result from the mutations of ENaC subunits. The predictable clinical phenotype is low-renin hypertension and suppressed aldosterone secretion. In 1963 Liddle et al. described a familial syndrome of severe hypertension, hypokalemia, and metabolic alkalosis that mimicked hyperaldosteronism.

The lack of down-regulation of the ENaC in the face of persistent volume expansion underlies the pathophysiology of this syndrome. Clinical studies revealed that affected patients had exceptionally low rates of aldosterone secretion, hyporeninemia, no response to spironolactone, and positive responses to both triamterene and salt restriction *(63)*. The characterization of the extended original pedigree of Liddle's syndrome reported that overnight urinary potassium excretion was high and urinary aldosterone excretion was low in affected individuals. Very low urinary aldosterone/potassium ratios are consistent with the physiological effect of ENaC activity at the potassium secretory site in the collecting tubule *(62)*.

Mutations were originally described in Liddle's syndrome as truncations or frame-shifts in the β or γ subunits of the ENaC *(69)*. These mutations delete a critical proline-rich region of the cytosolic tail, which interacts with a cytoskeletal protein called Nedd4 *(70)*. Several pedigrees with mutations of critical amino acids in this proline-rich region have been described.

Glucocorticoid-remediable aldosteronism (GRA) is an important autosomal dominant cause of human genetic hypertension. Initially described in 1966 by Sutherland et al. as a new hypokalemic hypertensive syndrome in a father and son *(71)*, today the genetic basis of this disorder is completely understood. GRA is relatively common, and the syndrome represents the first example of a successful application of new genetics to define an inherited human hypertensive syndrome. It is the result of a chimeric gene product that places 18-hydroxylase (aldosterone synthase) under the control of an adrenocorticotropic hormone (ACTH) promoter that regulates its level and cellular site of expression. As a consequence, ACTH-regulated 18-hydroxylase activity is aberrantly expressed in the zona fasciculata and acts on the cortisol that is normally produced in this zone to form 18-hydroxycortisol and 18-oxocortisol *(72)*. The continuing stimulation of adrenal steroidogenesis by ACTH and the suppressive effects of modest doses of dexamethasone are usual features of the syndrome.

The laboratory features of GRA include the following: serum potassium levels are normal to low, typically PRA levels are profoundly suppressed, and serum aldosterone and urine aldosterone levels are usually elevated. These levels, however, may be within the normal range and therefore are not reliable markers for GRA. Recent studies have used genetic testing prospectively to identify affected family members and to further define the clinical phenotype. Genetic testing is 100% sensitive and specific to diagnose GRA and requires only a single blood collection for leukocyte DNA assessment *(72)*.

Clinically, GRA is characterized by moderate to severe hypertension whose onset is early in life. Recent data indicate that GRA may emerge as an important etiology of pediatric hypertension. The hypertension varies in severity, is typically refractory to standard antihypertensive agents, and tends to become milder with age *(73)*. Children and adolescents with unexplained or refractory hypertension, with strong hypertensive family histories, and particularly those with suppressed PRA levels need to be screened for GRA. This syndrome is associated with high morbidity and mortality from early onset of hemorrhagic stroke and ruptured intracranial aneurysms *(74)*. Accordingly, screening of asymptomatic GRA patients with magnetic resonance angiography is recommended, beginning at puberty, and every 5 years thereafter.

Historically, GRA patients have been treated with steroids, dexamethasone or prednisone, in an attempt to suppress ACTH and thereby suppress ectopic aldosterone production. Of great importance is the potential toxicity associated with excessive doses of suppressive glucocorticoids. In children, if the clinician chooses to use glucocorticoid suppression, it is recommended that linear growth be measured by a stadiometer every 6 months to prevent overtreatment and growth retardation.

Given the abnormal aldosterone regulation in GRA, aldosterone antagonists such as spironolactone provide a useful therapeutic alternative to steroids. In addition, agents such as amiloride, which blocks sodium transport in the distal nephron, may also be an effective treatment option *(75)*. Accordingly, unless the clinician has experience with the use of GCs in children, treatment with spironolactone or antagonists of the aldosterone-regulated ENaC is probably safer and equally effective.

AME syndrome is a rare autosomal recessive disorder that was described in 1977 in a child with low-renin hypertension *(76)*, and fewer than 50 cases have been reported since *(77)*. This disorder is caused by 11 β-hydroxysteroid dehydrogenase isozyme deficiency, which converts cortisol to cortisone in many organs, including the kidney. Excessive cortisol in the kidney binds to the mineralocorticoid receptors, causing features of mineralocorticoid excess with low to undetectable aldosterone levels. Such patients excrete excessive amounts of cortisol metabolites, tetrahydrocortisol (THF) and allotetrahydrocortisol (aTHF), and there is a reduced excretion of the cortisone metabolite tetrahydrocortisone (THE) in the urine. An elevated THF plus aTHF/THE ratio in the urine is diagnostic of AME syndrome.

The clinical features of AME syndrome include hypertension, hypokalemia, alkalosis, polyuria, polidypsia, and a failure to thrive. These children can present the syndrome at different ages, and some have died in early infancy and childhood. In the fetus, the enzyme deficiency may lead to intrauterine growth retardation and low birth weight. Dexamethasone administration suppresses cortisol secretion and thereby corrects hypertension and hypokalemia. An alternative treatment is the administration of mineralocorticoid inhibitors such as spironolactone and such sodium channel inhibitors as amiloride and triamterene.

Recently, a novel form of human hypertension, MR hypersensitivity syndrome, caused by a gain-of-function mutation in the MR S810L has been described *(68)*. This mutation results in constitutive mineral receptor activity and alters receptor specificity, with progesterone and other steroids lacking 21-hydroxyl groups, normally MR antagonists, becoming potent agonists. Structural and biochemical studies indicate that the mutation results in the gain of the van der Waals interaction between helix 5 and helix 3 that substitutes for interaction of the steroid 21-hydroxyl group with helix 3 in the wild-type receptor.

Geller et al reported that a serine to leucine mutation at position 810 in the hormone binding domain of the mineralocorticoid receptor changes the affinity of the MR for a number of steroids; progesterone in particular has an exceptionally high affinity for the receptor *(68)*. This mutation was found in a boy with unexplained severe hypertension. Clinically, it is characterized in early onset hypertension that is markedly exacerbated in pregnancy. Women harboring the L810 mutation will develop sever pregnancy-induced hypertension owing to the 100-fold increase in circulating progesterone levels that accompanies pregnancy.

All pregnancies among mutation carriers have indeed been complicated by development of severe hypertension, requiring early termination of pregnancy. These findings define a new Mendelian form of hypertension and represent the first demonstration of a Mendelian form of pregnancy-induced hypertension, showing that this common disorder can result from the abnormal action of a normal hormone of pregnancy.

Although the distal nephron is recognized as the major site of action of mineralocorticoids, expression of mineral receptors in the hippocampus, heart, and endothelium suggests extrarenal activity. The early development of congestive heart failure in some patients affected by this syndrome suggest that MR might contribute to additional clinical effects due to its expression in other tissues.

Familial hyperkalaemic hypertension, also called pseudohypoaldosteronism type II or Gordon's syndrome, is characterized by an autosomal dominant transmission of metabolic abnormalities: hyperkalemia, hyperchloremia, and metabolic acidosis despite normal glomerular filtration and normal levels of aldosterone. Although sometimes absent, high BP can be an important feature, especially in young affected individuals. The pathophysiology of pseudohypoaldosteronism type II remains obscure, and several possible causal mechanisms have been proposed: defect of the renal potassium secretory mechanisms, cellular defect in transmembrane potassium transport, increased rate of chloride reabsorption by the tubule, altered sensitivity to mineralocorticoids, and excessive renal sodium reabsorption proximal to the site of aldosterone action *(67)*.

Recently, the cause has been linked to mutations in the genes codifying for serine-threonine kinases (WNK1 and WNK4) *(66)*. Both are located in the distal convoluted tubule and collecting duct. But while WNK1 is cytoplasmic, WNK4 is located at intercellular junctions, within the tight junction complex. An increase in the expression of these kinases may explain the abnormalities observed in Gordon's syndrome.

## CONCLUSIONS

Secondary hypertension is associated with a broad spectrum of diseases that changes from childhood through adolescence. A rational approach based on a careful clinical evaluation and simple algorithms permits a direct evaluation, saving time and avoiding unnecessary tests. Since the definable causes of hypertension vary according to age, the approach to diagnosis may differ slightly at different ages. Diagnosis of the most frequent causes—parenchymal renal diseases, which account for more than 70% of the hypertension causes—is easy, but many of the other remaining causes are difficult to diagnose. Furthermore, the recognition of genetic causes of hypertension and the use of simple tests permit a fast diagnosis where a wide workup would have failed to lead to an adequate diagnosis. Surgical correction or intravascular manipulation may result in a permanent improvement of BP levels in some patients with coarctation of the aorta, renal artery stenosis, or tumors. Specifically targeted treatments may ameliorate other secondary causes of hypertension. The majority of patients, however, need permanent antihypertensive treatment in order to control BP levels and avoid further end-organ damage.

# REFERENCES


1. Lauer RM, Anderson AR, Beaglehole R, Burns TL. Factors related to tracking of blood pressure in children. Hypertension 1984;6:307–314.
2. National Heart, Lung and Blood Institute. Report of the task force on blood pressure control in children. Pediatrics 1977;59:797–820.
3. National Heart, Lung and Blood Institute. Report of the second task force on blood pressure control in children: 1987. Pediatrics 1987;79:1–25.
4. Update on the 1987 task force report on high blood pressure in children and adolescents: a working group report from the national high blood pressure education program. Pediatrics 1996;98:649–658.
5. Rocella EJ, Bowler AE, Horan M. Epidemiologic considerations in defining hypertension. Med Clin North Am 1987;71:785–801.
6. Burke GL, Cresanta JL, Shear CL, Miner MH, Berenson GS. Cardiovascular risk factors and their modification in children. Cardiol Clin 1986;4:33–46.
7. Sinaiko AR, Gomez-Marin O, Prineas RJ. Prevalence of "significant" hypertension in junior high school-aged children: the children and adolescent blood pressure program. J Pediatr 1989;114:664–669.
8. Adrogue H, Sinaiko A. Prevalence of hypertension in junior high school-aged children: effect of new recommendations in the 1996 update task force report. Am J Hypertens 2001;14:412–414.
9. Gardner LS, Heady JA. Some effects of within-person variability in epidemiological studies. J Chronic Dis 1973;26:781–795.
10. Sorof JM, Portman RJ. White-coat hypertension in children with elevated casual blood pressure. J Pediatr 2000;137:493–497.
11. Sorof JM, Poffenbarger T, Franco K, Portman RJ. Evaluation of white-coat hypertension in children: importance of the definitions of normal ambulatory blood pressure and the severity of casual hypertension. Am J Hypertens 2001;14:855–860.
12. Lurbe E, Redon J, Liao Y, Tacons J, Cooper R, Alvarez V. Ambulatory blood pressure monitoring in normotensive children. J Hypertens 1994;12:1417–1423.
13. Lurbe E, Thijs L, Redón J, Alvarez V, Tacons J, Staessen J. Diurnal blood pressure curve in children and adolescents. J Hypertens 1996;14:41–46.
14. Middeke M, Schrader J. Nocturnal blood pressure in normotensive subjects and those with white-coat, primary and secondary hypertension. BMJ 1994;308: 630–632.
15. Imai Y, Abe K, Munakata M, et al. Does ambulatory blood pressure monitoring improve the diagnosis of secondary hypertension? J Hypertens 1990;8(suppl): S71–S75.
16. Vogt BA. Hypertension in children and adolescents: definition, pathophysiology, risk factors and long-term sequelae. Curr Therap Res 2001;62:283–297.
17. Goonasekera CDA, Dillon MJ. Measurement and interpretation of blood pressure. Arch Dis Child 2000;82:261–265.
18. Arar MY, Hogg RJ, Arant BS, Seikaly MG. Etiology of sustained hypertension in children in the Southwestern United States. Pediatr Nephrol 1994;8:186–189.
19. Lieberman E. Hypertension in childhood and adolescence. In: Kaplan N, ed. Clinical Hypertension, 5th ed. Baltimore: Williams and Wilkins, 1990, pp. 407–433.
20. Yiu V, Dluhy RP, Lifton RP, Guay-Woodford LM. Low-peripheral plasma renin activity as a critical marker in pediatric hypertension. Pediatr Nephrol 1997;11: 343–346.
21. Zubrow AB, Hulman S, Kushner H, Falkner B. Determinants of blood pressure in infants admitted to neonatal intensive care units: a prospective multicenter study. J Perinatol 1995;15:470–479.

22. Flynn J. Neonatal hypertension: diagnosis and management. Pediatr Nephrol 2000;14:332–341.
23. Kay JD, Sinaiko AR, Daniels SR. Pediatric hypertension. Am Heart J 2001;142: 422–432.
24. Torra R, Badenas C, Darnell D, et al. Linkage, clinical features and prognosis of ADPKD types 1 and 2. J Am Soc Nephrol 1996:7:2142–51.
25. Pacack K, Linehan M, Eisenhofer G, Walther MM, Goldstein DS. Recent advances in genetics, diagnosis, localization, and treatment of pheochromocytoma. Ann Intern Med 2001;134:315–329.
26. Warnock, DG. Genetic forms of human hypertension. Curr Opin Nephrol Hypertens 2001;10:493–499.
27. Loggie, JMH. Systemic hypertension in children and adolescents. Pediatr Clin North Am 1971;18:1273–1310.
28. Londe S. Causes of hypertension in the young. Pediatr Clin North Am 1978;25: 55–65.
29. Galla JH, Luke RG. Hypertension in renal parenchymal disease. In: Brenner BM, ed. The Kidney: Diagnosis and Treatment, 5th ed. Philadelphia: Saunders, 1996, pp. 2126–2147.
30. Kaplan BS, Fay J, Shah V, Dillon MJ, Barrat TM. Autosomal recessive polycystic kidney diseases. Pediatr Nephrol 1989;3:43–49.
31. Brod J, Bahlmann J, Cachovan M, Pretschner P. Development of hypertension in renal disease. Clin Sci 1983;64:141–152.
32. Arant Jr. Vesicoureteric reflux and renal injury. Am J Kidney Dis 1991;17:491–511.
33. Goonasekera CDA, Shah V, Wade AM, Barrat TM, Dillon MJ. 15-year follow-up of renin and blood pressure in reflux nephropathy. Lancet 1996;347:640–643.
34. Lama G, Salsano ME, Pedulla M, Grassia C, Ruocco G. Angiotensin converting enzyme inhibitors and reflux nephropathy: 2-year follow-up. Pediatr Nephrol 1997;11:714–718.
35. Mailloux LU, Haley WE. Hypertension in the ESRD patient: pathophysiology, therapy, outcomes and future directions. Am J Kidney Dis 1998;32:705–719.
36. Broyer M, Guest G, Gagnadoux MF, Beurton D. Hypertension following renal transplantation in children. Pediatr Nephrol 1987;1:16–21.
37. Baluarte HJ, Gruskin AB, Ingelfinger JR, Stablein D, Tejani A. Analysis of hypertension in children post renal transplantation: a report of the North American Pediatric Renal Transplant Cooperative Study (NAPRTCS). Pediatr Nephrol 1994;8:570–573.
38. Petterson JC, Adler S, Bukart JM, et al for the Modification of Diet in Renal Disease Study. Blood pressure control, proteinuria, and the progression of renal disease: the modification of diet in renal disease study. Ann Intern Med 1995;123:754–762.
39. Cottone S, Panepinto N, Vadala A, et al. Sympathetic overactivity and 24 hour blood pressure pattern in hypertensives with chronic renal failure. Ren Fail 1995;17: 751–758.
40. Covic A, Goldsmith DJ. Ambulatory blood pressure monitoring in nephrology: focus on BP variability. J Nephrol 1999;12:220–229.
41. Timio M, Venanzi S, Lolli S, et al. "Non dipper" hypertensive patients and progressive renal insufficiency: a 3 year longitudinal study. Clin Nephrol 1995;43: 382–387.
42. Goldsmith DJ, Covic AC, Venning MC, Ackrill P. Ambulatory blood pressure monitoring in renal dialysis and transplant patients. Am J Kidney Dis 1997;29: 593–600.

43. Luik AJ, Struijk DG, Gladziwa U, et al. Diurnal blood pressure variations in haemodialysis and CAPD patients. Nephrol Dial Transplant 1994;9:1616–1621.
44. Sorof JM, Sullivan EK, Tejani A, Portman RJ. Antihypertensive medication and renal allograft failure: a report of the North American Pediatric Renal Transplant Cooperative Study. J Am Soc Nephrol 1999;10:1324–1330.
45. Van der Dorpel MA, Van der Meiracker AH, Lameris TW, et al. Cyclosporin A impairs the nocturnal blood pressure fall in renal transplant recipients. Hypertension 1996;28:304–307.
46. Deal JE, Snell ME, Barrat TM, Dillon MJ. Renovascular disease in childhood. J Pediatr 1992;25:55–65.
47. Ingelfinger JR. Renovascular disease in children. Kidney Int 1993;43:493–505.
48. Martinez-Maldonado M. Pathophysiology of renovascular hypertension. Hypertension 1991;17:707–719.
49. Dillon MJ. Renovascular hypertension. J Hum Hypertens 1994;8:367–369.
50. Safian RD, Textor SC. Renal artery stenosis. N Engl J Med 2001;344:431–442.
51. McTaggart SJ, Gellati S, Walker RG, Powell HR; Jones CL. Evaluation and long-term outcome of pediatric renovascular hypertension. Pediatr Nephrol 2000;14: 1022–1029.
52. Marcus B, Hohn AR. Coarctation of the aorta. In: Loggie JMH, ed. Pediatric and Adolescent Hypertension. Boston: Blackwell Scientific Publications, 1992, pp. 288–300.
53. Parker FB Jr, Farrell B, Streeten DHP, Blackman MS, Sondheimer HM, Anderson GH Jr. Hypertensive mechanisms in coarctation of the aorta: further studies of the renin-angiotensin system. J Thorac Cardiovasc Surg 1980;80:568–573.
54. Sealy WC. Paradoxical hypertension after repair of coarctation of the aorta: a review of its causes. Ann Thorac Surg 1990;50:323–329.
55. Hayes FA, Smith EI. Neuroblastoma. In: Pizzo PA, Poplack DG, eds. Principles and Practice of Pediatric Oncology. Philadelphia: JB Lippincott, 1989, pp. 607–622.
56. Eisenhofer G, Lenders JW, Linehan WM, Walter MM, Goldstein DS, Keiser HR. Plasma normetanephrine and metanephrine for detecting pheochromocytoma in von Hippel-Lindau disease and multiple endocrine neoplasia type 2. N Engl J Med 1999;340:1872–1879.
57. Young WF Jr. Pheochromocytoma: 1926–1993. Trends Endocrinol Metab 1993;4:122–133.
58. Chesney RW, Freidman AL. Miscellaneous cases of hypertension in children. In: Loggie JMH, ed. Pediatric and Adolescent Hypertension. Boston: Blackwell Scientific Publications, 1992, pp. 314–322.
59. Schwertfeger E, Keller E, Grotz W, Schollmeyer P, Rump LC. Pharmacokinetic profile of cyclosporine A after conversion to Sandimmun Optoral. influence on ambulatory blood pressure in renal transplant patients. Clin Nephrol 1996;45: 349–351.
60. Taler SJ, Textor SC, Canzanello VJ, Wilson DJ, Wiesner RH, Krom RA. Loss of nocturnal blood pressure fall after liver transplantation during immunosuppressive therapy. Am J Hypertens 1995;8:598–605.
61. Lange RA, Hillis LD. Cardiovascular complication of cocaine use. N Engl J Med 2001;345:351–358.
62. Botero-Velez M, Curtis JJ, Warnock DG. Brief report: Liddle's syndrome revisited: a disorder of sodium reabsorption in the distal tubule. N Engl J Med 1994;330:178–181.
63. Baker EH, Dong YB, Sagnella GA, et al. Association of hypertension with T594M mutation in beta subunit of epithelial sodium channels in black people resident in London. Lancet 1998;351:1388–1392.

64. Dluhy RG, Lifton RP. Glucocorticoid-remediable aldosteronism. J Clin Endocrinol Metab 1999;84:4341–4344.
65. Lifton RP. Molecular genetics of human blood pressure variation. Science 1996;272:676–680.
66. Wilson FH, Disse-Nicodeme S, Choate KA, et al. Human hypertension caused by mutations in WNK kinases. Science 2001;293:1107–1112.
67. Disse-Nicodeme S, Desitter I, Fiquet-Kempf B, et al. Genetic heterogeneity of familial hyperkalaemic hypertension. J Hypertens 2001;19:1957–1964.
68. Geller DS, Farhi A, Pinkerton N, et al. Activating mineralocorticoid receptor mutation in hypertension exacerbated by pregnancy. Science 2000;289:119–123.
69. Meneton P, Oh Ys, Warnock DG. Genetic renal tubular disorders of renal ion channels and transporters. Semin Nephrol 2001;21:81–93.
70. Abriel H, Loffing J, Rebhun JF, et al. Defective regulation of the epithelial Na+ channel by Nedd4 in Liddle's syndrome. J Clin Invest 1999;103:667–673.
71. Sutherland DJ, Ruse JL, Laidlaw JC. Hypertension, increased aldosterone secretion and low plasma renin activity relieved by dexamethasone. Can Med Assoc J 1966;95:1109–1119.
72. Dluhy RG, Anderson B, Harlin B, Ingelfinger J, Lifton R. Glucocorticoid-remediable aldosteronism is associated with severe hypertension in early childhood. J Pediatr 2001;138:715–720.
73. Lurbe E, Chavez FJ, Torró I, Armengod ME, Alvarez V, Redón J. Hiperaldosteronismo remediable con glucocorticoides: diagnóstico genético. Med Clin 1999;113:579–582 (in Spanish).
74. Litchfield WR, Anderson BF, Weiss RJ, Lifton RP, Dluhy RG. Intracranial aneurysm and hemorrhagic stroke in glucocorticoid remediable aldosteronism. Hypertension 1998;31:445–450.
75. Lifton RP. Genetic determinants of human hypertension. Proc Natl Acad Sci USA 1995;92:8545–8551.
76. Ulick S, Ramirez LC, New M. An abnormality in reductive metabolism in a hypertensive syndrome. J Clin Endocrinol Metab 1977;44:799–802.
77. White Pc, Mune T, Agarval AK. 11 β-Hydroxysteroid dehydrogenase and the syndrome of apparent mineralocorticoid excess. Endocrin Rev 1997;18:135–156.

# VI Sleep Apnea and Hypertension

# 17 Sleep Apnea and Hypertension

*Thomas G. Pickering,* MD, DPHIL
*and Mona Yacoub,* MD

*Contents*



Sleep-disordered breathing (SDB) and the related clinical syndrome, obstructive sleep apnea (OSA), have for many years been associated with hypertension in clinical reports, but it is only recently that a causal association linking SDB to the development of hypertension has been established, and most clinicians who manage hypertensive patients do not pay much attention to it. In the Joint National Committee on Prevention, Detection, Evaluation, and Treatment of High Blood Pressure (sixth report) (JNC VI), which is the standard guideline for the evaluation of hypertension in the United States, sleep apnea is not mentioned as a possible cause of hypertension *(1)*, and many major textbooks on hypertension also pay no attention to it. In this chapter, we review the physiology of sleep; circulatory changes during sleep; and associations between sleep apnea, hypertension, and obesity. We also discuss the effects of treating OSA, and controlling hypertension and its clinical implications.

From: *Secondary Hypertension: Clinical Presentation, Diagnosis, and Treatment*
Edited by: G. A. Mansoor © Humana Press Inc., Totowa, NJ

## PHYSIOLOGY OF SLEEP AND CIRCULATORY CHANGES

### *Normal Sleep Patterns*

Sleep is an active process regulated by centers in the brainstem and composed of distinct cycles that recur regularly throughout the course of the night *(2)*. States and stages of human sleep are defined on the basis of characteristic patterns in the electroencephalogram (EEG), the electro-oculogram (EOG) (a measure of eye-movement activity), and the surface electromyogram ( EMG), measured on the chin and neck. The continuous recording of this array of electrophysiological parameters to define sleep and wakefulness is termed polysomnography (PSG). Two basic varieties are recognized: nondreaming, or slow-wave sleep (so called because of low-frequency, high-amplitude waves on the EEG), and dreaming, or rapid eye movement (REM), sleep, which occurs when the EEG shows low-voltage, high-frequency activity similar to the pattern of wakefulness. Non-REM (NREM) sleep is divided into four stages, characterized by increasing arousal threshold and slowing of the cortical EEG. The deepest stages of slow-wave sleep (stages 3 and 4) occur in the first 2 hours of sleep; periods of REM sleep occur in 90-minute cycles, with episodes that last longer during the latter part of the night. REM sleep is characterized by a low-amplitude, mixed-frequency EEG similar to that of NREM stage 1 sleep. The first REM sleep episode usually occurs in the second hour of sleep. NREM and REM alternate through the night with an average period of 90 to 110 minutes (the "ultradian" sleep cycle). Overall, REM sleep constitutes 20 to 25% of total sleep, and NREM stages 1 and 2 comprise 50 to 60% (increasing in elderly subjects).

Most adults sleep 7 to 8 hours per night, although the timing, duration, and internal structure of sleep vary among healthy individuals and as a function of age.

Age has a profound impact on sleep-state organization. Slow-wave sleep is most prominent and intense during childhood, decreasing sharply at puberty and across the second and third decades of life.

### *Blood Pressure Changes During Sleep*

Blood pressure (BP) changes are closely linked to the level of arousal. During the first hour of sleep there is normally a progressive fall of BP, which usually shows its maximal decrease of 15 to 20% two hours after sleep onset *(3–8)*, as shown in Fig. 1. This coincides with the deepest stages of slow-wave sleep (stages 3 and 4). During REM sleep, the BP is at about the same level as in stage 2 (approximately 10% less than during wakefulness) but is much more variable, with fluctuations of as

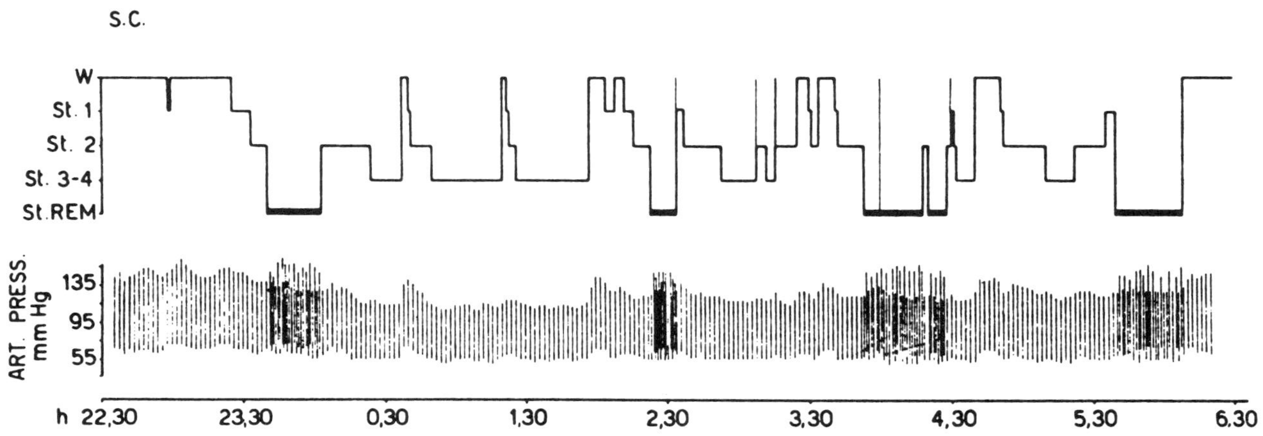


**Fig. 1.** Typical BP changes during sleep in a normal subject. Upper trace shows sleep stages. Blood pressure is plotted every 60 seconds, and every 30 seconds during REM sleep, to show increased variability. (Reproduced with permission from ref. *4*.) REM, rapid eye movement sleep; St. 1, 2, 3, 4, stages 1–4 of sleep; W, waking.

much as 30 mmHg over a few minutes *(3)*. BP rises immediately on waking.

## Is There a Circadian Rhythm of BP?

Recordings made over 24 hours in ambulatory subjects, using either invasive *(9)* or noninvasive recorders *(10)* have typically shown that BP tends to be highest in the morning, with a gradual decrease over the course of the day, and lowest during the night (Fig. 2A). This observation led to the suggestion that there might be an intrinsic circadian rhythm of BP analogous to the circadian pattern of cortisol or body temperature. The case for an intrinsic sinusoidal pattern of BP variation has been argued most forcefully by Halberg, who found that such curves fitted the BP pattern of a subject kept in a confined environment for a period of several days *(11)*. It has also been proposed that there is a gradual increase of BP during the early morning hours (3 AM to 6 AM) before the time of wakening, and that this increase could contribute to the high incidence of cerebral hemorrhage and myocardial infarction in the early morning. Other workers, however, have presented data that indicate that the apparently sinusoidal pattern of BP is most probably an artifact attributable to the averaging of records from individuals who wake at different times: when the recordings are synchronized to the time of waking rather than the time of day, the early morning rise of pressure is no longer seen *(12)*. Instead, BP remains relatively stable during the hour before waking but rises abruptly at the moment of waking (Fig. 2B).

The question of whether there is an endogenous circadian rhythm of BP or whether the changes can be accounted for by variations in activity can best be answered by removing the influence of external stimuli, so that if the rhythm persists, it can be attributed to endogenous factors. This was done in the study by Athanassiadis et al. *(8)*, in which BP was monitored noninvasively for 24 hours in patients in an orthopedic ward who were immobilized by plaster casts. In this situation, the BP showed no evidence of any sinusoidal change, being relatively constant during the day and decreasing during sleep. There were in effect two levels of pressure, one corresponding to waking, and the other to sleeping. Similar observations were made in hospitalized patients kept on bed rest *(13)*. In the latter study, diurnal variations of pressure became more pronounced when subjects were studied a second time, but while being physically active during the day. Studies of shift workers have also shown a close linkage between activity and BP. In general, when people change from working a day shift to a night shift, the BP rhythm adapts immediately to the new cycle of activity, but the heart rate takes longer to adapt *(14–16)*.

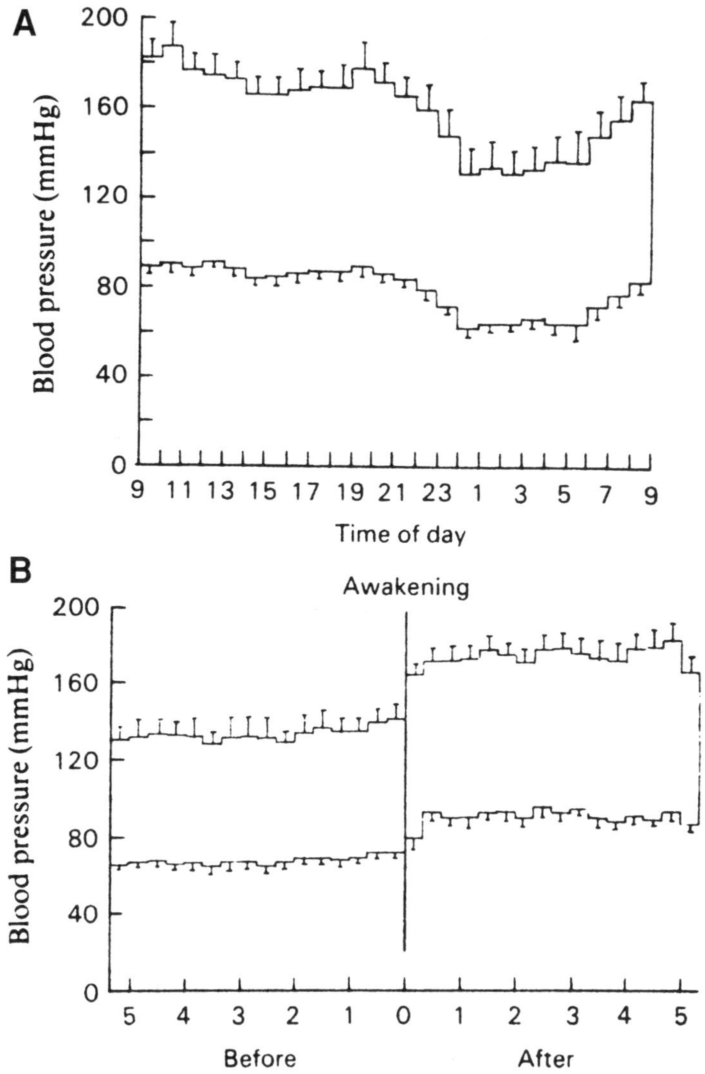


**Fig. 2.** Diurnal rhythm of blood pressure: **(A)** pooled data for 14 hypertensive subjects plotted according to clock time; **(B)** same data plotted according to time of waking. (Reproduced with permission from ref. *12*.)

**Dipping and Nondipping Patterns.** In patients with hypertension, the diurnal pattern of BP change is generally similar to the changes occurring in normotensive subjects, except that the entire BP profile is shifted upward. Thus, the differences between work and home pressures, and between home and sleep pressures, are approximately the same in normotensive and hypertensive subjects (about a 20% decrease during sleep in both cases) when expressed on a percentage basis, although in absolute terms they may be greater in hypertensives *(17)*.

### *Hemodynamic and Neurohormonal Changes During Sleep*

The fall of BP during sleep is accompanied by a decreased heart rate. Cardiac output decreases by a modest amount *(5)*, but there may also be vasodilation *(18)*. Renal blood flow and glomerular filtration rate (GFR) fall by as much as 20% *(19)*, but there is a much more pronounced decreased in urine flow, which has been attributed to increased tubular reabsorption *(19)*. The composition of the urine also changes: there are large decreases in the excretion of sodium and chloride but relatively small decreases of potassium and bicarbonate *(19)*.

Plasma and urinary catecholamine levels fall during sleep, which would be consistent with a diminished sympathetic activity *(20,21)*. This rhythm is still apparent in recumbent subjects who remain awake during the night, but it has a smaller amplitude *(21)*. Plasma renin and aldosterone levels have usually been found to rise steadily at the onset of sleep and reach their highest levels during the second half of the night *(22)*. There is a very close linkage with the stage of sleep: renin secretion is shut off during episodes of REM sleep *(26)*, which occur mainly during the second half of the night. When sleep is undisturbed, there is a marked rhythmicity of renin secretion, such that secretion increases during NREM sleep and stops during REM sleep. These findings suggest that there is a single central mechanism regulating both sleep cycles and renin secretion during the night. How it operates is far from clear; the most obvious neural influence on renin secretion is via the sympathetic nervous system (SNS), and yet sympathetic nervous activity increases on waking, while renin secretion is suppressed.

The decrease of BP during sleep is paralleled by increased secretions of growth hormone and prolactin *(23,24)*, whose release is stimulated by endogenous opioids, which also lower BP *(30)*. Naloxone, a specific opioid inhibitor, has been shown to prevent the fall of systolic BP (SBP) that accompanies the onset of sleep, without affecting diastolic BP (DBP) or heart rate *(25)*, suggesting that opioids may be involved in the regulation of BP during sleep. Antidiuretic hormone (ADH) levels rise during the night, which could contribute to the nocturnal oliguria *(26)*. Plasma atrial natriuretic factor (ANF) also rises at night but this does not occur if subjects remain recumbent and awake throughout the entire 24-hour period *(26)*.

## SLEEP-RELATED BREATHING DISORDERS AND HYPERTENSION

A wide spectrum of severe SDB has been recognized, with snoring at the benign extreme, and OSA at the other. These conditions are relevant to the present discussion not only because they affect the changes of BP occurring during sleep, but also because they are significant risk factors for cardiovascular disease. As a result of the compartmentalization of contemporary medical science, their significance has not been fully appreciated by researchers or clinicians in the field of cardiovascular disease.

### *Mechanisms of SDB*

OSA is a disorder in which there are repeated episodes of partial (hypopnea) or complete (apnea) cessation of breathing during sleep. Such episodes may be of central origin or caused by mechanical obstruction of the airways, or to a combination of the two. By definition apneas or hypopneas lasting at least 10 seconds are considered to be of clinical significance, although they usually last for 20 to 30 seconds and can last for more than a minute. The apnea/hypopnea index (AHI, also known as the respiratory distress index, or RDI) is the average number of apneas and hypopneas per sleep hour. If OSA is defined as an AHI of greater than or equal to 10, about 10% of the middle-aged population has OSA. Habitual snorers are defined as people who snore most of the night on most nights but have an AHI of less than 5 *(27)*.

Most, if not all, apneic episodes are caused by collapse of the pharyngeal airway *(28)*. This is the narrowest part of the airway and the most dependent on muscle tone to maintain its patency. Muscle tone relaxes during sleep, and this may result in narrowing of the upper airway during inspiration and hence snoring. This collapse of the airway also leads to increased respiratory effort and arousal. There is in fact a spectrum of airway collapse ranging from hypopnea, to complete apnea, where there is diminution but not cessation of respiratory movements, to the increased upper airway resistance syndrome, which is manifested by no diminution of airflow but increased respiratory effort and arousal during sleep. The arousal restores the muscle tone of the upper airways, allowing the subject to fall asleep once more. In this way, the cycle of sleep and arousal may be repeated throughout the night.

The hemodynamic changes occurring during the apneic episodes are initiated by systemic oxygen desaturation and an abrupt elevation of arterial pressure, without any accompanying tachycardia *(29)*. How-

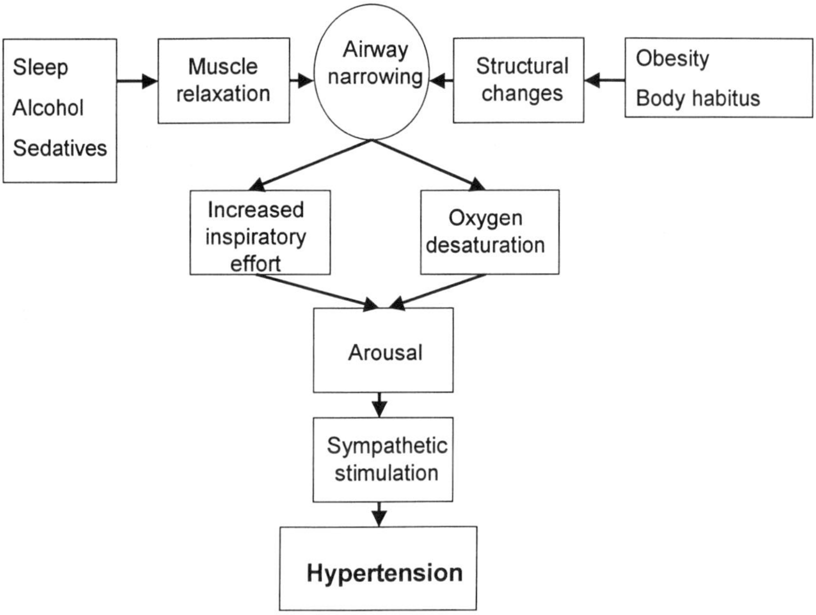


**Fig. 3.** Schematic illustration of mechanisms involved in the genesis of hypertension in patients with SDB.

ever, in elderly subjects, apneic episodes may be associated with hypotension *(30)*. The increases of BP during apneic episodes are almost certainly mediated by the SNS. Sympathetic nervous activity (which can be directly recorded from the peroneal nerve) increases markedly during the episodes *(31)*. Urine and plasma catecholamines are higher in patients with sleep apnea compared to normal controls *(32)*; furthermore, the usual nocturnal fall of catecholamine excretion is absent. After tracheostomy or continuous positive airway pressure (CPAP) treatment, the nocturnal catecholamine excretion falls to normal, along with the BP *(33)*. This sequence is illustrated thematically in Fig. 3.

The usual nocturnal decrease of urine and electrolyte excretion is also impaired in patients with sleep apnea but normalizes following treatment with CPAP *(34,35)*. This phenomenon could not be explained by changes in GFR or ADH secretion, or by changes in renin and aldosterone *(35)*, but may be attributable to high levels of ANF, which are lowered by CPAP *(36)*.

## *Epidemiology of OSA*

Because sleep apnea OSA often goes undiagnosed, studies of its epidemiology need to be population-based surveys. The Wisconsin Sleep

Cohort Study is the best example of such a study *(27)*, in which Young et al. estimated the prevalence of SDB in a cohort of working middle-aged adults aged 30–60 years. The main finding was that 2% of women and 4% of men in the middle-aged workforce (ages 30–60) have sleep apnea (defined as an AHI score of 5 or more and daytime sleepiness). The Wisconsin cohort study also suggests a lower prevalence of SDB among women *(27)*. The prevalence of an AHI of 5 or more increases with age, reaching a maximum at about age 70 *(37)*. The prevalence is higher in certain subgroups, including habitual snorers and obese persons. No studies specifically assessing the effect of race on sleep apnea syndrome have been published.

## *SDB and Hypertension*

Both SDB and hypertension are common, and, not surprisingly, there are many individuals who have both conditions. Furthermore, both are closely linked to obesity (particularly central obesity as seen in the metabolic syndrome), so there is a cluster of related syndromes: hypertension, SDB, diabetes, and the metabolic syndrome. There is a high prevalence of essential hypertension (EH) in OSA. About 50 to 60% of OSA patients have EH *(38)*. In the Wisconsin Sleep Cohort Study, Young et al. found a linear relationship between 24-hour BP and AHI that was independent of confounding factors such as body mass index (BMI) *(39,40)*. There is a high prevalence of OSA in EH, which has been estimated to be about 30% *(41–44)*. One of the issues is the causal linkage between SDB and hypertension. The largest study of the association between SDB and hypertension is the Sleep Heart Health Study (SHHS), which is a prospective study of the relationship between SDB and cardiovascular morbidity. In an initial cross-sectional study of 6132 subjects aged 40 or more *(45)*, there was a dose–response relationship between the AHI score and the prevalence of hypertension, although some of it was attributable to the effects of increased BMI (Fig. 4). Nevertheless, after adjusting for other factors such as BMI, neck circumference, and waist–hip ratio, the odds ratio for hypertension comparing an AHI of 30/hour with the lowest level (<1.5/hour) was 1.37. The association between SDB and hypertension was seen in both sexes, at older and younger ages, and among normal and overweight groups. Another survey of 2677 patients who were referred to a sleep clinic, who not surprisingly tended to have more advanced SDB than the SHHS cohort, also found a strong relationship between SDB and AHI that was independent of measures of obesity *(46)*.

To establish that SDB is an independent risk factor for the development of EH, it is necessary to be able to demonstrate that SDB precedes

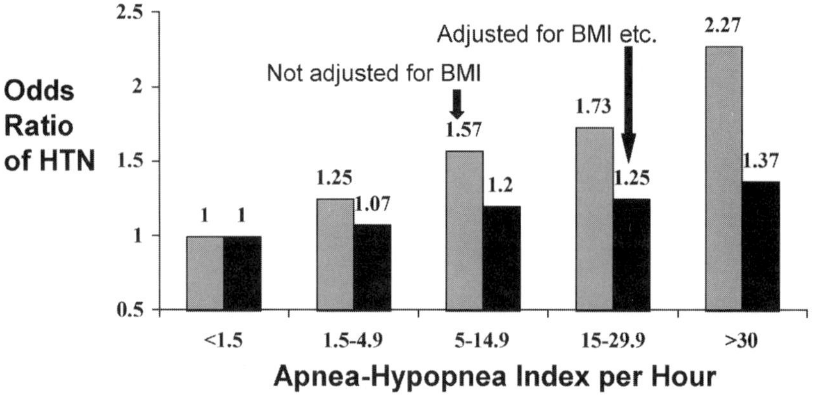


**Fig. 4.** Relationships between AHI and prevalence of hypertension, with and without adjustment for obesity, from the SHHS. (Data plotted from ref. *45*.)

and predicts the onset of hypertension and that there is a dose–response relationship between the severity of SDB and the prevalence and severity of the hypertension. This has been achieved most convincingly by the Wisconsin Sleep Cohort Study. Young et al. found a consistent dose–response relationship, even after controlling for age, sex, BMI, and antihypertensive medications *(47)* (Fig. 5). A second, but much smaller, prospective study was performed by Wright et al.*(48)* in 82 normotensive subjects, who were evaluated at baseline with an Edentec (Eden Prairie, MN) device that evaluates nasal airflow, oximetry, and chest movements, but not EEG. Both the RDI at baseline and the change of RDI over 5 years predicted the 24-hour BP level, which was measured at 5 years followup but not at baseline. Another dose–response relationship that has been found is between the prevalence of nondipping BP and the severity of OSA. The prevalence of nondipping decreases with treatment of the associated OSA.

Whether SDB is related to systolic hypertension of the elderly, which is generally thought to be unrelated to obesity and other causes of hypertension in younger people, is unclear, but what evidence there is makes this doubtful. One study found a significant correlation between AHI and mean arterial pressure *(49)*, but not with pulse pressure.

### *SDB and Dipping*

It might be expected that repeated interruptions of breathing during the night, together with the arousals from sleep, would result in an absence of the normal dipping pattern of BP. It is certainly true that nocturnal BP is more variable in patients with SDB during the night *(40)*,

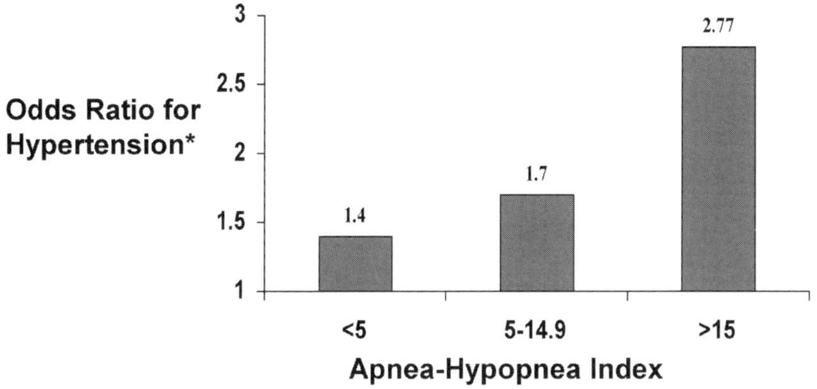


**Fig. 5.** Odds ratio of developing hypertension over a 4-year followup period based on AHI at baseline. (Data plotted from ref. *47*.)

and some studies have reported an absence of any decrease of BP during the night or even an increase *(50)*. However, the correlation between SDB and nondipping is not close: Suzuki et al. found that 50% of normotensive subjects with SDB were nondippers, and 43% of hypertensives were. Those with higher AHIs were more likely to be nondippers.

### *Snoring As an Independent Risk Factor for EH*

It has often been claimed that snoring is associated with an increased risk of hypertension, coronary heart disease (CHD), and cerebral infarction, independently of BP. Snoring is commoner in men than in women and is also associated with increasing age, obesity, and smoking. Young et al. *(51)* in a study of SDB in the community, found that when all their data were adjusted for age, sex, BMI, and antihypertensive medications, habitual snorers without OSA have a higher morning and evening SBP/DBP than normal nonapneic simple snorers, on the average 4/2 mmHg higher. In fact, the BP of habitual snorers was identical to that of people with mild OSA (AHI 5–15). Many habitual snorers, like many OSA patients, fail to reduce their BP normally during sleep *(52)*. This is consistent with the fact that habitual snorers who have hypertension have a far greater number of arousals during sleep than normotensive habitual snorers *(53)*. These short arousals, usually lasting only a few seconds, may represent episodes of marked increases in upper airway resistance during sleep and are associated with sudden increases in BP.

Snorers with a normal AHI may have the upper airway resistance syndrome, which has also been associated with hypertension *(54)*.

### *Sleep Apnea As a Cause of Drug-Resistant Hypertension*

To determine the prevalence of OSA in patients with drug-resistant hypertension, defined as a clinic BP of 140/90 mmHg or more, while taking a sensible combination of three or more antihypertensive drugs, titrated to maximally recommended doses, Logan et al. *(55)* studied 41 patients, all of whom completed an overnight polysomnographic study and all but two of whom had a 24-hour ambulatory BP measurement. The prevalence of OSA, defined as an AHI of 10 or more, was 83%. Patients were generally late middle aged (mean age 57.2 years), predominantly white (85%), obese (BMI = 34.0 kg/m$^2$), and taking a mean of 3.6 different antihypertensive medications. OSA was more prevalent in men than in women (96 vs 65%, $p = 0.014$) and more severe (mean AHI of 32.2 vs 14.0 events/hour, $p = 0.004$). There was no gender difference in BMI or age. In another study *(56)*, sleep apnea was found to be an independent predictor of uncontrolled hypertension in patients under 50 years of age.

## MORBIDITY ASSOCIATED WITH SLEEP-DISORDERED BREATHING

As reviewed above, epidemiologic studies suggest that individuals with SDB are at greater risk of daytime hypertension, even after controlling for other risk factors. OSA syndrome is a chronic disease without evidence of spontaneous remission or improvement without treatment. It is generally thought that sleep apnea is an independent risk factor for both coronary and cerebrovascular morbidity, although prospective data on this is relatively limited at the present time. For example, some of the earlier studies indicating an increased morbidity in OSA were retrospective analyses that had incomplete followup *(57)* or many of the patients had a diagnosis of cardiovascular disease (CVD) at baseline *(58)*. It is the goal of the prospective SHHS, a multicenter study funded by the National Institutes of Health (NIH), to provide some answers.

### *Stroke*

A cross-sectional analysis of data from the 6424 subjects in the SHHS found that the presence of OSA was associated with an increase of stroke by 1.58 times in subjects with an AHI greater than 11 *(59)*. A Swedish prospective study of 408 patients with known CHD found that an AHI greater than 10 was associated with an increased risk of stroke with an odds ratio of 2.62 *(60)* Sleep apnea is also very common (in 43–91% of patients) following a stroke and is obstructive rather than central in origin. To what extent this is a consequence as opposed to a cause of the strokes is unclear.

### *CHD*

As might be expected from the frequent occurrence of hypoxic episodes during the night in patients with OSA, silent ischemia is communally seen and has been related both to the hypoxic episodes and to the increase in double product during the ensuing surge of BP and heart rate. The cross-sectional analysis of the SHHS data found a modest association between CHD and sleep apnea, with an odds ratio of 1.27 for those in the highest AHI quartile (>11). Prospective data are few. One small study of 62 patients with CHD found that those with OSA had a higher mortality (38%) than those without (11%). One prospective Swedish study of 408 patients with known CHD found that an AHI greater than 10 was associated with an increased risk of cardiovascular events (death, stroke, and myocardial infarction) *(60)*. A second Swedish cohort *(61)* was followed for 7 years and found that sleep apnea at baseline (defined as 30 or more episodes of desaturation per night) was independently associated with a 4.9-fold increased risk of cardiovascular events (including new onset of hypertension, coronary, and cerebrovascular events). Of particular interest was the finding that this increased risk was confined to patients whose OSA was inadequately treated in the interim; in these patients, the overall odds ratio for any cardiovascular event was 11.1, and for coronary heart disease events was 5.4.

### *Congestive Heart Failure (CHF)*

As with stroke, there is evidence to suggest that CHF may be both a cause and a consequence of sleep apnea. In the cross-sectional analysis of the SHHS, the presence of sleep apnea (AHI > 11) was associated with a 2.38-fold increase in the occurrence of CHF *(59)*. Although sleep apnea may contribute to pulmonary and systemic hypertension, sleep apnea alone does not appear to be a cause of right heart failure.

## ETIOLOGIC/PREDISPOSING FACTORS

### *Structural Factors*

It is well established that structural abnormalities, including obesity-related fat deposits that narrow the normal upper airway lumen can cause and/or exacerbate SDB episodes. In support of this hypothesis, SDB activity has been induced by experimentally produced nasal obstruction in normal subjects *(62)* and in patients with epistaxis treated with anterior and posterior nasal packs *(63)*.

### *Genetic Factors*

Several published case series have suggested a role for genetic inheritance in OSA syndrome *(64)*. In the only analytic study designed to assess familial OSA syndrome, Redline et al. *(65)* assessed the role of inheritance in OSA by quantitating the degree of familial clustering of symptoms associated with sleep-related breathing disorders. The unadjusted odds ratios of habitual or disruptive snoring, breathing pauses, and excessive daytime sleepiness in subjects with a single relative with the same symptom were 1.40 to 1.53 ($p < 0.05$). Odds ratios increased progressively for subjects with increasing numbers of symptomatic relatives. Adjustment for BMI, age, and gender modestly reduced these odds ratios to 1.33 to 1.42. These data suggest a significant familial aggregation of symptoms associated with SDB that appears independent of familial similarities in weight.

### *Endocrine Disorders*

Conditions that increase soft tissue growth theoretically can cause narrowing and obstruction of the upper airway and subsequent OSA syndrome. For example, several case series have suggested an association between acromegaly *(66)* and hypothyroidism and OSA syndrome *(67)*. Since sleep apnea is more common in men, a hormonal basis for sleep apnea has been suggested, although the mechanism of action of the female hormones has not been established. Several case series have suggested an androgen/progesterone imbalance contributing to the development of OSA syndrome. A related condition is the polycystic ovary syndrome, characterized by increased androgenic hormones, insulin resistance, and central obesity. It has been reported that women with this condition have an increased prevalence of OSA, even after controlling for obesity *(68)*. If menopausal status has an impact on sleep apnea, progesterone might be expected to have an effect on SDB. However, although there were some studies that were moderately encouraging *(69,70)*, this mode of treatment has fallen out of favor.

### *Alcohol and Sedatives*

Alcohol, even in moderate amounts, has been demonstrated to exacerbate existing OSA syndrome and to induce apneic activity in asymptomatic individuals *(71,72)*. Benzodiazapines have also been demonstrated to exacerbate existing OSA syndrome, mainly by increasing the duration of the apneic events and the degree of oxygen desaturation *(72,73)*.

### *Animal Models of Sleep Apnea and Its Effects on BP*

A series of animal studies in rats and dogs has identified possible mechanisms by which SDB might lead to hypertension. Fletcher et al. have described a rat model in which repetitive episodes of hypoxia administered for 7 hours a day result in a persistent increase of BP and left ventricular mass *(74)*. A role for the carotid chemoreceptors as the afferent stimulus was demonstrated by showing that surgical denervation of the chemoreceptors prevented the increase of BP *(75)*. In addition, the role of the SNS as the efferent mediator was shown by sympathectomy using adrenal demedullation and 6-hydroxy dopamine, which also prevented the increase of BP *(75,76)*. The renin-angiotensin system (RAS) may also play a role, because when it is suppressed by a high-salt diet, the hypoxia-induced hypertension no longer occurs *(77)*.

In dogs, obstructing a tracheostomy to simulate apnea causes an acute increase of BP of about 20 mmHg, which lasts for several hours and is exacerbated by prior sleep deprivation *(78)*. The same model has been used to investigate the relative contributions of arousal and chemoreceptor stimulation on BP. When partial airway obstruction is induced that is sufficient to produce hypoxia but not arousal on the EEG, there is a rise of mean BP of about 8 mmHg, but this increases to 17 mmHg when there is arousal as well *(78)*. The BP increase can be blocked by pharmacological blockade of the autonomic nervous system with hexamethonium, which shows that it is mediated by the SNS rather than by mechanical factors related to changes of intrathoracic pressure.

### *Role of Excessive Sympathetic Drive As a Mediator of Higher BP in Sleep Apnea*

The SNS is a key contributor to the increases in BP. The association between high sympathetic traffic and increased BP may also be especially relevant to patients with OSA who exhibit both high levels of sympathetic traffic and an increased incidence of hypertension. Figure 6 shows an example of sympathetic nerve activity in a patient with OSA during an apneic episode. The chemoreceptors respond to hypoxia and hypercapnia, which elicit marked increases in peripheral sympathetic vasoconstrictor activity with consequent increases in BP *(79)*. Increased minute ventilation during chemoreceptor activation inhibits the sympathetic response; thus, apnea during hypoxia or hypercapnia results in a potentiated sympathetic vasoconstrictor response.

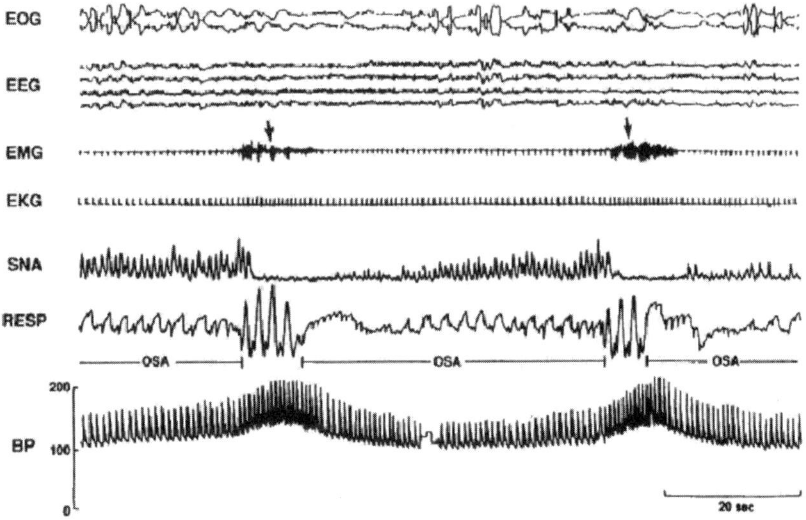


**Fig. 6.** Apneic episodes during REM sleep in a patient with OSA. Arrows show increase of muscle tone and cessation of rapid eye movements characteristic of REM sleep toward the end of the apneic period. BP, intra-arterial BP; EEG, electroencephalogram; EKG, electrocardiogram; EMG, electromyogram; EOG, electro-oculogram; RESP, respiration; SNA, muscle sympathetic nerve activity. (Reproduced with permission from ref. *50*.)

During normal sleep, as described above, sympathetic nerve activity decreases, reechoing its lowest level during stage 4 sleep, but during periods of arousal (such as K complexes) and REM sleep, there is an acute increase *(80)*. In patients with SDB there is extensive evidence for increased sympathetic tone during both the day and night (Fig. 7). Thus, 24-hour urine catecholamine levels are increased *(32)* as are plasma levels measured during the day *(81;82)*. Sympathetic nerve activity is also increased even while awake *(50,82,83)* and may increase further during sleep, along with the BP *(50)*.

Remarkably, the high sympathetic drive is present even during daytime wakefulness when subjects are breathing normally and no evidence of hypoxia or chemoreflex activation is apparent. It has been proposed that tonic activation of the chemoreflex contributes to the increased sympathetic drive *(84)*. Patients with OSA show an increased muscle sympathetic nerve activity (MSNA) while at rest, but when the chemoreflex is deactivated by breathing 100% oxygen, there is a decrease of both MSNA and BP in the OSA patients, but not in normal controls. Treatment of OSA with tracheostomy reduces the elevated urinary catecholamine levels *(33)*.

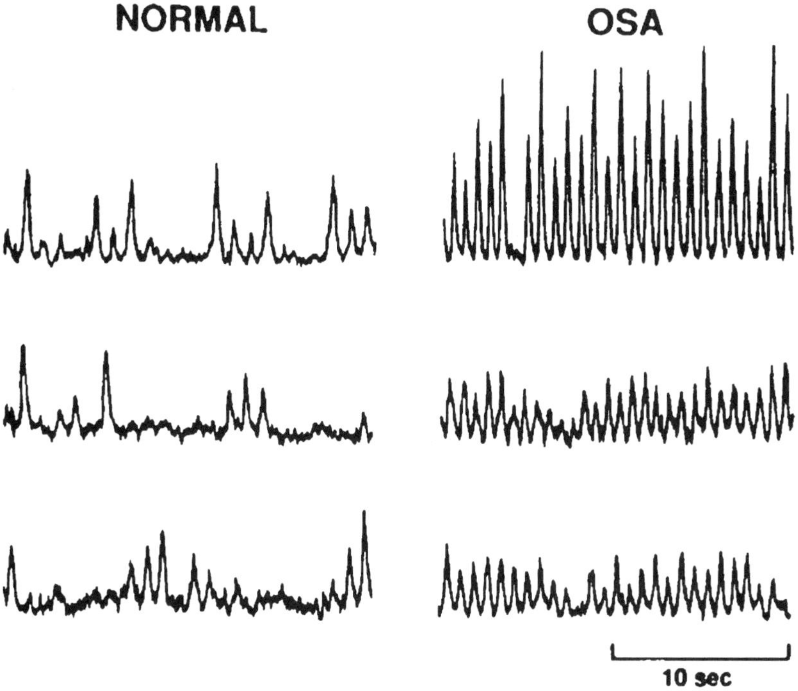


**Fig. 7.** Recordings of MSNA during wakefulness in three patients with OSA and matched normotensive controls. (Reproduced with permission from ref. *50*.)

### *Endothelin*

A causal relationship between endothelin levels and BP in OSA has been suggested by Narkiewicz et al. *(85)*, who found that after 4 hours of untreated sleep apnea in patients with OSA, BP increased and was correlated with a parallel increase of circulating endothelin-1, but there was no correlation with changes in plasma norepinephrine (NE) of renin. After 5 hours of CPAP, both BP and endothelin decreased.

## CLINICAL EVALUATION

The cardinal manifestations of the OSA syndrome are snoring and daytime sleepiness *(86)*. However, both may be denied or minimized by the patient. Snorers may be unaware of the sounds of their nightly battle to breathe unless there is a listener to tell them. There are at least two problems with sleepiness as a symptom. One is that patients may develop sleepiness so slowly over years that they forget what normal alertness is like. The other is that sleep deprivation is so common in our society that sleepiness is ubiquitous and thus nonspecific. The observation of some-

Table 1
Clinical Clues Suggesting SDB

| |
|---|
| Male sex |
| Central obesity |
| Increased neck circumference |
| Hypertension that is difficult to control |
| Snoring |
| Daytime sleepiness |

one who has seen the patient's sleep behavior (and daytime alertness) can be very helpful to the clinician. Witnessed obstructive events during sleep in a habitual snorer are a strong predictor of clinically important sleep apnea.

Morning headaches are characteristic of SDB and are usually of relatively short duration (less than 30 minutes) *(87)*. They are related to the severity of AHI and may be relieved by CPAP or surgery.

## *Physical Examination*

Examination of the prototypical patient with OSA reveals a hypertensive, obese, middle-aged male with a large neck. Although obstruction in the upper airway is the critical factor, the loci of obstruction are not easily assessed by the clinician while the patient is awake. Clues may include severe nasal obstruction, a low-hanging soft palate and large uvula, enlarged tonsils/adenoids, and retrognathia or micrognathia. It is important to note the patient's neck circumference. Neck size appears to be a stronger predictor of sleep apnea than body mass index, presumably because that is where additional tissue can influence the size of compliance of the upper airway. The clinical clues are summarized in Table 1.

## *Initial Laboratory Evaluation*

Routine laboratory data are generally not helpful. However, screening for hypothyroidism should be performed, particularly in older patients after the diagnosis of OSA is established.

## *Diagnostic Tests*

### Epworth Sleepiness Scale (ESS)

Sleepiness is most commonly evaluated using questionnaires such as the ESS. This is a self-administered, eight-question test that measures sleep propensity and correlates reasonably well with the RDI. The patient rates from 0 to 3 the likelihood of falling asleep, and a total score is obtained, ranging from 0 to 24. As the RDI increases, the ESS score becomes progressively higher.

### PSG

At present, PSG is the test of choice for suspected OSA. Patients with excessive daytime sleepiness and the constellation of risk factors described above are candidates for testing. Traditionally, patients undergo diagnostic polysomnographic study over a full night, with a subsequent study for nasal CPAP titration. However, in an effort to reduce costs, many centers have been encouraged by insurance carriers to combine diagnostic and therapeutic nasal CPAP studies into one split-night study. Data are now emerging to support this approach, particularly in patients with more significant sleep apnea (>20 events per hour), and algorithmic approaches are being formulated. However, caution is necessary if a patient with a high pretest suspicion for OSA has a negative one-night study. Despite the fact that PSG is considered the gold standard diagnostic study, there can be considerable night-to-night variability.

#### Screening Techniques

There is now a broad interest in developing accurate and less costly portable diagnostic techniques than PSG. A number of monitors have been developed that measure variables such as respiratory effort and airflow, heart rate, and oxygen saturation. Actigraphy is one such technique; it records body movements during the night but, like other screening techniques, has insufficient sensitivity to be fully reliable *(88)*.

## TREATMENT

There are two general issues when it comes to treating hypertensive patients who have SDB: first, treatment of the underlying condition, and second, treating the hypertension itself. Since many of these patients will have the metabolic syndrome, attention should be paid to general hygienic measures such as weight loss and exercise. Although lip service is traditionally paid to these interventions, no controlled trials of their value appear to have been done *(89)*. Gastric bypass surgery, which can produce dramatic weight loss in the morbidly obese, has been reported to produce equally marked improvements in the RDI (from 96.9 to 11.3 in one study *[90]*), and other studies have shown a reduction of BP *(91)*. Another major issue concerns the effects of relieving the apneic episodes by surgery or nasal CPAP on BP.

### *Acute and Chronic Effects of CPAP on BP Control*

Effective treatment of sleep apnea by CPAP has been shown to markedly and acutely decrease BP and sympathetic traffic during sleep. Chronic effects of CPAP treatment are less clear. Silverberg et al. *(38)* reviewed 23 prospective studies published since 1989, of which 21 used CPAP, one used surgery (uvulopalato-pharyngoplasty), and one "positional therapy" (a tennis ball placed in the middle of the back at night to keep patients on their sides rather than their backs). Nineteen of these studies showed a reduction in daytime BP as a result of treatment. Since then, a number of other studies have appeared. Three studies have been double blind, comparing CPAP with either placebo pills or with antihypertensive drugs. One *(92)* showed a small but significant fall of BP from CPAP, particularly in patients with nocturnal hypoxemia; however, most of the patients were not hypertensive. A second study showed no net effect on BP, but again, only 25% of the patients were hypertensive *(93)*. The third study used subtherapeutic (sham) CPAP *(94)* and found a reduction of 3.4/3.3 mmHg (slightly larger during the day than during the night). In patients taking antihypertensive drugs, the 24-hour mean BP fall was about twice as large (6.7 mmHg vs 3.3).

### *Effects of Antihypertensive Drugs on Sleep Apnea*

It is likely that antihypertensive drugs will have different effects in patients with sleep apnea, but there are few systematic data on this. Clonidine has been reported to suppress REM sleep and hence the apneas occurring during REM, which resulted in a lessened nocturnal hypoxemia *(95)*. Cilazapril, an angiotensin-converting enzyme inhibitor (ACEI), had no effect of the RDI but lowered BP during sleep *(96)*, whereas celiprolol, a β-blocker, decreased daytime BP but had relatively little effect during the night *(97)*.

## CLINICAL IMPLICATIONS AND RECOMMENDATIONS

It is clear from the above considerations that SDB is an important and generally unrecognized cause of EH. Physicians who treat hypertensive patients need to raise their level of awareness for the condition and incorporate questions regarding snoring, sleep problems, and daytime sleepiness into the routine history. Patients who have put on a lot of weight or who have features suggestive of the metabolic syndrome are at particularly high risk. Those with apparently refractory hypertension are another important group. Apart from central obesity, a stocky build with a short thick neck is also suggestive.

Unfortunately, there is no reliable screening test at the present time, so the diagnosis can only convincingly be established by doing a full PSG in an accredited sleep lab. Such is the interest in these tests now that there is often a long waiting list. If the diagnosis is confirmed, there are several therapeutic options. Although CPAP is the definitive treatment, it is poorly tolerated by many patients, and other modalities of treatment include weight loss and sleeping on the side as opposed to the back, in some cases by wearing a belt with a tennis ball in the small of the back. Surgery has its advocates, but the results are disappointing.

## REFERENCES

1. The sixth report of the Joint National Committee on Prevention, Detection, Evaluation, and Treatment of High Blood Pressure. Arch Intern Med 1997;157(21): 2413–2446.
2. Kleitman N. Sleep and wakefulness. Chicago, IL: University of Chicago Press, 1963.
3. Snyder F, Hobson JA, Morrison DF, et al. Changes in respirations, heart rate, and systolic blood pressure in human sleep. J Appl Physiol 1964;19:417–422.
4. Coccagna G, Mantovani M, Brignani F, Manzini A, Lugaresi E. Arterial pressure changes during spontaneous sleep in man. Electroencephalogr Clin Neurophysiol 1971;31(3):277–281.
5. Khatri IM, Fries ED. Hemodynamic changes during sleep. J Appl Physiol 1967;22:867–873.
6. Richardson DW, Honour AJ, Goodman AC. Changes in arterial pressure during sleep in man. Hypertension 1968;16:62–78.
7. Pickering TG. Sleep, circadian rhythms and cardiovascular disease. Cardiovasc Rev Rep 1980;1:37–47.
8. Athanassiadis D, Draper GJ, Honour AJ, Cranston WI. Variability of automatic blood pressure measurements over 24 hour periods. Clin Sci 1969;36(1):147–156.
9. Millar-Craig MW, Bishop CN, Raftery EB. Circadian variation of blood-pressure. Lancet 1978;1(8068):795–797.
10. Clark LA, Denby L, Pregibon D, et al. A quantitative analysis of the effects of activity and time of day on the diurnal variations of blood pressure. J Chronic Dis 1987;40(7):671–681.
11. Halberg F, Ilhamdjanova DC, Carandente O, et al. The chronobiology of blood pressure in 1994. Chronobiologia 1994;21(1–2):1–6.
12. Floras JS, Jones JV, Johnston JA, Brooks DE, Hassan MO, Sleight P. Arousal and the circadian rhythm of blood pressure. Clin Sci Mol Med Suppl 1978;4: 395s–397s:395s–397s.
13. Mann S, Craig MW, Melville DI, Balasubramanian V, Raftery EB. Physical activity and the circadian rhythm of blood pressure. Clin Sci 1979;57 Suppl 5:291s–294s.
14. Sundberg S, Kohvakka A, Gordin A. Rapid reversal of circadian blood pressure rhythm in shift workers. J Hypertens 1988;6(5):393–396.
15. Baumgart P, Walger P, Fuchs G, Dorst KG, Vetter H, Rahn KH. Twenty-four-hour blood pressure is not dependent on endogenous circadian rhythm. J Hypertens 1989;7(4):331–334.
16. Chau NP, Mallion JM, de Gaudemaris R, et al. Twenty-four-hour ambulatory blood pressure in shift workers. Circulation 1989;80(2):341–347.

17. Pickering TG, Harshfield GA, Kleinert HD, Blank S, Laragh JH. Blood pressure during normal daily activities, sleep, and exercise: comparison of values in normal and hypertensive subjects. JAMA 1982;19;247(7):992–996.
18. Bristow JD, Honour AJ, Pickering TG, Sleight P. Cardiovascular and respiratory changes during sleep in normal and hypertensive subjects. Cardiovasc Res 1969;3(4):476–485.
19. Sirota JH, Baldwin DW, Villareal H. Diurnal variations of renal function in man. J Clin Invest 1950;29:187–192.
20. Watson RD, Hamilton CA, Reid JL, Littler WA. Changes in plasma norepinephrine, blood pressure and heart rate during physical activity in hypertensive man. Hypertension 1979;1(4):341–346.
21. Bing RF, Harlow J, Smith AJ, Townshend MM. The urinary excretion of catecholamines and their derivatives in primary hypertension in man. Clin Sci Mol Med 1977;52(3):319–323.
22. Modlinger RS, Sharif-Zadeh K, Ertel NH, Gutkin M. The circadian rhythm of renin. J Clin Endocrinol Metab 1976;43(6):1276–1282.
23. Van Cauter E, Leproult R, Plat L. Age-related changes in slow wave sleep and REM sleep and relationship with growth hormone and cortisol levels in healthy men. JAMA 2000;284(7):861–868.
24. Spiegel K, Follenius M, Simon C, Saini J, Ehrhart J, Brandenberger G. Prolactin secretion and sleep. Sleep 1994;17(1):20–27.
25. Rubin P, Blaschke TF, Guilleminault C. Effect of naloxone, a specific opioid inhibitor, on blood pressure fall during sleep. Circulation 1981;63(1):117–121.
26. Richards AM, Tonolo G, Fraser R, et al. Diurnal change in plasma atrial natriuretic peptide concentrations. Clin Sci (Lond) 1987;73(5):489–495.
27. Young T, Palta M, Dempsey J, Skatrud J, Weber S, Badr S. The occurrence of sleep-disordered breathing among middle-aged adults. N Engl J Med 1993;328(17): 1230–1235.
28. Douglas NJ, Polo O. Pathogenesis of obstructive sleep apnoea/hypopnoea syndrome. Lancet 1994;344(8923):653–655.
29. Tilkian AG, Guilleminault C, Schroeder JS, Lehrman KL, Simmons FB, Dement WC. Hemodynamics in sleep-induced apnea: studies during wakefulness and sleep. Ann Intern Med 1976;85(6):714–719.
30. McGinty D, Beahm E, Stern N, Littner M, Sowers J, Reige W. Nocturnal hypotension in older men with sleep-related breathing disorders. Chest 1988;94(2): 305–311.
31. Hedner J, Ejnell H, Sellgren J, Hedner T, Wallin G. Is high and fluctuating muscle nerve sympathetic activity in the sleep apnoea syndrome of pathogenetic importance for the development of hypertension? J Hypertens Suppl 1988;6(4): S529–S531.
32. Clark RW, Boudoulas H, Schaal SF, Schmidt HS. Adrenergic hyperactivity and cardiac abnormality in primary disorders of sleep. Neurology 1980;30(2):113–119.
33. Fletcher EC, Miller J, Schaaf JW, Fletcher JG. Urinary catecholamines before and after tracheostomy in patients with obstructive sleep apnea and hypertension. Sleep 1987;10(1):35–44.
34. Warley AR, Stradling JR. Abnormal diurnal variation in salt and water excretion in patients with obstructive sleep apnoea. Clin Sci (Lond) 1988;74(2):183–185.
35. Krieger J, Imbs JL, Schmidt M, Kurtz D. Renal function in patients with obstructive sleep apnea: effects of nasal continuous positive airway pressure. Arch Intern Med 1988;148(6):1337–1340.

36. Krieger J, Laks L, Wilcox I, et al. Atrial natriuretic peptide release during sleep in patients with obstructive sleep apnoea before and during treatment with nasal continuous positive airway pressure. Clin Sci (Lond) 1989;77(4):407–411.
37. Young T, Shahar E, Nieto FJ, et al. Predictors of sleep-disordered breathing in community-dwelling adults: the Sleep Heart Health Study. Arch Intern Med 2002;162(8):893–900.
38. Silverberg DS, Oksenberg A, Iaina A. Sleep-related breathing disorders as a major cause of essential hypertension: fact or fiction? Curr Opin Nephrol Hypertens 1998;7(4):353–357.
39. Young T, Peppard P, Palta M, et al. Population-based study of sleep-disordered breathing as a risk factor for hypertension. Arch Intern Med 1997;157(15): 1746–1752.
40. Hla KM, Young TB, Bidwell T, Palta M, Skatrud JB, Dempsey J. Sleep apnea and hypertension: a population-based study. Ann Intern Med 1994;120(5):382–388.
41. Kales A, Bixler EO, Cadieux RJ, et al. Sleep apnoea in a hypertensive population. Lancet 1984;2(8410):1005–1008.
42. Williams AJ, Houston D, Finberg S, Lam C, Kinney JL, Santiago S. Sleep apnea syndrome and essential hypertension. Am J Cardiol 1985;55(8):1019–1022.
43. Lavie P, Ben Yosef R, Rubin AE. Prevalence of sleep apnea syndrome among patients with essential hypertension. Am Heart J 1984;108(2):373–376.
44. Fletcher EC, DeBehnke RD, Lovoi MS, Gorin AB. Undiagnosed sleep apnea in patients with essential hypertension. Ann Intern Med 1985;103(2):190–195.
45. Nieto FJ, Young TB, Lind BK, et al. Association of sleep-disordered breathing, sleep apnea, and hypertension in a large community-based study. Sleep Heart Health Study. JAMA 2000;283(14):1829–1836.
46. Lavie P, Herer P, Hoffstein V. Obstructive sleep apnoea syndrome as a risk factor for hypertension: population study. BMJ 2000;19;320(7233):479–482.
47. Peppard PE, Young T, Palta M, Skatrud J. Prospective study of the association between sleep-disordered breathing and hypertension. N Engl J Med 2000342(19): 1378–1384.
48. Wright JT, Jr., Redline S, Taylor AL, et al. Relationship between 24-H blood pressure and sleep disordered breathing in a normotensive community sample. Am J Hypertens 2001;14(8 Pt 1):743–748.
49. Grote L, Hedner J, Peter JH. Mean blood pressure, pulse pressure and grade of hypertension in untreated hypertensive patients with sleep-related breathing disorder. J Hypertens 2001;19(4):683–690.
50. Somers VK, Dyken ME, Clary MP, Abboud FM. Sympathetic neural mechanisms in obstructive sleep apnea. J Clin Invest 1995;96(4):1897–1904.
51. Young T, Finn L, Hla KM, Morgan B, Palta M. Snoring as part of a dose-response relationship between sleep-disordered breathing and blood pressure. Sleep 1996;19(10 Suppl):S202–S205.
52. Mateika JH, Mateika S, Slutsky AS, Hoffstein V. The effect of snoring on mean arterial blood pressure during non-REM sleep. Am Rev Respir Dis 1992;145(1): 141–146.
53. Lofaso F, Coste A, Gilain L, Harf A, Guilleminault C, Goldenberg F. Sleep fragmentation as a risk factor for hypertension in middle-aged nonapneic snorers. Chest 1996;109(4):896–900.
54. Guilleminault C, Stoohs R, Shiomi T, Kushida C, Schnittger I. Upper airway resistance syndrome, nocturnal blood pressure monitoring, and borderline hypertension. Chest 1996;109(4):901–908.

55. Logan AG, Perlikowski SM, Mente A, et al. High prevalence of unrecognized sleep apnoea in drug-resistant hypertension. J Hypertens 2001;19(12):2271–2277.
56. Grote L, Hedner J, Peter JH. Sleep-related breathing disorder is an independent risk factor for uncontrolled hypertension. J Hypertens 2000;18(6):679–685.
57. He J, Kryger MH, Zorick FJ, Conway W, Roth T. Mortality and apnea index in obstructive sleep apnea: experience in 385 male patients. Chest 1988;94(1):9–14.
58. Partinen M, Guilleminault C. Daytime sleepiness and vascular morbidity at seven-year follow-up in obstructive sleep apnea patients. Chest 1990;97(1):27–32.
59. Shahar E, Whitney CW, Redline S, et al. Sleep-disordered breathing and cardiovascular disease: cross-sectional results of the Sleep Heart Health Study. Am J Respir Crit Care Med 2001;163(1):19–25.
60. Mooe T, Franklin KA, Holmstrom K, Rabben T, Wiklund U. Sleep-disordered breathing and coronary artery disease: long-term prognosis. Am J Respir Crit Care Med 2001;164(10 Pt 1):1910–1913.
61. Peker Y, Hedner J, Norum J, Kraiczi H, Carlson J. Increased incidence of cardiovascular disease in middle-aged men with obstructive sleep apnea: a 7-year follow-up. Am J Respir Crit Care Med 2002;166(2):159–165.
62. Zwillich CW, Pickett C, Hanson FN, Weil JV. Disturbed sleep and prolonged apnea during nasal obstruction in normal men. Am Rev Respir Dis 1981;124(2):158–160.
63. Wetmore SJ, Scrima L, Hiller FC. Sleep apnea in epistaxis patients treated with nasal packs. Otolaryngol Head Neck Surg 1988;98(6):596–599.
64. Strohl KP, Saunders NA, Feldman NT, Hallett M. Obstructive sleep apnea in family members. N Engl J Med 1978;299(18):969–973.
65. Redline S, Tosteson T, Tishler PV, Carskadon MA, Millman RP, Milliman RP. Studies in the genetics of obstructive sleep apnea: familial aggregation of symptoms associated with sleep-related breathing disturbances. Am Rev Respir Dis 1992;145(2 Pt 1):440–444.
66. Perks WH, Horrocks PM, Cooper RA, et al. Sleep apnoea in acromegaly. BMJ 1980;280(6218):894–897.
67. Rajagopal KR, Abbrecht PH, Derderian SS, et al. Obstructive sleep apnea in hypothyroidism. Ann Intern Med 1984;101(4):491–494.
68. Vgontzas AN, Legro RS, Bixler EO, Grayev A, Kales A, Chrousos GP. Polycystic ovary syndrome is associated with obstructive sleep apnea and daytime sleepiness: role of insulin resistance. J Clin Endocrinol Metab 2001;86(2):517–520.
69. Orr WC, Imes NK, Martin RJ. Progesterone therapy in obese patients with sleep apnea. Arch Intern Med 1979;139(1):109–111.
70. Strohl KP, Hensley MJ, Saunders NA, Scharf SM, Brown R, Ingram RH, Jr. Progesterone administration and progressive sleep apneas. JAMA 1981;245(12):1230–1232.
71. Issa PG, Sullivan CE. Alcohol, snoring and sleep apnea. J Neurol Neurosurg Psychiatry 1982;45:353–359.
72. Guilleminault C, Silvestri R, Mondini S, Coburn S. Aging and sleep apnea: action of benzodiazepine, acetazolamide, alcohol, and sleep deprivation in a healthy elderly group. J Gerontol 1984;39(6):655–661.
73. Dolly FR, Block AJ. Effect of flurazepam on sleep-disordered breathing and nocturnal oxygen desaturation in asymptomatic subjects. Am J Med 1982;73(2):239–243.
74. Fletcher EC, Lesske J, Qian W, Miller CC, III, Unger T. Repetitive, episodic hypoxia causes diurnal elevation of blood pressure in rats. Hypertension 1992;19(6 Pt 1):555–561.

75. Lesske J, Fletcher EC, Bao G, Unger T. Hypertension caused by chronic intermittent hypoxia: influence of chemoreceptors and sympathetic nervous system. J Hypertens 1997;15(12 Pt 2):1593–1603.
76. Fletcher EC, Lesske J, Culman J, Miller CC, Unger T. Sympathetic denervation blocks blood pressure elevation in episodic hypoxia. Hypertension 1992;20(5):612–619.
77. Fletcher EC, Orolinova N, Bader M. Blood pressure response to chronic episodic hypoxia: the renin-angiotensin system. J Appl Physiol 2002;92(2):627–633.
78. O'Donnell CP, Ayuse T, King ED, Schwartz AR, Smith PL, Robotham JL. Airway obstruction during sleep increases blood pressure without arousal. J Appl Physiol 1996;80(3):773–781.
79. Narkiewicz K, van de Borne PJ, Pesek CA, Dyken ME, Montano N, Somers VK. Selective potentiation of peripheral chemoreflex sensitivity in obstructive sleep apnea. Circulation 1999;99(9):1183–1189.
80. Somers VK, Dyken ME, Mark AL, Abboud FM. Sympathetic-nerve activity during sleep in normal subjects. N Engl J Med 1993;328(5):303–307.
81. Ziegler MG, Nelesen R, Mills P, Ancoli-Israel S, Kennedy B, Dimsdale JE. Sleep apnea, norepinephrine-release rate, and daytime hypertension. Sleep 1997;20(3): 224–231.
82. Carlson JT, Hedner J, Elam M, Ejnell H, Sellgren J, Wallin BG. Augmented resting sympathetic activity in awake patients with obstructive sleep apnea. Chest 1993;103(6):1763–1768.
83. Leuenberger U, Jacob E, Sweer L, Waravdekar N, Zwillich C, Sinoway L. Surges of muscle sympathetic nerve activity during obstructive apnea are linked to hypoxemia. J Appl Physiol 1995;79(2):581–588.
84. Narkiewicz K, van de Borne PJ, Montano N, Dyken ME, Phillips BG, Somers VK. Contribution of tonic chemoreflex activation to sympathetic activity and blood pressure in patients with obstructive sleep apnea. Circulation 1998;97(10): 943–945.
85. Phillips BG, Narkiewicz K, Pesek CA, Haynes WG, Dyken ME, Somers VK. Effects of obstructive sleep apnea on endothelin-1 and blood pressure. J Hypertens 1999;17(1):61–66.
86. Young T, Hutton R, Finn L, Badr S, Palta M. The gender bias in sleep apnea diagnosis: are women missed because they have different symptoms? Arch Intern Med 1996;156(21):2445–2451.
87. Loh NK, Dinner DS, Foldvary N, Skobieranda F, Yew WW. Do patients with obstructive sleep apnea wake up with headaches? Arch Intern Med 1999; 159(15):1765–1768.
88. Aubert-Tulkens G, Culee C, Harmant-Van Rijckevorsel K, Rodenstein DO. Ambulatory evaluation of sleep disturbance and therapeutic effects in sleep apnea syndrome by wrist activity monitoring. Am Rev Respir Dis 1987;136(4):851–856.
89. Shneerson J, Wright J. Lifestyle modification for obstructive sleep apnoea. Cochrane Database Syst Rev 2001;(1):CD002875.
90. Scheuller M, Weider D. Bariatric surgery for treatment of sleep apnea syndrome in 15 morbidly obese patients: long-term results. Otolaryngol Head Neck Surg 2001;125(4):299–302.
91. Cowan GS, Jr., Buffington CK. Significant changes in blood pressure, glucose, and lipids with gastric bypass surgery. World J Surg 1998;22(9):987–992.
92. Faccenda JF, Mackay TW, Boon NA, Douglas NJ. Randomized placebo-controlled trial of continuous positive airway pressure on blood pressure in the sleep apnea-hypopnea syndrome. Am J Respir Crit Care Med 2001;163(2):344–348.

93. Barnes M, Houston D, Worsnop CJ, et al. A randomized controlled trial of continuous positive airway pressure in mild obstructive sleep apnea. Am J Respir Crit Care Med 2002;165(6):773–780.
94. Pepperell JC, Ramdassingh-Dow S, Crosthwaite N, et al. Ambulatory blood pressure after therapeutic and subtherapeutic nasal continuous positive airway pressure for obstructive sleep apnoea: a randomised parallel trial. Lancet 2002;19;359(9302): 204–210.
95. Issa FG. Effect of clonidine in obstructive sleep apnea. Am Rev Respir Dis 1992;145(2 Pt 1):435–439.
96. Grote L, Wutkewicz K, Knaack L, Ploch T, Hedner J, Peter JH. Association between blood pressure reduction with antihypertensive treatment and sleep apnea activity. Am J Hypertens 2000;13(12):1280–1287.
97. Planes C, Foucher A, Leroy M, et al. Effect of celiprolol treatment in hypertensive patients with sleep apnea. Sleep 1999;22(4):507–513.

# Index

## A

## D



## E

## H